Pathophysiology and Techniques of Cardiopulmonary Bypass

Volume II

This volume is one of the Cardiothoracic Surgery Series,
Edited by Joe R. Utley

Pathophysiology and Techniques of Cardiopulmonary Bypass

Volume II

Editor

Joe R. Utley, M.D.

Professor of Surgery
University of California
San Diego

Editorial Associate

Rosanne Betleski, B.A.

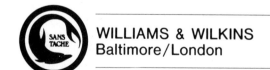

WILLIAMS & WILKINS
Baltimore/London

Made in the United States of America

Library of Congress Cataloging in Publication Data

(Revised for vol. 2)

Main entry under title:

Pathophysiology and techniques of cardiopulmonary bypass.

  (Cardiothoracic surgery series)
  Includes bibliographies and indexes.
  1. Cardiopulmonary bypass. 2. Aortocoronary bypass. 3. Postoperative complications. I. Utley, Joe R. II. Ashleigh, E. Alexandra (Elizabeth Alexandra) [DNLM: 1. Aortocoronary—Bypass. 2. Postoperative— Complications. WG 169 P297 1982]
  RD598.P37 1982   617'.412   82-21752
  ISBN 0-683-08501-8 (v. 1)
  ISBN 0-683-08502-6 (v. 2)

Composed and printed at the
Waverly Press, Inc.
Mr. Royal and Guilford Aves.
Baltimore, MD 21202, U.S.A.

Series Editor's Foreword

In the second volume of the Cardiothoracic Surgery series, we again address topics related to cardiopulmonary bypass. The response to Volume I by cardiac surgeons, perfusionists, cardiac anesthesiologists, cardiologists, intensivists, and nurse specialists has been very gratifying. In this volume of the Cardiothoracic Surgery series, some of the practical problems related to postperfusion syndromes, gastrointestinal complications, lung function, potassium kinetics, pulsatile flow, ventricular venting, and air embolus are reviewed. In addition, we explore the areas of vasomotor activity and venous compliance, fluid balance, carbon dioxide transport and acid base balance, complement activation, cardioplegic additives, and deep hypothermia. Other chapters are concerned with the problems related to conducting a clinical trial of an investigational device and the medical-legal implications of cardiopulmonary bypass. The influence of nonsurgeons on surgical practice is obvious when exploring these topics. It is the series' goal that the knowledge, capability, standard of practice, and performance of the reader will be enhanced by the information presented in this monograph.

In keeping with the goal of the series to publish monographs that will deal in a broad sense with information related to the care of the cardiac and thoracic surgery patient, forthcoming volumes will deal with perioperative cardiac dysfunction and cardiothoracic trauma.

Preface

The topics presented in this monograph were discussed at the Second Annual Cardiothoracic Symposium in San Diego, California in February, 1982. The interest of surgeons, perfusionists, anesthesiologists, cardiologists, intensivists, operating room and ICU nurses, and representatives of the medical device industry was obvious at that time. The information presented here includes material related to basic science, organ function, total organism and organ physiology, biochemistry, immunology, physical chemistry, practical use of devices and components of the heart-lung machine, as well as the legal implications of clinical trials and use of cardiopulmonary bypass.

Acknowledgments

This monograph is the result of the efforts of a great number of peoaple. The editor wishes to acknowledge the efforts of the members of the Division of Cardiothoracic Surgery, University of California, San Diego and the authors who contributed so willingly to this volume. The efforts of editorial associate, Rosanne Betleski, cannot be underestimated. Others whose efforts contributed greatly to the monograph include Christine Johnson, Cleonice Y. Gordon, Michelle Brown, Nanci Anderson, Suzanne Seigal, Elizabeth A. Ashleigh, Linny Sarnecki, Dorothea Rehman, and Judith Bohannan.

Contributors

Dennis E. Chenoweth, Ph.D., M.D., Assistant Professor of Pathology, University of California, San Diego

Richard E. Clark, M.D., Professor of Surgery, Washington University, St. Louis, Missouri

Donald B. Doty, M.D., Professor of Surgery, The University of Iowa, Iowa City

G. Duke Duncan, Ph.D., Associate Director, Heineman Medical Research Laboratories, Charlotte Memorial Hospital, North Carolina

L. Henry Edmunds, Jr., M.D., Professor of Surgery, University of Pennsylvania, Philadelphia

Michael H. Hall, M.D., Assistant Attending Professor of Surgery, North Shore University Hospital, Cornell University Medical College, Manhasset, New York

William B. Long, III, M.D., Assistant Professor of Surgery, University of California, San Diego

Thomas N. Masters, Ph.D., Director, Heineman Medical Research Laboratories, Charlotte Memorial Hospital, North Carolina.

Carmine G. Moccio, M.D., Assistant Attending Professor, North Shore University Hospital, Cornell University Medical College, Manhasset, New York

William Y. Moores, M.D., Assistant Professor of Surgery, University of California, San Diego

Ricardo J. Moreno-Cabral, M.D., Clinical Assistant Professor of Cardiovascular Surgery, Stanford University, Stanford, California

Roy L. Nelson, M.D., Assistant Attending Professor of Surgery, North Shore University Hospital, Cornell University Medical College, Manhasset, New York

Witold Niesluchowski, M.D., Surgery Resident, Charlotte Memorial Hospital, North Carolina

Richard M. Peters, M.D., Professor of Surgery and Bioengineering, University of California, San Diego

Allen K. Ream, M.D., Assistant Professor of Anesthesia, Stanford University, Stanford, California

Bruce A. Reitz, M.D., Associate Professor of Cardiovascular Surgery, Stanford University, Stanford, California

Francis Robicsek, M.D., Clinical Professor of Surgery, University of North Carolina, Chapel Hill

Benson B. Roe, M.D., Professor of Surgery, University of California, San Francisco.

Gerald D. Silverberg, M.D., Assistant Professor of Neurosurgery, Stanford University, Stanford, California

Joseph M. Sindell, L.L.B., J.D., La Jolla, California

D. Barton Stephens, C.C.P., University of California, San Diego

Julie A. Swain, M.D., Assistant Professor of Surgery, University of California, San Diego

Yehuda Tamari, M.S., Biostatistician, North Shore University Hospital, Manhasset, New York

Anthony J. Tortolani, M.D., Assistant Attending Professor of Surgery, North Shore University Hospital, Cornell University Medical College, Manhasset, New York

Joe R. Utley, M.D., Professor of Surgery, University of California, San Diego

Yitzhak Weinstein, Ph.D., Postdoctoral Fellow, Physiological Research Laboratory, Scripps Institution of Oceanography, University of California, San Diego

Fred N. White, Ph.D., Professor of Medicine (Physiology), Director, Physiological Research Laboratory, Scripps Institution of Oceanography, University of California, San Diego

William Williams, C.C.P., University of Pennsylvania, Philadelphia

Steven R. Wyte, M.D., Associate Clinical Professor of Anesthesiology, University of California, San Diego

John C. Yeager, Ph.D., Associate Professor of Physiology, East Carolina University School of Medicine, Greenville, North Carolina

Contents

CHAPTER 1

VASOMOTOR ACTIVITY DURING CARDIOPULMONARY BYPASS

FRANCIS ROBICSEK, M.D.
THOMAS N. MASTERS, PH.D.
WITOLD NIESLUCHOWSKI, M.D.
JOHN C. YEAGER, PH.D.
G. DUKE DUNCAN, PH.D.

The purpose of this essay is to provoke, not to prescribe.

Fred N. White (31)

Differences between "normal" hemodynamics and the hemodynamics of cardiopulmonary bypass are significant and multifold: 1. The heart and the lungs are temporarily eliminated and replaced by a mechanical pump and oxygenator, which unlike the patient's own organs, have no autoregulation to compensate for some of the deficiencies of extracorporeal circulation. 2. The physiological systolic-diastolic pressure variation is absent. 3. Some basic physiological factors which under normal conditions are conveniently accepted as constants (hematocrit, viscosity of the blood, temperature, pH, P_{O_2}, P_{CO_2}, etc.) suddenly arise as significant variants. 4. Probably the most important difference is, however, that the intent of nature to provide an optimal perfusion and gas exchange is replaced by our own capitulating attitudes of being content with the acceptable minimum.

This very abnormal situation existing during cardiopulmonary bypass does not insinuate that the same physical forces which govern the circulation under the normal circumstances do not act the same way while the patient is connected to the heart-lung machine. The basic function of cardiopulmonary bypass is to provide an adequate *flow* of oxygenated blood to the tissues in need. It is affected by three primary factors: *velocity*, a force which acts in the direction of the flow; the *pressure*, the force-vector of which is perpendicular to the direction of the flow; and the *circulatory resistance*, which is opposition to these forces. Accordingly, the basic equation of hemodynamics is $F = \dfrac{P}{R}$; flow is directly proportional with pressure and is in an inverse proportion with resistance. Blood flow is regarded as adequate during normothermic cardiopulmonary bypass if it is close to the patient's own prebypass cardiac output. "Normal" flows of 3.1 liter/min/m^2 can be achieved indeed but at the expense of somewhat increased risk of high arterial line pressure, platelet aggregation, micro-airbolism, etc. Bypass flows of 2.2 to 2.4 liter/min/m^2 are generally considered to be an acceptable compromise.[1-3] "Safe" levels for hypo-

1

thermic perfusions are lower, but have not been established with certainty. The reason for this may be that such attempts included primarily the degree but not the duration of the hypothermia and also that additional factors, such as variable degree of ischemia of different organs, such as the heart, has not been properly evaluated. Blood flow is not a unified entity, because the different organs of the body require it disproportionally to their mass. The striated muscle and the skin require much lower flow rates than the vital organs, such as the brain, the heart, and the kidneys. To complicate the matter further, it has to be realized that the majority of patients undergoing open heart surgery suffer from diffuse arteriosclerotic changes and often have different degrees of narrowing or even complete occlusion of major visceral arteries. Such patients are more sensitive to low flow rates and can easily suffer irreversible organ injuries.

Exactly what is optimal or even acceptable perfusion pressure is also a matter of discussion. It is also debated whether or not it is necessary to maintain a pulsatile pressure difference. Generally speaking, experience has shown that the function and protection of vital organs depend on flow rather than on pressure, and the efficiency of perfusion is not assured by a seemingly adequate pressure alone. It is generally agreed though that a minimal perfusion pressure of 35 to 40 mm Hg mean is necessary to maintain capillary patency.

Besides the adequacy of the blood flow and an assured perfusion pressure, the most important hemodynamic information during cardiopulmonary bypass is the total systemic vascular resistance, or more properly called the total systemic circulatory resistance. In 1841, Poiseuille presented his basic law that governs flow through cylindrical pipes. This law states that the head of pressure is directly proportional to tube length, rate of flow, and viscosity, and inversely proportional to the fourth power of the internal radius. Applying this concept for the determination of circulatory resistance:

$$R = \frac{8\eta L}{\pi r^4}$$

where R is circulatory resistance, η is vicosity, L is length, and r equals the internal radius. Evidently the diameter of the tube is the prime determinant of resistance in most clinical conditions.

In hemodynamics, it is customary to equate peripheral circulatory resistance with the resistance represented by the arterioles. While this approach is practical, indeed, in most conditions, it also has to be realized[4] that other components of the vascular bed may also contribute sometimes most significantly to the resistance to blood flow, as seen in Table 1.1.

In 1960[5] we were among the first to describe the seemingly mysterious behavior of systemic circulatory resistance. We found that due to changes in resistance during cardiopulmonary bypass, if flow rates are set constant, the pressure will significantly fluctuate. On the other hand, if an effort was made to keep the pressure constant, the flow rate had to be readjusted repeatedly. There were also unexplained shifts in the blood volume and significant changes in the circulatory resistance corresponding with underperfusion and hypoxemia. Since then, a wealth of observations have been added to our own investigations, but the origin of these changes remained a mystery.

Trying to establish some kind of a system in these hemodynamic events occurring during cardiopulmonary bypass which involve primarily the circulatory resistance,

Table 1.1

Relative Resistance to Blood Flow in Different Segments of the Vascular System*

Aorta	4%	Venules	4%
Large arteries	5%	Terminal veins	0.3%
Main arterial branches	10%	Main venous branches	0.7%
Terminal branches	6%	Large veins	0.5%
Arterioles	41%	Vena cava	1.5%
Capillaries	27%		
Total arterial + capillary	93%	Total venous	7%

* From A. C. Burton: *Physiology and Biophysics of the Circulation*, Ed. 2, Chap. 8. Copyright © 1972 by Year Book Medical Publishers, Inc., Chicago.

we can divide them into two basic phenomena (Fig. 1.1): 1) An initial severe drop in peripheral circulatory resistance at the beginning of bypass (Phenomenon A); and 2) a gradual recovery and progressive increase in peripheral circulatory resistance as the bypass progresses (Phenomenon B).

PHENOMENON A

Originally, *Phenomenon A* was attributed to the adjustment of the body to inadequate perfusion. Soon, however, it became apparent that a severe drop in total peripheral circulatory resistance occurs even if the perfusion rate is set at or even in excess of the patient's own cardiac output as measured before the initiation of cardiopulmonary bypass. It usually lasts from 5 to 10 minutes,

after which there is a gradual return of peripheral resistance and arterial mean pressure (with appropriate flow) to prebypass levels. A possibility, which initially appeared to be plausible to us, was that Phenomenon A represents a shock-like situation caused by the very unnatural state of the extracorporeal circulation itself. It is certainly without doubt that the induced cardiac arrest, the cessation of respiration, the artificial perfusion and oxygenation of the tissues represents a trauma of considerable magnitude. Such traumatic states could easily evoke the release of histamine and histamine-like substances and cause massive vasodilatation and drop in the perfusion pressure. This theory held on for quite a while, but it could not be supported with objective demonstration of increased hista-

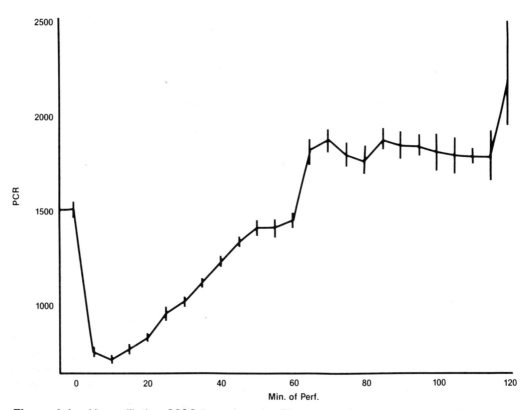

Figure 1.1. Hemodilution 20°C hypothermia. Diagrammatic representation of circulatory resistance (*PCR*) changes during 120 minutes of cardiopulmonary bypass in 20 patients at tympanic temperatures of 20°C with crystalloid prime. *Vertical bar*, standard error of the mean.

mine levels in the blood. Another hypothesis to explain the mechanism of Phenomenon A was just the opposite; the drop of systemic circulatory resistance is not due to liberation of vasoactive substances but to dilution of normal amount of catecholamines circulating in the blood. Again, this theory was studied, but the findings revealed that although the priming fluid may dilute the patient's circulating blood volume and with it the circulating catecholamines as much as 1:2, the restoration of catecholamine level is so fast that it is usually back to normal within 2 minutes. The initial shock-like reaction of cardiopulmonary bypass has also been attributed to reaction to blood prime[6–8] and was named by Gadboys et al.[6] as "homologous blood syndrome," characterized by drop in circulatory resistance and perfusion pressure, severe acidosis, pooling of the blood in the splanchnic area, coagulopathy, renal and cerebral dysfunction and was caused by an incompatibility reaction between the blood elements of the donor and the recipient.[32] While occasional incompatibility reactions during extracorporeal circulation are indeed a possibility if blood prime is used, the commonly occurring Phenomenon A cannot be explained by this theory alone. As a matter of fact, in our own clinical observations, we found that the most efficient way *to avoid* Phenomenon A was to use full blood instead of crystalloid prime.

Someone may also consider Phenomenon A to be invoked simply by the aggravated trauma of sudden inundation of the vascular system with cold priming solution. Theoretically, this may indeed cause a temporary partial or total paralysis of the smooth muscle of the vascular wall resulting in excessive drop in circulatory resistance. The concomitant drop in mean perfusion pressure (unless it is compensated for with excessively high flow rates) will persist until the vessels recover from this initial cold insult and regain appropriate vascular tone. Again this was tested, and we found that the events of Phenomenon A occurred regardless of the temperature of the priming fluid (Figs. 1.2 and 1.3).

At the present stage of our knowledge, it appears to us that the primary reason that we could not appreciate exactly the hemodynamic events of Phenomenon A was that we kept thinking in the traditional way of peripheral circulatory resistance, namely that it is a direct indication of the vascular tone. While this is indeed true in almost all situations in off-perfusion hemodynamics, it is certainly not valid for the patients on cardiopulmonary bypass where the total circulatory resistance depends on not a single, but on two primary factors: (a) the vascular resistance representing the state of the arterioles, and (b) the viscosity of the blood. Typically, the serum viscosity of a normal

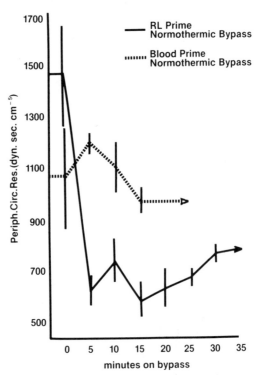

Figure 1.2. Changes in circulatory resistance (*solid line*) in 15 patients with crystalloid prime (*RL*, Ringers Lactate) during tympanic temperatures maintained at 35 to 37°C. The *dotted line* represents changes in eight patients who received blood prime and throughout bypass were maintained at tympanic temperatures of 35 to 37°C. *Vertical bar*, standard error of the mean.

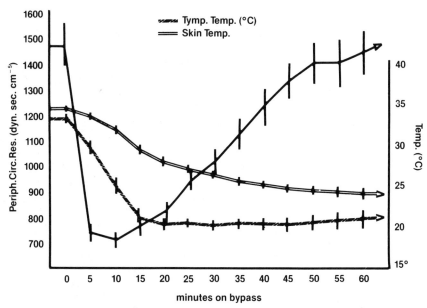

Figure 1.3. Alterations in circulatory resistance (*solid line*) in 25 patients with crystalloid prime. Accompanying skin and tympanic temperature changes are also displayed. *Vertical bar*, standard error of the mean.

individual is approximately 1.4 to 1.8 times that of the water. If the blood is diluted with an excess of crystalloid priming solution (as it may occur at the initiation of bypass) its viscosity and consequently the total circulatory resistance may drop appreciably, causing the shock-like situation of Phenomenon A. This hypothesis was tested in a number of clinical observations in which we found that: (1) Phenomenon A occurs regularly if crystalloid prime was used, regardless of the temperature of the priming liquid (Figs. 1.2 and 1.3); (b) The occurrence of Phenomenon A can be prevented by using full blood prime, regardless of the temperature of the blood.

PHENOMENON B

A second interesting hemodynamic event we had the opportunity to observe in the course of open heart operations performed with the aid of extracorporeal circulation was the progressive increase in the total peripheral circulatory resistance: *Phenomenon B*. This rise in resistance usually began

shortly after the subsidence of Phenomenon A became significant if the procedure was done in hypothermia, and it appeared to be proportional with both the time period and the degree of cooling (Figs. 1.1 to 1.3).

Following the line of reasoning that we observed at the beginning of this chapter, it appears to be logical to examine Phenomenon B in the light of viscosity as a potential factor. As it has been mentioned in connection with Phenomenon A, at the beginning of perfusion, blood viscosity takes a nose dive due to hemodilution by crystalloid prime. As time progresses, however, there is a regression of this process due to diuresis and shifts of fluid from the vascular space to the cellular and intracellular spaces. Besides this process of hemoconcentration, there are two additional reasons for the gradually increasing blood viscosity. The first reason is that blood being a non-Newtonian fluid, its viscosity changes with the velocity gradient. As the body temperature of the patient decreases, it is customary to cut back the flow rate. When the velocity drops below a critical level, intense aggregation and rouleaux formation of the corpuscular elements occur. This creates a rather thick material and leads to increased viscosity. The second mechanism by which blood becomes more viscous is the hypothermia itself (Figs. 1.4 and 1.5). At a shear rate of 213/second, the blood viscosity increases by 5% for every 1C° drop in temperature.

According to the above, Phenomenon B could be well explained by the gradual increase in viscosity alone. The evidence for

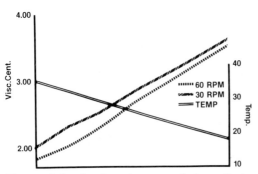

Figure 1.4. *In vitro* changes of viscosity in human whole blood with varying temperatures. The measurements were made with two different revolutions per minute (RPM) on the viscometer.

this would be the demonstration that Phenomenon B does not develop if the factor of viscosity is maintained constant. This, however, did not prove to be the case. As we do routinely during myocardiac revascularization procedures, we placed patients on cardiopulmonary bypass and gradually lowered body temperature down to 20C°. After the temperature dropped to this level, we assured unchanged viscosity by maintaining the composition and temperature of the blood constant. In some patients the perfusion pressure (Figs. 1.6 and 1.7), in others the flow rate, was kept unchanged (Fig. 1.8). In either case, there was further increase in total peripheral circulatory resistance, clearly indicating that in the genesis of Phenomenon B changes in vascular status indeed play a significant role.

Vasoconstrictive response during cardiopulmonary bypass has long been suspected and thought to be mediated through the increase of circulating catecholamines. Tan et al.[9] measured the level of serum catecholamines during total body perfusions performed in moderate hypothermia and were unable to document an increase in the levels of epinephrine and norepinephrine, nor did they observe a reduction—an observation which agrees with our findings

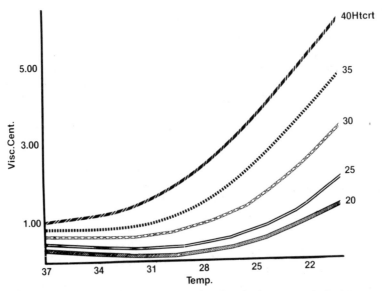

Figure 1.5. Changes in viscosity measured *in vitro* in human whole blood with varying temperatures and hematocrit (*Htcrt.*)

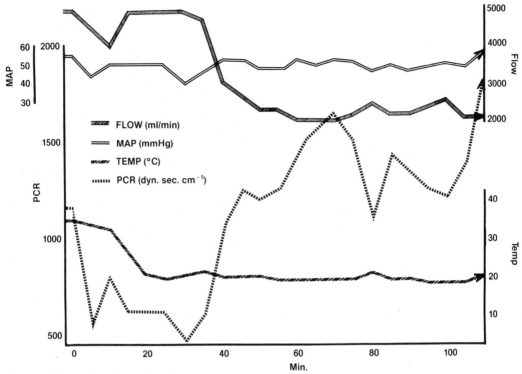

Figure 1.6. Alterations in circulatory resistance (*PCR*) and flow during hypothermia with constant mean arterial pressure (*MAP*) in one representative patient.

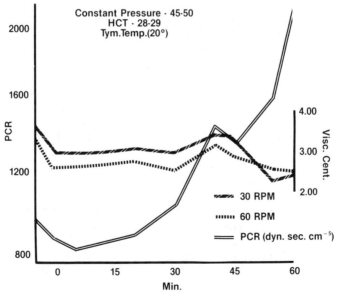

Figure 1.7. Circulatory resistance (*PCR*, dyn.sec.cm^{-5}) changes determined during hypothermic cardiopulmonary bypass, with arterial mean pressure and viscosity maintained constant in one representative patient.

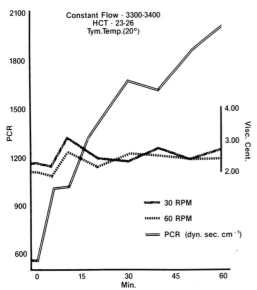

Figure 1.8. Changes in circulatory resistance (*PCR*) during hypothermia (20°C), with pump flow and viscosity maintained constant in one representative patient.

(Fig. 1.9). Tan reasoned that the catecholamine level in the circulating blood did not decrease, despite the introduction of 2 liters of crystalloid prime which would suggest that these amines have been added to the circulation to compensate for the dilution. The sources for this, they suggested, were the adrenals and the sympathetic nerve terminals to which Ngai et al.[10] refer to as the "re-uptake process." The theory of vasoconstriction has been further supported by the experimental observation of Lopez-Belio and associates[11] who found that the drug chlorpromazine, if given in sufficient amounts, is capable of maintaining peripheral circulatory resistance at near normal levels even during hypothermic perfusions. These findings are again in accord with our own observations[12] that the regularly occurring gradual increase of peripheral circulatory resistance (Phenomenon B) can be easily and promptly counteracted by the administration of different vasodilators, such as nitroprusside or intravenous nitroglycerine.

The next question which naturally arises is: What is the cause of this vasoconstric-

tion? The role of pulsatile versus nonpulsatile flow in the origin of elevated peripheral circulatory resistance during cardiopulmonary bypass has been implicated by several authors.[1, 13, 14] The "high resistance acidosis syndrome" has been reported by Dunn et al.,[15] Replogle et al.,[16] and Sanderson et al.[17] in connection with nonpulsatile bypass. Interestingly enough, others[18–21] did not confirm these observations. These divergent views have been correlated by Harrison,[22, 23] who demonstrated that in normothermic perfusions, acidosis, organ failure, and elevated peripheral circulatory resistance occur below a critical level of less than 70 ml/min/kg flow rates with both pulsatile and nonpulsatile bypass. Similarly, this syndrome would not manifest regardless of the type of perfusion if the flow rates are kept above 130 ml/min/kg. At the interim rates of 80 to 120 ml/min/kg, however, pulsatile flow prevents the development of high peripheral circulatory resistance, but nonpulsatile flow does not.

In hypothermic perfusions, though, the situation is radically different. While we are using significantly lower flow rates, we believe that the tissues are adequately perfused due to the lowering of metabolic needs by hypothermia. This view is certainly supported by the fact that the venous pH and P_{CO_2} is in a well acceptable range (Figs. 1.10 and 1.11). Looking at the bright red blood entering the body through the arterial line and at the bright red blood leaving the patient through the venous line (Fig. 1.12), the question naturally arises: Are we overoxygenating our patients during hypothermia? Could this be the cause of an extensive vasoconstrictive response?

That the O_2 tension may be an important moderator of blood flow to the skeletal muscle has already been suggested by several investigators.[24–26] The most notable experiments were those of Berne et al.[27] who demonstrated that high P_{O_2} levels caused significant constriction; low P_{O_2} levels induced appreciable dilatation of the arterioles of the hamster pouch, as well as in the coronary circulation of the open-chested dog.[27] In 1960, we performed somewhat similar experiments[5] on dogs placed on car-

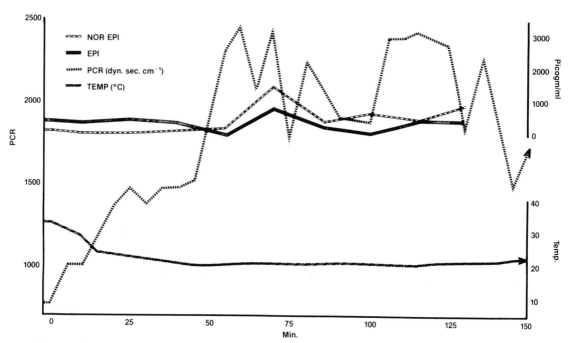

Figure 1.9. Hemodilution .20°C hypothermia. Diagrammatic representation of changes in norepinephrine and epinephrine during hypothermic cardiopulmonary bypass. Changes in circulatory resistance (*PCR*) are also displayed in three patients.

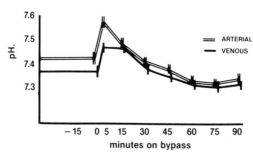

Figure 1.10. Hemodilution .20°C hypothermic bypass. Changes in arterial and venous pH during hypothermic bypass. The first sample was taken 5 minutes into the bypass procedure and 15 minutes thereafter. *Double vertical bar and vertical bar*, standard error of the mean.

diopulmonary bypass. We found that hypoxemia, induced by decreasing the O_2 flow to the oxygenator, caused a severe and immediate fall in both perfusion pressure and peripheral circulatory resistance. The possibility that hyperoxygenation of the blood could have unwanted hemodynamic seque-

lae during cardiopulmonary bypass is certainly not a comforting one because we traditionally consider overoxygenation by the heart-lung machine as "staying on the safe side." If, in deep hypothermia we follow closely the oxygen saturation and the oxygen tension of the arterial and venous blood (Fig. 1.12), it is evident that there is practically no difference in the oxygen saturation,[28] and the very moderate oxygen consumption seems to come almost entirely from the physically dissolved gas. And even this might be excessive for the cold tissues which barely need any oxygen at all. Or do they?

There is, however, another possibility, namely that instead of tissue hyperoxia, we are faced with tissue hypoxia amidst overoxygenated blood. This could occur by several mechanisms. One of such is the opening of numerous arteriovenous shunts which could divert the lion's share of the arterial blood flow away from the tissues and directly into the venous circulation. Another possibility is that the affinity of hemoglobin

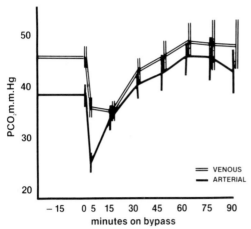

Figure 1.11. Alterations in P_{CO_2} during hypothermic bypass in arterial and venous blood. The first sample was taken 5 minutes into the bypass procedure and 15 minutes thereafter. *Double vertical bar and vertical bar*, standard error of the mean.

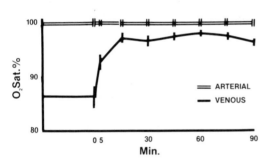

Figure 1.12. Hemodilution .20 hypothermia. Arterial and venous blood O_2 saturation during hypothermic cardiopulmonary bypass. *Double vertical bar and vertical bar*, standard error of the mean.

for oxygen is greatly increased as the temperature drops, so although the same or even greater amounts of oxygen are available in the blood, less will be released to the tissues. In other words, hypothermia may shift the oxygen-hemoglobin dissociation curve to the left to such a degree that the cells may remain hypoxic, despite the fact that the blood is well oxygenated, just as the ship-wrecked sailor thirsts in the lifeboat floating in the ocean.

When such a hypoxia occurs, the cells are forced to survive on anerobic metabolism, resulting in a buildup of lactic acid and metabolic acidosis; and the already serious situation can be further aggravated by arteriolar constriction. The latter may be the only clinically manifested indicator of the intracellular events.

The influence of pH upon the total systemic circulatory resistance during cardiopulmonary bypass is not clear. The combination of metabolic acidosis with elevated values of circulatory resistance is well recognized,[18, 19, 21, 29] but is generally regarded as coincidental rather than causative.

In normothermic perfusions, pH and P_{CO_2} levels close to or at normal are generally regarded as optimal by most surgeons. The opinions, however, are less than equivocal regarding cardiopulmonary bypass performed in combination with hypothermia, especially if the perfusion is carried out in deep (<22C°) cooling. Because the hemoglobin-oxygen dissociation curve is more favorable during hypothermia in the acidotic range, most authors recommend that the level of the arterial pH should indeed be kept moderately (7.30 to 7.35) acidotic. This is accomplished by using an oxygen-carbon dioxide mixture instead of pure oxygen gas in the oxygenator. The advisability of this protocol has been recently challenged by Becker et al.[30] who, using the analogy of ectotherms, such as reptiles hibernating under hypothermic conditions, now recommend that the arterial pH during hypothermic perfusions should be maintained alkalotic. They found in animal experiments that by assuring an alkalotic arterial pH of 7.7 to 7.9, they obtained not only better protection of the myocardium, improved cerebral flow, and a normal lactate metabolism, but also a systemic vascular resistance 90% below the level of that observed in the control animal perfused with normal pH of 7.4.

CONCLUSION

In conclusion, hypothermic cardiopulmonary bypass has permitted a prolongation of more complicated cardiac surgical procedures, allowing greater safety, more favorable metabolic parameters and less postoperative complications. However, maintaining a warm-blooded temperature-regulated species at subnormal frigid environments may evoke dormant reactions which lost their importance on the tree of evolution. Our experiences, along with those of others, establish similar responses to hypothermia and emphasize the need for a better understanding of the human species subjected to lowered temperatures. There are presumably questions unasked in this vast area due to our naivety which, once answered, will provide a safer application of this necessary technique during cardiac surgical procedures.

References

1. Bartlett RH, Gazzaniga AB: Physiology and pathophysiology of extracorporeal circulation. In *Techniques in Extracorporeal Circulation*, edited by MI Ionescu. London, Butterworths, 1981.
2. Replogle RL: Use of corticosteroids during cardiopulmonary bypass. Possible lyosome stabilization. *Circulation* 33 and 34(Suppl I):86, 1966.
3. Tarham S, Moffitt EA: Anaesthesia and supportive care during and after cardiac surgery. Ann Thorac Surg 11:64, 1971.
4. Haddy FJ: Effect of histamine on small and large vessel pressure in the dog foreleg. Am J Physiol 198:161, 1960.
5. Sanger PW, Robicsek F, Taylor FH, Rees TT, Stam RE: Vasomotor regulation during extracorporeal circulation and open-heart surgery. J Thorac Cardiovasc Surg 40:355, 1960.
6. Gadboys HT, Slonim R, Litwak RS: Homologous blood syndrome. I. Preliminary observations on its relationship to clinical cardiopulmonary bypass. Ann Surg 156:793, 1962.
7. Ankeney JS, Murphy SK: A study of peripheral (IVC and SVC) and central (splanchnic) venous flow rates during extracorporeal bypass. J Thorac Cardiovasc Surg 44:589, 1962.
8. Dow JW: The shock state in heart-lung bypass in dogs. Trans Am Soc Artif Intern Organs 5:240, 1959.
9. Tan CK, Glissin SN, El-Etr AA, Ramakishmaiah KB: Levels of circulatory norepinephrine and epinephrine before, during and after cardiopulmonary bypass in man. J Thorac Cardiovasc Surg 71:928, 1976.
10. Ngai SH, Dairman W, and Marchelle M: Effects of lidocaine and etidocaine on the axoplasmic transport of catecholamine-synthesizing enzymes. Anesthesiology 41(6):542–548, 1974.
11. Lopez-Belio M, Tasaki G, Balagot R, Sanchez L, Gomez F, Julian OC: Effect of hyperthermia during

cardiopulmonary bypass on peripheral resistance. Alteration by diluate blood perfusate and by chlorpromazine. Arch Surgery 81:283, 1960.
12. Arora MV, Partney KL, Ferrari HA, Robicsek F, Masters TN: Thermographic evidence of the effects of nitroglycerin on myocardial perfusion. Crit Care Med 6:99, 1978.
13. Trinkle JK, Helton NE, Bryant LR, Gridden WO: Pulsatile cardiopulmonary bypass: Clinical evaluation. Surgery 68:1074, 1970.
14. Trinkle JK, Helton NE, Wood RE, Bryant LR: Metabolic comparison of a new pulsatile pump and a roller pump for cardiopulmonary bypass. J Thorac Cardiovasc Surg 58:562, 1969.
15. Dunn F, Kirsch M, Harness J, Carroll M, Strokes J, Sloan H: Haemodynamic, metabolic and haemotologic effects of pulsatile cardiopulmonary bypass. J Thorac Cardiovasc Surg 68:138, 1974.
16. Replogle RL, Levy M, DeWall RA, Lillehei RC: Catecholamine and serotonin response to cardiopulmonary bypass. J Thorac Cardiovasc Surg 44:638, 1962.
17. Sanderson JM, Wright G, Simms FW: Brain damage in dogs immediately following pulsatile and nonpulsatile blood flow in extracorporeal circulation. Thorax 27:275, 1972.
18. Boucher JK, Rudy LW, Edmunds LH: Organ blood flow during pulsatile cardiopulmonary bypass. J Appl Physiol 36:86, 1974.
19. Harken AH: The influence of pulsatile perfusion in oxygen uptake by the isolated canine hind limb. J Thorac Cardiovasc Surg 70:237, 1975.
20. Rudy LW, Heymann MA, Edmunds LH: Distribution of systemic blood flow during cardiopulmonary bypass. J Appl Physiol 34:194, 1970.
21. Wesolowski·SA, Sauvage LR, Pine RD: Extracorporeal circulation: The role of the pulse in maintenance of the systemic circulation during heartlung bypass. Surgery 37:663, 1954.
22. Harrison TS, Charola RC, Seton JF, Robinson BH: Carotid sinus origin of adrenergic responses compromising the effectiveness of artificial circulatory support. Surgery 68:20, 1970.
23. Harrison TS, Seton JF: An analysis of pulse frequency as an adrenergic excitant in pulsatile circulatory support. Surgery 73:868, 1973.
24. Guyton AC, Ross JM, Carrier O Jr, Walker JR: Evidence for tissue oxygen demand as the major factor causing autoregulation. Circ Res(Suppl I, 14–15):I-60–I-69, 1964.
25. Vane JR, McGiff JC: Possible contributions of endogenous prostaglandins to the control of blood pressure. Circ Res(Suppl I, 36–37):68, 1975.
26. Detar R, Bohr DF: Oxygen and vascular smooth muscle contraction. Am J Physiol 214(2):241, 1968.
27. Berne RM, Blackmon JR, Gardner TH: Hypoxemia and coronary blood flow. J Clin Invest 36(7):1101, 1957.
28. Padhi RK, Ko ES, Rainbow RLG, Lynn RB: Some observations on deep hypothermia using extracorporeal circulation. Angiology 12:12–16, 1961.
29. Rudy LW, Heymann MA, Edmunds LH: Distribution of systemic blood flow during total cardiopul-

monary bypass in rhesus monkeys. Surg Forum 21:149, 1970.

30. Becker H, Vinten-Johansen F, Buckerberg GD, Robertson JM, Leaf FD, Lazar HL, Manganaro AF: Myocardial damage caused by keeping pH 7.40 during systemic deep hypothermia. J Thorac Cardiovasc Surg 82:810, 1981.

31. White FN: A comparative physiological approach to hypothermia. J Thorac Cardiovasc Surg 82:821, 1981.

32. Litwak RS, Slonim R, Wisoff BG, Cadboys HL: Homologous blood syndrome during extracorporeal circulation in man. N Engl J Med 268:1377, 1963.

CHAPTER 2

VENOUS COMPLIANCE DURING CARDIOPULMONARY BYPASS

DONALD B. DOTY, M.D.

Most of the emphasis in the study of the circulatory system has been placed on the heart and the arterial circulation. The heart serves as the pump or energy source to propel the blood through the arteries which serve as the conduits to bring the blood to the body tissues. The physiologic dynamics of this "delivery" side of the circulatory system has received considerable attention while the "return" or venous system has not been extensively studied. The role of the venous system in circulatory control is generally considered to be passive. The venous system, however, contains 70 to 80% of the blood volume and has the ability to make rapid adjustments in vascular dimensions to provide sufficient blood to maintain adequate pressure to fill the cardiac chambers between cardiac contractions.[1] Furthermore, in sympathetic discharge states which accompany hemorrhage, vasoconstriction of the venous vascular bed occurs rapidly and actually precedes constriction in the arterial circulation.[2] Thus, the venous system is of major importance in general circulatory system control and responds rapidly and actively to the altered circulatory states.

VASOMOTOR DYNAMICS OF THE NORMAL VENOUS SYSTEM

The systemic veins are important in maintaining filling of the right atrium and maintenance of the central blood volume. The systemic veins hold the major portion of the blood volume and serve a reservoir function, which by dynamic alteration of capacity provides availability of blood for cardiac filling. The dampening effect of this large and dynamic capacitance system exerts an evening or smoothing effect on the function of the circulatory system. The venous capacitance system throughout the body functions as a unit to regulate cardiac filling and is not affected by local changes in tissues or individual organs. The arterial or resistance vessels, on the other hand, respond to supply local needs for blood flow to meet metabolic demand. The coordination of the venous system in relation to total circulatory control is accomplished mainly through the sympathetic nerves to the smooth muscle in veins.

Neural Effects

Shepherd and Vanhoutte[1] have reviewed the dynamics of the venous system detailing the variations of density of innervation and the quantity of smooth muscle cells in veins in various areas in the body. Sympathetic innervation and smooth muscle are plentiful in cutaneous and splanchnic veins, while the veins in skeletal muscle have little or no sympathetic innervation and only a small amount of smooth muscle in their walls (Fig.

2.1). The sympathetic nervous system, therefore, may exert active control over the capacity of the splanchnic and cutaneous veins, while the role of veins in skeletal muscle will generally be passive, having little response to sympathetic nervous system circulatory control. Norepinephrine liberated at sympathetic nerve endings is the essential neurotransmitter causing contraction of the smooth muscle cells in the vein wall resulting in venoconstriction. Norepinephrine effect is removed by various mechanisms, including breakdown within smooth muscle cells by catechol-o-methyltransferase and monoamine oxidase, uptake by adrenergic nerve endings, and outflow into the bloodstream or extracellular fluid. Various drugs and anesthetic agents alter adrenergic neurotransmission and may affect venomotor control. Outstanding among these agents are halothane, local anesthetics, digitalis analogs, morphine and its derivatives, and various antidepressants or tranquilizer drugs.

Smooth Muscle

Active changes in capacity of the venous system occur in response to contraction or relaxation of the venous smooth muscle cells, causing expulsion from or uptake of blood to the venous bed. The activity or tone of the smooth muscle cells of the vein wall may be determined by the presence of norepinephrine either liberated by sympathetic nerve endings or circulating in the blood in response to central nervous system sympathetic control. The splanchnic vascular bed, including the liver, spleen, and mesenteric veins contains about 20% of the total body blood volume and is a major regulator in maintenance of cardiac filling. The splanchnic venous bed responds actively and is controlled by cardiovascular reflexes. Pressoreceptors in the carotid sinus and the aortic arch are key regulators which in response to low arterial pressure cause increased sympathetic outflow, resulting in constriction of the splanchnic venous bed

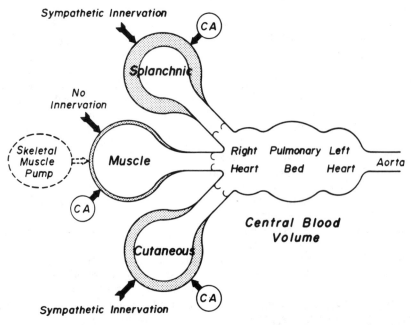

Figure 2.1. Splanchnic and cutaneous veins have an abundance of smooth muscle (*dotted areas*) and a rich sympathetic innervation. Muscle veins have little smooth muscle and few if any sympathetic nerves. (Reproduced with permission from J. T. Shepherd and P. M. VanHoutte.[1])

and increased availability of blood for cardiac filling. Cardiopulmonary receptors located at the junction of the great veins and the atria may also initiate similar reflexes in response to low pressure which cause splanchnic venous constriction and increased blood flow to the heart. Low pressure baroreceptors also produce venoconstrictor response in the extremities.[3] Active venoconstriction of skeletal muscle veins may occur to a lesser degree than splanchnic or cutaneous veins but by virtue of the large mass of skeletal muscle may exert major potential to decrease venous capacity for availability of a substantial volume of blood. Cutaneous veins actively respond to reduced body temperature by vasoconstriction mediated by increased sympathetic stimulation and as a local effect of cold which makes these veins more reactive to stimulation.[1] Venoconstriction of cutaneous veins transfers blood from superficial veins to deep veins in the extremities where countercurrent heat exchange occurs with the accompanying arteries in order to conserve body heat. Similar venoconstrictive response occurs following increase in depth of respiration and any strong emotional stimulus.

Passive Effects

Passive changes in venous capacity are the result of the distensible and compliant nature of the elastin and collagen fibers which lie between the smooth muscle cells in vein walls. Small changes of intraluminal distending pressure, therefore, may cause significant changes in vein diameter and the amount of blood contained in the venous system. The venous system may respond passively in harmony to active changes in the arterial system. Active constriction of precapillary arterioles resulting in decreased intraluminal venous pressure causes compliant reduction of venous diameter with passive expulsion of blood from the affected venous bed. This passive venous capacity change may be important during generalized arteriolar constriction associated with hypotension, making blood available for the maintenance of cardiac output. Passive changes in veins of skeletal muscle beds of

the extremities are especially important in maintaining hemodynamic steady states in upright posture. Operations using cardiopulmonary bypass are usually performed with the patient in the supine position so that hydrostatic forces affecting passive venous changes are not evoked unless there are changes of body position by elevation or lowering of the legs during surgery. Elevation of leg position reduces hydrostatic inflow pressure to the limb, resulting in passive reduction of venous volume and transfer of blood to the central circulation. Lowering the legs produces the opposite effect, with accumulation of blood in the compliant veins. Principles of passive venous compliance as a source for transfer of blood to the central circulation by external compression of the legs and abdomen has been utilized to assist the circulation following trauma and after cardiac surgical procedures which exclude the right ventricle.[4]

Resistance in Veins

In addition to the capacitance function of veins, there is also a resistance function of the veins. The venous contribution to blood flow resistance is quite small in magnitude compared to arteriolar resistance factors, but the functional importance of venular resistance in the overall maintenance of circulatory system integrity may be great.[2] The capillary vessels of the vascular system, where nutritional filtration and diffusion processes occur between the blood and tissues of the body, are situated between arterioles and venules. These blood vessels are both capable of adjusting resistance to blood flow by means of smooth muscle cells in the vascular wall. Total blood flow through a vascular bed is adjusted by the total resistance of the vascular bed, with arterioles the major resistance factor. Hydrostatic pressure of the capillaries, however, is dependent on adjustment of the balance or ratio of the inflow (arteriole) and outflow (venular) resistances. If the inflow/outflow resistance ratio increases, capillary hydrostatic pressure falls, leading to net inflow of fluid from the extravascular tissue space to the circulation. The opposite situation occurs with loss of fluid from the circulation to the extravascular space when inflow/outflow resistance ratio decreases. Changes in this resistance ratio may be a major factor in controlling nutritional diffusion exchange and the maintenance of steady states in relationships of plasma volume to other fluid spaces of the body. Alterations of this ratio depend not only on arteriolar resistance or tone but also on venous tone, which in this ratio presumably has equal importance and influence. Postcapillary venular resistance changes, while by no means the magnitude of the arteriolar resistive function, assume great potential importance when considered in terms of the balance of resistive forces.

Methods of Study

Methods to study the capacitative and resistive functions of the venous system are not as precise as methods used to study the function of the heart or arterial circulation. As a consequence, very little is known about the physiologic function of veins in health and disease states. Most of the useful information about veins has come from plethysmographic or volume studies of the vascular beds of the limbs. The technology for plethysmography using strain gauge or impedance techniques is quite refined, however, and reproducible, reliable extremity volume studies may be obtained. A strain gauge is placed around the calf or forearm for determination of limb circumference, or electrodes for changes in electrical impedance are used to estimate changes in extremity volume in response to venous outflow obstruction which is produced by circumferential cuff pneumatic compression of the thigh or arm. A standard thigh or arm blood pressure cuff is inflated to 50 mm Hg for 45 seconds and then rapidly deflated. This pressure should leave arterial flow to the extremity unimpaired while totally obstructing venous outflow. Venous capacitance is measured as the height or deflection of the strain gauge or electrical impedance as extremity volume is increased by blood trapped in the venous system compared to (divided by) a 1% volume change standard[5] (Fig. 2.2). The result is expressed cc/100 cc tissue (normal range = 2.0 to 3.0 cc/100 cc).

The slope of rise is taken to represent the muscle blood flow and is standardized from limb to limb by dividing the slope by the 1% volume calibration (normal approximately 3.5 cc/100 cc/min) Maximum venous outflow is determined during the initial 3 seconds after the release of outflow obstruction.

VASOMOTOR STATE BEFORE AND AFTER SURGERY

Venous capacitance response to general surgical procedures was established by Tripolitis and associates.[6] In this study of 50 patients having a variety of general operations, venous capacitance was normal preoperatively (2.96 ± 0.10 cc/100 cc) and fell significantly (2.17 ± 0.10 cc/100 cc, $p < 0.001$) when observed 1 day after surgery. This reduction of venous capacitance was not observed in patients who became fully ambulatory during the study period (Fig. 2.3). None of the patients in the study group had obvious cardiac disease and only 5 of the 50 had peripheral vascular disease.

Cardiac Diseases

Studies of venous tone in patients with cardiac disease provide an interesting comparison and demonstrate that significant alterations in vasomotor dynamics may exist prior to operation.[7] The operation produces additional alterations of venous tone, which is an accentuated vasoconstrictive response. Comparing the hemodynamic and vasomotor response in patients with coronary artery disease to mitral valve stenosis, it can be seen that preoperative vasomotor tone is more affected in patients with mitral valve disease (Table 2.1). In these patients, with reduced cardiac performance there is increased calculated peripheral vascular resistance, presumably due to arteriolar constriction and reduced venous capacitance, probably due to active and passive venous constriction as a compensatory measure to displace blood volume into the central circulation to provide high left atrial pressure to overcome mitral valve stenosis. Preoperative changes are less pronounced in the coronary artery disease patients, owing to

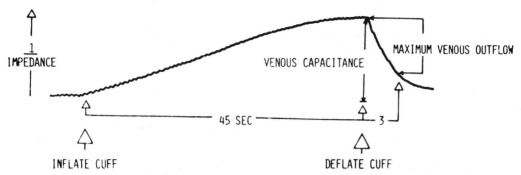

Figure 2.2. Venous impedance plethysmograph tracing. A standard pneumatic thigh blood pressure cuff is inflated to 50 mm of mercury for 45 seconds. Steady uniform increase of impedance during the 45-second occlusion of venous outflow is noted to a plateau which occurs prior to deflation of the cuff. Venous capacitance is measured as the height of deflection compared to a 1% impedance volume change standard. The slope of rise is taken to represent muscle blood flow. Maximum venous outflow is determined during the initial 3 seconds after release of outflow obstruction. (Reproduced with permission from A. E. Young et al.[5])

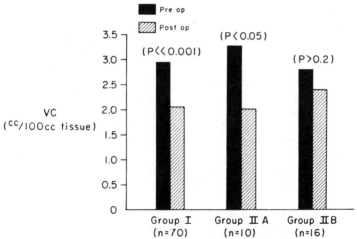

Figure 2.3. Pre- and postoperative mean venous capacitance (VC) in three groups of patients having general surgical procedures. Group I are patients who remained at bed rest following surgery and showed a significant reduction of venous capacitance following surgery. Group II A was minimally ambulatory and also showed reduction of mean venous capacitance following surgery with less degree of statistical significance. Patients in group II B, who were fully ambulatory, had no change in venous capacitance following surgery. (Reproduced with permission from A. J. Tripolitis et al.[6])

the fact that cardiac performance was near normal.

Cardiac Surgery

Postoperatively, a general vasoconstrictive state is noted following either mitral valve replacement or coronary artery bypass graft procedures, with the patients having the former operation showing a more profound response than the latter. There is an equivalent reduction of cardiac output (23%) in both types of patients, but since

Table 2.1

Vasomotor Tone and Hemodynamics before and One Hour after Mitral Valve Replacement and Coronary Artery Bypass Graft*

	VC/50 cc/100 cc	MBF cc/100 cc	CI liters/min/m^2	TPVR (units)	LA (mm Hg)
Preoperative					
Coronary artery bypass grafts	2.0 ± 0.1	1.5 ± 0.2	2.6 ± 0.2	34 ± 3	9 ± 2
Mitral valve replacements	1.5 ± 0.1	2.0 ± 0.2	2.2 ± 0.2	42 ± 3	24 ± 2
Postoperative					
Coronary artery bypass grafts	0.5 ± 0.1†	1.2 ± 0.2	2.0 ± 0.2†	44 ± 3†	19 ± 2†
Mitral valve replacements	0.3 ± 0.1†	1.6 ± 0.2	1.7 ± 0.2†	62 ± 3†	29 ± 2†

* Abbreviations used are VC$_{50}$, venous capacitance; MBF, muscle blood flow; CI, cardiac index; TPVR, total peripheral vascular resistance; LA, left atrial pressure.
† Statistically significant ($p = <0.05$).

the mitral valve replacement patients have lower initial level of cardiac output, this group drops to postoperative levels of cardiac performance (cardiac output mean 1.7 ± 0.2 liters/min/m^2) which would be expected to be associated with profound vasoconstriction. Reduction of extremity muscle blood flow is equivalent (20%) in both groups and of the same order of magnitude as reduction in cardiac output, so that reduction of arterial input to the limb may be the major cause of reduced venous capacitance as suggested by Tripolitis and associates.[6] Compensatory venous constriction is marked following cardiac surgery, with 75 to 80% reduction of venous capacitance in the early postoperative period. Intraoperative factors contributing to reduced cardiac performance and vasomotor constriction following cardiac surgery include the use of cardiopulmonary bypass, anesthetics and other medications, operative tissue trauma, as well as complex undefined factors.

EFFECT OF CARDIOPULMONARY BYPASS ON VENOUS TONE

Operations utilizing cardiopulmonary bypass cause major alterations of vasomotor tone and distribution of organ blood flow. Complex neurohumoral mechanisms are activated with the onset of nonpulsatile blood flow, reduced mean arterial pressure, and rapid reduction of atrial pressure which accompany initiation of cardiopulmonary bypass. These hemodynamic changes should provide strong stimulus to vasoconstrictive reflexes mediated through low pressure baroreceptors in the right and left atria and in the carotid sinus and aortic arch. In addition, body temperature is usually lowered by perfusion with blood at reduced temperatures, which should also produce a vasoconstrictive response, especially of cutaneous veins. In spite of these maximal stimuli to venous constriction, with the onset of cardiopulmonary bypass very little change in venous capacitance is actually observed.[8]

The hemodynamics and venous capacitance changes associated with cardiopulmonary bypass are shown in Figure 2.4. Left and right atrial pressures fall to zero as the heart is emptied to the reservoir of the oxygenator by gravity drainage. Mean arterial pressure drops approximately 40%, and there is usually no more than 10 to 15 mm Hg of pulse pressure. Subsequently, arterial pressure gradually increases 5 to 10 mm Hg every 15 minutes on bypass but usually remains 15 to 20 mm Hg below prebypass levels. Cardiac output assumes the level fixed by pump rates commonly used clinically at 2.0 to 2.5 liters/min/m^2. This may or may not represent a change in cardiac output, depending on individual patient cardiac output under anesthesia prior to cardiopulmonary bypass. In our studies, this was not a change in patients having aorto-coronary bypass graft operations for coronary artery disease. While usual cardiopulmonary bypass flow rates are below accepted lower limits for resting cardiac out-

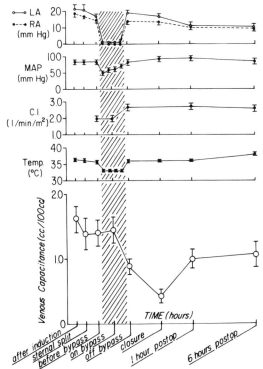

Figure 2.4. Hemodynamic response during operations utilizing cardiopulmonary bypass. Left atrial (*LA*) and right atrial (*RA*) pressures were reduced during bypass as the heart emptied. Mean arterial pressure (*MAP*) was initially markedly reduced and later rose under influence of neurohumoral compensatory mechanisms. Cardiac output (*C.I.*) was little changed by conditions of cardiopulmonary bypass used in this study. Moderate hypothermia was evident by reduction of body temperature (Temp.). Venous capacitance was reduced by general effects of the operation, especially under conditions of light anesthesia following bypass and during wound closure. Venous tone was not changed by cardiopulmonary bypass. (Reproduced with permission from D. B. Doty et al.[8])

put, these flow rates may actually be nearly the same as usual cardiac output for patients with cardiac disease under effects of anesthesia and operation. Thus, pressure hemo-

dynamic changes with initiation of cardiopulmonary could evoke reflex mechanisms, even though total blood flow may not change acutely.

Cardiopulmonary bypass as practiced clinically does not appear to cause significant reduction of venous capacitance. As shown in Figure 2.4, mean venous capacitance just prior to cardiopulmonary bypass of 1.40 ± 0.19 cc/100 cc remained at 1.44 ± 0.20 cc/100 cc during bypass. Venoconstriction already present before bypass is not intensified during the period of extracorporeal circulation. Induction of anesthesia is associated with venoconstriction to a reduced capacitance of 1.62 ± 0.22 cc/100 cc, and the stimulus of wound closure further reduces venous capacitance to 0.43 ± 0.10 cc/100 cc. These were more important determinants of venous tone than use of cardiopulmonary bypass during cardiac surgery.

The explanation for the apparent lack of venous constriction during cardiopulmonary bypass is probably related to the fact that venous tone is already quite high and cardiopulmonary bypass can add little further stimulus. Initial observations of venous capacitance after induction of anesthesia show values below expected normal of 2.0 to 3.0 cc/100 cc tissue. Operative manipulation and division of the sternum add further stimulus for venoconstriction which is likely part of a general vasoconstriction response, with arterial hypertension and increased plasma renin documented by Bailey and associates.[9] Reduced blood temperature stimulus to cutaneous venous constriction provided by cardiopulmonary bypass may be blunted by prior maximal cutaneous vein contraction in response to the unusually cool operating room environment (commonly <65°C) and resultant drop in body temperature (35.6 ± 1°C). Profound venous constriction associated with cardiac surgery appears to be a general response related to many facets of the operation, and the use of cardiopulmonary bypass, while providing major stimulus to sympathoadrenal reflexes, may have little effect on an already contracted venous capacitance bed.

EFFECTS OF VASODILATORS ON VENOUS TONE AFTER CARDIOPULMONARY BYPASS

Patients having operations for cardiac disease often require vasodilator drugs to treat the vasoconstrictive response which naturally accompanies this type of surgery. About one-third of patients having coronary artery bypass grafts have significant hypertension requiring medical treatment in the postoperative period. Most normotensive patients have elevation of calculated peripheral arterial vascular resistance which may also be treated to obtain more optimal hemodynamics. Sequential changes in peripheral resistance, cardiac output, and left atrial pressure in patients after coronary artery bypass and the effects of nitroprusside and nitroglycerine are shown in Figure 2.5, and venous capacitance and muscle blood flow studies are shown in Figure 2.6. Nitroprusside was given to patients having arterial hypertension, and nitroglycerine was given prospectively to some of the patients as soon as possible after cardiopulmonary bypass and continued postoperatively to reduce and maintain left atrial pressure at 7 to 8 mm Hg in order to modify venous tone. Elevation of peripheral resistance early after surgery in the nitroprusside group reflects the conditions of the hypertensive subgroup which had not received any medical treatment. The hypertensive patients had profound elevation of peripheral arterial resistance until treated with nitroprusside, while reduced venous capacitance changes were equivalent to normotensive patients demonstrating that the hypertensive response is nearly a pure arterial resistance change rather than a generalized vasomotor response. When nitroglycerine was given immediately after cardiopulmonary bypass to alter venous tone it also affected the arterial resistance in that none of the patients were hypertensive. Nitroglycerine, with primary effects on venous capacitance, effected venodilation and return of venous capacitance to normal. Nitroglycerine and nitroprusside had equivalent effects on reducing arterial resistance and increasing cardiac output presumably by afterload reduction, but only nitroglycerine had any real effect on reduc-

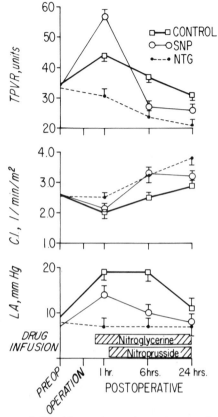

Figure 2.5. Hemodynamics in patients having coronary artery bypass graft operations with mean values and confidence limits (standard error) plotted as a function of time. *Top panel* shows total peripheral vascular resistance (*TPVR*). At 1 hour postoperative control group showed increased arterial resistance while hypertensive group which later received nitroprusside (*SNP*) had even greater increase in TPVR. Patients receiving nitroglycerine (*NTG*) and nitroprusside had equivalent reduction of TPVR and left atrial pressure (*LA, lower panel*) and increase in cardiac index (*C.I., middle panel*) at the 6-hour observation. (Reproduced with permission from W. E. Gall et al.[7])

ing profound postoperative vasoconstriction of the venous capacitance vascular bed.

Manipulation of Venous Capacitance

Should anything be done to alter the vasoconstrictive response affecting both arte-

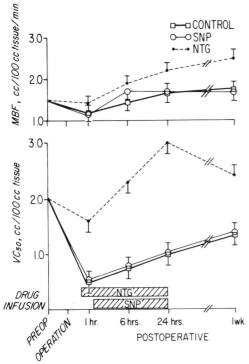

Figure 2.6. Muscle blood flow (*MBF, top panel*) and venous capacitance (*VC₅₀, lower panel*) in patients having coronary artery bypass graft with mean values and confidence limits (standard error) plotted as a function of time. Operation is associated with marked reduction of VC_{50}. Nitroglycerine (*NTG*) infusion produced sustained venodilation, while nitroprusside (*SNP*) had little measurable effect on venous circulation. (Reproduced with permission from W. E. Gall et al.[7])

rial resistance and venous capacitance beds during and after operations requiring the use of cardiopulmonary bypass? The answer to this debatable question remains for interpretation of when the degree of vasoconstriction representing normal compensatory response to major surgery and the altered hemodynamic state of cardiopulmonary bypass becomes an abnormal and undesirable determinant of blood flow. The risk of vasodilator medications to reduce arterial blood pressure while on cardiopulmonary bypass is the possibility of alteration of central organ blood flow distribution which

may adversely affect cerebral oxygen and nutrient delivery. In the postoperative period, reduction of arterial blood pressure may reduce cardiac afterload at the expense of reduced coronary blood flow. Kaplan and Jones[10] have shown that nitroprusside and nitroglycerine have equivalent dose-related effects on afterload reduction and decrease of myocardial oxygen demand, while nitroprusside tends to reduce coronary perfusion pressure and occasionally aggravate ischemic patterns on electrocardiogram. According to Kerber et al.,[11] any deleterious effects of vasodilators on coronary blood flow should be eliminated when arterial pressure reduction is limited to between 7 and 15% of pretreatment mean arterial pressure.

Alteration of venous tone following cardiac surgery could be considered simply cosmetic as constricted cutaneous veins are the rule after any major operation as part of generally increased sympathetic nervous system activity. Tripolitis and associates[6] suggest that postoperative contracted venous capacitance involves not only cutaneous but also deep veins of the extremities and accompanies reduced arterial inflow to the limb. This overall venous constriction may be important in the generalized increased resistance or impedance to blood flow as detailed earlier. Hence, venular resistance alteration may be of considerable importance when attempting to favorably influence the hemodynamic state in the postoperative period.

Nitroglycerine may be used as a vasodilator to increase venous capacitance in the postoperative period. Nitroglycerine will increase muscle blood flow and total cardiac output while reducing atrial pressure or cardiac preload as a consequence of pharmacologic venous dilation.[8, 12–14] Maximum increase of cardiac output requires maintenance of adequate cardiac preload by fluid infusion sufficient to maintain atrial pressure during venous dilation. It could be argued that large volume fluid infusion in the postoperative period is less desirable than accepting some venous constriction. Marco and associates[15] thought it is best to use a pure arteriolar vasodilator to reduce left ventricular impedance without altering preload and that agents which affect both arterial and venous dilation may be inappropriate in the postoperative period because of volume replacement necessary to maintain cardiac filling. This viewpoint ignores the contribution of venous resistance to total circulatory impedance. It could even be argued that vasodilation of either arteries or veins in the postoperative period may do very little for central organ blood flow effecting increased flow to muscle and cutaneous vascular beds in the limbs with what appears to be favorable increase of total cardiac output at the expense of increased cardiac work. Current trends in management, however, favor use of vasodilator drugs to effect return of the peripheral circulation from a postoperative vasoconstricted state toward normal. As such, treatment must include consideration of not only the arterial resistar.ce blood vessels but also the venous capacitance vascular bed.

References

1. Shepherd JT, Vanhoutte PM: Role of the venous system in circulatory control. Mayo Clin Proc 53:247, 1978.
2. Folkow B, Mellander S: Veins and venous tone. Am Heart J 68:397, 1964.
3. Zoller RP, Mark AL, Abboud FM, Schmid PG, Heistad DD: The role of low pressure baroreceptors in reflex vasoconstrictor responses in man. J Clin Invest 51:2967, 1972.
4. Heck HA, Doty DB: Assisted circulation by phasic external lower body compression. Circulation 64(Suppl):II–118, 1981.
5. Young AE, Henderson BA, Phillips DA, Couch NP: Impedance plethysmography: Its limitations as a substrate for phlebography. Cardiovasc Radiol 1:223, 1978.
6. Tripolitis AJ, Bodily KC, Blackshear WM, Cairols M, Milligan EB, Thiele BL, Strandness DE: Venous capacitance and outflow in the postoperative patient. Ann Surg 190:634, 1979.
7. Gall WE, Clarke WR, Doty DB: Vasomotor dynamics associated with cardiac surgery. I. Venous tone and the effects of vasodilators. J Thorac Cardiovasc Surg 83:724, 1982.
8. Doty DB, Montanaro GD, Carter JG, Moyers JR: Vasomotor dynamics associated with cardiac surgery. II. Effect of cardiopulmonary bypass on venous tone. J Thorac Cardiovasc Surg 83:732, 1982.
9. Bailey DR, Miller ED Jr, Kaplan JA, Rogers PW: The renin-angiotensin-aldosterone system during cardiac surgery with morphine-nitrous oxide anesthesia. Anesthesiology 42:538, 1975.
10. Kaplan JA, Jones EL: Vasodilator therapy during coronary artery surgery. J Thorac Cardiovasc Surg 77:301, 1979.
11. Kerber RE, Martins JB, Marcus ML: Effect of acute ischemia, nitroglycerin and nitroprusside on regional myocardial thickening, stress and perfusion. Circulation 60:121, 1979.
12. Mason OT, Braunwald E: The effect of nitroglycerin and amyl nitrate on anteriolar and venous tone in the human forearm. Circulation 32:755, 1965.
13. Hempelmann G, Peipenbrock S, Seitz W, Karliczek G: Changes in hemodynamic parameters, inotropic state, and myocardiac oxygen consumption owing to intravenous application of nitroglycerin. J Thorac Cardiovasc Surg 73:836, 1977.
14. Miller RR, Vismara LA, Williams DO, Amsterdam EA, Mason DT: Pharmacologic mechanisms for left ventricular unloading in clinical congestive heart failure: Differential effects of nitroprusside, phentolamine, and nitroglycerin on cardiac function and peripheral circulation. Circ Res 39:127, 1976.
15. Marco JD, Standeven JW, Barner HB: Afterload reduction with hydralazine following valve replacement. J Thorac Cardiovasc Surg 80:50, 1980.

CHAPTER 3

FLUID BALANCE DURING CARDIOPULMONARY BYPASS

JOE R. UTLEY, M.D.
D. BARTON STEPHENS, C.C.P.

Intraoperative fluid shifts in patients subjected to cardiopulmonary bypass differ significantly from that of patients having major surgical procedures without cardiopulmonary bypass. Fluid accumulation during cardiopulmonary bypass may contribute to postoperative organ dysfunction. The patient's preoperative cardiac status may have a profound effect on the total blood volume and may significantly effect the fluid shifts during and after cardiopulmonary bypass. Diuresis to achieve negative fluid balance may be a high priority in postoperative care. The factors which may affect fluid shifts during cardiopulmonary bypass include temperature, flow rates, hemodilution, plasma colloid oncotic pressure, interstitial fluid pressure, capillary permeability, and urine output. The accumulation of fluid during cardiopulmonary bypass is greater in some organs than others. The amount of fluid accumulation during cardiopulmonary bypass may determine the need for postoperative use of diuretics, osmotic agents, and vasoactive drugs.

GENERAL EFFECTS

Early attempts to perform cardiac surgery with cardiopulmonary bypass without gain in patient weight led to significant postoperative hypovolemia and poor cardiac performance.[1-4] The deficit in blood volume and plasma volume following perfusion described in 1961 is probably attributable to failure to appreciate the interstitial fluid accumulation during bypass.[5] The intravascular volume deficit was correlated with a suboptimal postoperative recovery or death. Many patients have a "puffy" appearance after cardiopulmonary bypass which may appear more pronounced in the face, periorbital areas, neck, and abdomen rather than in the ankles or sacral area. Adult patients may gain from 1 to 15 pounds during the operation. Analysis of total fluid intake and output during cardiopulmonary bypass shows that patients gain from 0 to 150 cc fluid per kilogram body weight and up to 2500 cc/m^2 body surface area.[6] Several studies of blood volume before and after cardiac surgery show that despite a calculated blood volume excess postoperatively there existed significant "concealed blood loss." Ecchymoses and hemorrhage in the area of the wound and fluid in transit in the pleural space were suggested as the cause of the "concealed blood loss."[7]

Breckenridge et al.[8] studied patients before and after cardiopulmonary bypass and found the extracellular fluid space to be expanded after cardiopulmonary bypass. Extracellular fluid volume was assessed by determining the distribution spaces of inulin and bromide with moderate hemodilution techniques. Cardiopulmonary bypass produced 33% increase in inulin space and 18% increase in bromide space. They concluded that the increased extracellular volume developed during cardiopulmonary bypass.

Cleland et al.[9] compared the blood volume and body fluid compartment changes in patients after cardiac surgical procedures with and without cardiopulmonary bypass. The authors determined the volume of dilution of ^{51}Cr-labeled red cells, ^{125}I-labeled albumin, ^{82}Br, Na^{35}SO$_4$, and tritiated water. They found a variable response of plasma volume and red cell mass among groups of patients with left to right shunts, and valve disease with and without heart failure. Extracellular fluid volume was increased in all groups, but the interstitial fluid volume (extracellular fluid minus plasma volume) was greatly increased. They found the shape of the ^{82}Br and ^{35}S curve to be different after cardiopulmonary bypass, suggesting a more slowly equilibrating pool of extracellular fluid. They postulated this slow equilibrating fluid to be in the wound or pleural space.[9]

Hematocrit rises progressively postoperatively because of diminishing plasma volume. Plasma volume may be shifted into interstitial space or excreted as urine output. Cleland et al.[9] found the increase in interstitial fluid to be correlated with duration of cardiopulmonary bypass and presence of preoperative congestive failure. He found no increase in total body water, suggesting that intracellular fluid is decreased. Berger et al.[10] confirmed that plasma volume progressively fell in the 24 hours following cardiopulmonary bypass.

The general principle that intravascular volume tends to fall with associated increase in extracellular volume was confirmed by Beattie et al. as well. Beattie et al.[11, 12] determined ^{82}Br space, tritiated water space, ^{125}I albumin space, and calculated oncotic pressure before and after cardiopulmonary bypass. His studies were performed 2 days and 6 to 8 days postoperatively. The decrease in blood volume was greatest on the 2nd postoperative day but still diminished on the 6th to 8th postoperative day. Similarly, the increase in extracellular fluid volume and total body water was increased more on day 2 than on days 6 to 8. On the 2nd postoperative day the extracellular space was increased 33%, and total body

water increased 13%. He showed a strong correlation ($r = 0.82$) between the extracellular volume and total body water. The line of regression intercepts the total body water axis above zero, suggesting that intracellular volume is increased. Beattie believed the principal cause of the fluid shift was diminished colloidal oncotic pressure. He also postulated that factors released from damaged white cells and platelets increased capillary permeability. Plasma volume decrease and extracellular volume increase with no change in intracellular volume was found by Reid et al.[13] Beall et al.[14] performed studies of total body water and extracellular water and intracellular water with tritiated water and sodium sulfate dilutional studies before, immediately after, and 7 to 10 days after cardiopulmonary bypass and showed the greatest change to be in expansion of extracellular volume. The expanded extracellular volume persisted for 7 to 10 days in his patients. Lilleaasen and Stokke[15] compared patients perfused at Hct 27% and 18% and found the total fluid excess 24 hours postoperatively to be 2.0 and 1.5 liters, respectively.[15]

The studies of late changes in fluid distribution 2 weeks postoperatively in patients with preoperative congestive failure show increased plasma volume, decreased red cell volume, and no change of blood volume. Total body water was unchanged, but interstitial and extracellular fluid excess persisted. Patients with no cardiac failure preoperatively had had much less increase in plasma volume, interstitial and extracellular volume at 2 weeks postoperatively. Patients with left to right shunts without congestive failure had diminished plasma volume and interstitial and extracellular volume postoperatively. The ability to clear the excess interstitial fluid postoperatively may be related to increasing rates of urinary sodium excretion.[16]

Decreasing water content of plasma has been observed during cardiopulmonary bypass. Possible causes of water loss are wound surfaces, pump oxygenator, skin, kidneys; one study concluded that the wound surface accounted for a greater amount of insensible water loss than the pump oxygenator, skin, or kidneys.[17] They found no fall in serum water concentration when the pump oxygenator was circulated alone but a fall in patient serum water concentration during the period before the onset of cardiopulmonary bypass. The rise in serum osmolarity observed by Dordoni et al.[18] may be related to water vapor loss.

PREOPERATIVE FACTORS

The patient's preoperative blood volume and body fluid composition may be important determinants of the changes in fluid balance during cardiopulmonary bypass. Patients with congestive heart failure have increased total body water, extracellular and intrastitial fluid, plasma volume, and red cell volume. Total exchangeable sodium is increased.[19–21] If heart failure is chronic, red cell mass is also increased. Patients with cardiac cachexia have reduced body mass and extracellular water. They typically have an increase in exchangeable sodium and decreased exchangeable potassium.[22] Patients with congenital heart disease with increased or decreased pulmonary blood flow have increased blood volume. The expanded blood and plasma volumes of patients with congestive failure is in contrast to the contracted plasma volumes in patients with coronary artery disease and normal ventricular function. These patients have less than normal predicted blood volume, plasma volume, and red cell volume. These abnormalities persist despite the relief of myocardial ischemia by coronary revascularization. Cohn et al.[23] postulates that the contraction of plasma volume observed in patients with coronary disease is in response to increased sympathetic activity which has been observed in these patients. Infusion of catecholamines has been shown to decrease plasma volume. Wigboldus et al.[24] termed the plasma volume deficit in coronary artery patients the "empty heart" phenomenon and found the postoperative fluid balance to be greatly positive in these patients. These patients tend to have a fall in hematocrit during induction of anesthesia presumably due to fluid shifts from interstitial space to intravascular space. They are more prone to hypotension and arrhythmia during induc-

tion and preparation for cardiopulmonary bypass. Wigboldus et al. indicated that increased sympathetic tone causing increased ventricular ejection was the probable cause rather than hypovolemia. He recommended fluid infusion to manage the "empty heart" phenomena.

We calculated the patient's blood volume at the time of onset of cardiopulmonary bypass from the prebypass hematocrit of the patient and the oxygenator priming solution, the known volume of the priming solution, and the hematocrit after equilibration on cardiopulmonary bypass. These determinations of blood volume showed that coronary artery disease patients with poor ventricular function (ejection fraction less than 0.4) had greater blood volume than patients with higher ejection fractions. Furthermore, the blood volume was increased with valve disease and was related to the number of valves diseased. Patients with congenital heart disease also had increased blood volume[25] (Fig. 3.1).

The surgical correction of valve and ventricular abnormalities and closure of intracardiac shunts may relieve congestive failure and lower filling pressures and increase

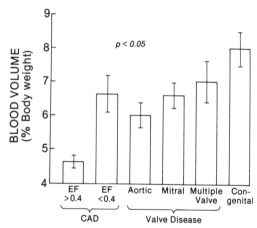

Figure 3.1. Blood volume expressed as percent body weight varies with different cardiac diseases. This variation is important in planning blood conservation and in understanding variations in fluid accumulation during cardiopulmonary bypass. *EF*, ejection fraction; *CAD*, coronary artery disease.

cardiac output. The preoperative and postoperative filling pressures may be important determinants of fluid accumulation. Closure of large left to right shunts may diminish central blood volume and decrease the accumulation of fluid perioperatively.[16] Our studies show that fluid accumulation during cardiopulmonary bypass is significantly related to the preoperative cardiac disease. The fluid accumulation was least in patients who underwent closure of left to right shunts, intermediate in patients with coronary disease, single valve disease, or cyanotic congenital heart disease, and greatest in patients with multiple valve disease (Fig. 3.2).[6] The mean positive fluid accumulation ranged from 727 cc/m² in patients with left to right shunts to 2077 cc/m² in patients with multiple valve disease. The reasons for these differences are undoubtedly complex and related to preoperative body fluid composition and altered hemodynamics following surgical correction. Accumulation of fluid during cardiopulmonary bypass has been found to be a function of duration of bypass in several studies. In a group of patients having coronary artery surgery the

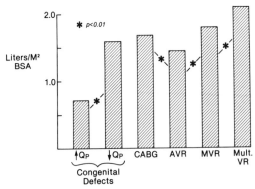

Figure 3.2. Accumulation of fluid during cardiopulmonary bypass is related to the cardiac disease. The reasons for this variation are undoubtedly complex and related to preoperative and postoperative hemodynamics and duration of cardiopulmonary bypass. Qp, pulmonary blood flow; CABG, coronary bypass grafts; AVR, aortic valve replacement; MVR, mitral valve replacement; Mult VR, multiple valve replacement; BSA, body surface area.

patients were found to accumulate 20 to 30 cc per bypass graft. Greater weight gain was observed in patients with lower serum albumin and hemodilution.[26]

Our studies of patients having surgery for coronary valve and congenital heart lesions show a significant relationship between duration and fluid accumulation (Fig. 3.3). Although the correlation coefficient was 0.51, 25% of the variation in fluid accumulation was attributable to duration of cardiopulmonary bypass. The mean accumulation per hour of cardiopulmonary bypass was 800 cc/m² body surface area.[6]

HEMODILUTION AND DIMINISHED PLASMA COLLOIDAL ONCOTIC PRESSURE

Although hemodilution has been implicated as the cause of fluid retention during cardiopulmonary bypass, its relative role compared to other factors, especially hypothermia and the effect of the pump oxygenator, was recently determined experimentally.[27] This study shows that hemodilution is the main cause of fluid retention during cardiopulmonary bypass when compared to the effect of hypothermia or the pump oxygenator. The most obvious effect of hemodilution which would contribute to fluid accumulation and edema is decrease in plasma colloidal oncotic pressure. Other effects of hemodilution which may be important are diminished viscosity of blood, diminished oxygen-carrying capacity, and vasodilation.

The decrease in plasma colloidal oncotic pressure with hemodilution is correlated with fall in plasma proteins.[28] The changes in colloidal oncotic pressure were more closely correlated with changes in albumin concentration than with concentration of globulin fractions. The plasma colloidal oncotic pressure fell from 34 to 27 cm water in the study of Webber and Garnett.[28] Webber and Garnett found that plasma colloidal oncotic pressure rose during the period of bypass, in contrast to the study of English et al.[29] which found it to remain relatively constant.[29] Webber found that the colloidal oncotic pressure and albumin levels remained at 80% of normal during the week

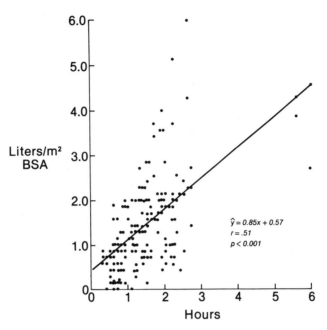

Figure 3.3. The duration of cardiopulmonary bypass is a significant factor determining accumulation of fluid.

following operation. English found the colloidal oncotic pressure fell from 29 mm Hg to 19 mm Hg with the onset of bypass but returned to 26 mm Hg in 24 hours. The diminished colloidal oncotic pressure correlates with the intravascular volume deficit observed postoperatively.[11]

Gollub et al.[30] studied five Jehovah's Witness patients who underwent cardiac repair without the use of blood or albumin. They retained 650 to 4731 cc of fluid intraoperatively, most of which was extravascular. They found that for every volume of blood lost postoperatively, 3.5 volumes of crystalloid solution must be given and 2.5 volumes were retained in the interstitial space. Their calculation suggested that significant amounts of extravascular protein was mobilized intraoperatively and that postoperatively protein was transferred to the intravascular space. They calculated that 6.5 gm protein was mobilized intraoperatively, and 20.9 gm protein was mobilized during the first 18 hours postoperatively. They noted excellent renal function, absence of pulmonary edema, and prominence of pleural effusions in these patients.[30]

The safety of hemodilution is well established.[31–33] The improvement in blood coagulation, lung function, renal function, and myocardial function attributed to hemodilution is probably related to the absence of homologous blood in the priming solution rather than the effect of decreased plasma colloidal osmolar pressure or viscosity. The reduction in perfusion pressure with hemodilution cardiopulmonary bypass is correlated with fall in blood viscosity.[34, 35]

In experimental studies hemodilution causes a significant increase of blood flow to myocardium, outer cortex of kidney, cerebral cortex, spleen, and intestine. The diminished oxygen-carrying capacity of hemodilution is compensated by increased flow to maintain normal oxygen delivery in all areas except kidney and spleen. Hemodilution produces increased water content in myocardium, medulla of kidney, liver, stomach, and intestine (Fig. 3.4). The increased water content is correlated with increased flow in myocardium and intestine. Edema is not correlated with diminished blood flow or diminished oxygen delivery in any area. The regions of increased water

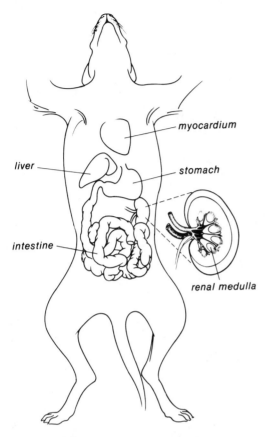

Figure 3.4. Experimental studies in dogs have shown that hemodilution is the principal cause of fluid accumulation. The organs which accumulate significant amounts of water are the myocardium, liver, stomach, intestine, and renal medulla.

content do not correlate with the organs which commonly demonstrate postoperative dysfunction except for myocardium.[27]

HYPOTHERMIA

Although hypothermia is a less potent cause of tissue edema than hemodilution it has been implicated in some of the fluid shifts which occur with cardiopulmonary bypass.[27] The principal goal of hypothermia is to decrease oxygen consumption and demand during cardiopulmonary bypass. The increased viscosity and red blood cell sludging which accompanies hypothermia may

have adverse effects on flow.[36] Investigators have repeatedly observed a decrease in plasma volume during hypothermia.[37–39] The hemoconcentration which occurs is due to plasma loss plus the mobilization of sequestered red blood cells especially from the spleen.[40] Hypothermia produces a "slow" circulation of 25% of red cells which do not equilibrate rapidly with the central circulation.[41] Others have observed an increase in plasma colloid oncotic pressure during cooling. The change in plasma colloidal oncotic pressure is not explained by the fluid shifts calculated from the changes in hematocrit. Either a change in the configuration of plasma proteins or a change in the concentration of plasma proteins from tissue stores is postulated.[42] Other components of the mechanism may be a shift of fluid into the intracellular space or trapping of fluid in the peripheral vascular bed.[43] Hepatic and visceral congestion as well as bloody ascites have been observed with hypothermic cardiopulmonary bypass.[44] The increased vascular resistance with hypothermia may be due to increased viscosity, vasoconstriction, or both. These effects are reversed by hemodilution.[45] Experimental study of the effect of hypothermia on regional blood flow and water content shows that hypothermia causes diminished flow to kidney cortex, cerebral cortex, and skin, and these flow changes are not accompanied by any changes in water content.[27] Although hypothermia protects the ischemic or injured brain from edema, no effect of hypothermia on the water content of the normal brain has been demonstrated.[46, 47]

PUMP OXYGENATOR

The pump oxygenator produces changes in the serum proteins and cellular elements which may affect the distribution of body fluids. The denaturation of serum proteins and the destabilization of soluble fats may affect the colloidal properties of blood and contribute to edema.[48]

The postulated changes in capillary permeability with cardiopulmonary bypass may be related to the effect of pump oxygenator foreign surfaces on circulating complement levels.[49] The release of kinins and other vasoactive substances from the destruction of platelets, and white blood cells by the pump oxygenator may also contribute to tissue edema during cardiopulmonary bypass. Microemboli may produce areas of ischemia leading to edema, especially in the central nervous system.[50] The diminished flow to the subendocardium of the left ventricle and the cortex of the kidney produced by the pump oxygenator may be related to the selective delivery of particles to the terminal arteries of the coronary and renal circulation because of axial migration of particles within arteries.[27] The increased flow to intestines produced by the pump oxygenator may be related to nonpulsatile flow.

INTERSTITIAL FLUID PRESSURE

The clinical and experimental studies show that fall in plasma colloidal oncotic pressure and rise in interstitial fluid volume are important factors in the development of tissue edema during cardiopulmonary bypass.[51] Studies of the interstitial hydrostatic pressure of tissues during hemodilution cardiopulmonary bypass show strong correlations with plasma colloidal oncotic pressure. Studies of the intramuscular and subcutaneous interstitial fluid pressure in patients undergoing valve replacement or coronary bypass grafting show that interstitial pressure of muscle rose more than that of subcutaneous tissue (Fig. 3.5). Muscle interstitial pressure rose faster than subcutaneous interstitial pressure with the sudden fall in plasma colloidal oncotic pressure at the onset of cardiopulmonary bypass.[52]

In experiments performed on dogs, significant increases in interstitial fluid pressure were observed in subcutaneous tissue, muscle and myocardium but not in stomach (Fig. 3.6). The greatest water content occurs in myocardium and stomach, rather than muscle or subcutaneous tissue; thus, the rise in interstitial fluid pressure does not correlate with the rise in water content. This is probably related to the compliance of the interstitial space. If the interstitial space is compliant, fluid can accumulate without significant rises in interstitial fluid pressure, such as we observed in the stomach. Other

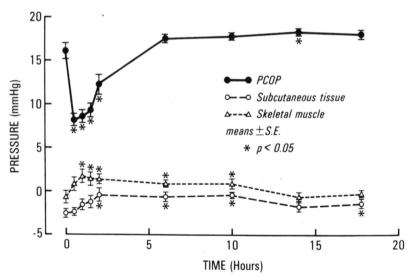

Figure 3.5. PCOP and interstitial fluid pressure changes due to cardiopulmonary bypass in patients. Studies of patients show that hemodilution hypothermic cardiopulmonary bypass is associated with a rapid fall in plasma colloidal osmotic pressure (*PCOP*). The rise of interstitial fluid is most rapid in muscle and more delayed in subcutaneous tissue. Plasma colloidal osmotic pressure returns to normal rapidly, following cardiopulmonary bypass. Interstitial fluid pressure in skeletal muscle and subcutaneous tissue returns to normal more slowly.

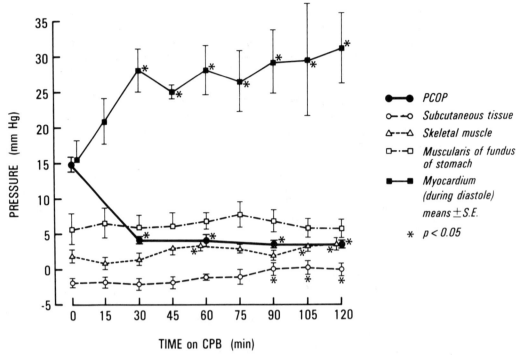

Figure 3.6. PCOP and interstitial fluid pressure changes during cardiopulmonary bypass (CPB) in dogs. During a 2-hour period of cardiopulmonary bypass in dogs plasma colloidal osmotic pressure (PCOP) falls rapidly and remains low. Diastolic intramyocardial pressure rises rapidly and progressively. Interstitial fluid pressure in muscle and subcutaneous tissue rises more slowly. No increase in interstitial fluid pressure in the function of the stomach was observed.

less compliant interstitial spaces may have a significant rise in interstitial fluid pressure with the development of interstitial edema, such as we observed in the myocardium. Tissue with noncompliant interstitial spaces may develop rising interstitial pressures with a fall in plasma colloidal oncotic pressure without measurable increase in water content. This is consistent with our observations of interstitial fluid pressure in muscle and subcutaneous tissue. The different rates of rise of interstitial pressure in muscle and subcutaneous tissue may be related to pressure volume curves of the interstitial space of the two tissues and could be related to the rigid fascia compartment of skeletal muscle.[53] Guyton's studies[51] of the compliance of the interstitial space of muscle shows that pressure rise occurs very quickly with less that 5% change in tissue weight.

CAPILLARY PERMEABILITY

Increased capillary permeability has been suspected as a contributing factor in the development of interstitial edema during cardiopulmonary bypass.[11, 12] Studies of the serial changes in plasma proteins during cardiopulmonary bypass show that albumin, alpha-2, and gamma globulins progressively fall during cardiopulmonary bypass. The alpha-1 and beta globulins tend to rise; the tendency of heavier globulins to rise suggests increased capillary permeability to smaller molecules.[54] The injury of platelets and release of serotonin and other vasoactive amines may be a factor in deterioration in capillary integrity.[55] Other studies show the preservation of capillary integrity with use of serotonin antagonists.[56] Reactions known to produce increased capillary permeability that are produced by cardiopulmonary bypass include platelet aggregation, leukocyte adherence reactions, membrane damage, complement activation, and formation of anaphylactoxins and kinins.[49]

The reduction in complement levels observed did not return to normal 44 hours after cardiopulmonary bypass but was normal 8 days after cardiopulmonary bypass. Diminished complement levels produce increased capillary permeability.[49] A later study showed that complement conversion occurs with cardiopulmonary bypass. The conversion of complement occurred only after the conclusion of cardiopulmonary bypass when pulmonary circulation was restored. Parker et al.[49, 57] postulated that damaged platelets and leukocytes produced the complement conversion rather than the presence of immune complexes.[54]

OSMOTICALLY ACTIVE COMPONENTS IN OXYGENATOR PRIMING SOLUTION

Investigations have studied, in a variety of ways, the concept that restoring the colloidal oncotic pressure toward normal while maintaining a low hematocrit during hemodilution cardiopulmonary bypass would reverse the tendency to gain interstitial fluid while preserving the rheological advantage of a low hematocrit. The osmotically active components which have been used include whole blood, albumin, dextran and starch solutions, and mannitol. An analysis of fluid accumulation during cardiopulmonary bypass in patients with or without albumin, mannitol, or whole blood added to the oxygenator prime solution showed that patients whose prime contained albumin or mannitol accumulated significantly less fluid. No diminished accumulation was found in patients with whole blood in the priming solution[6] (Figs. 3.7 to 3.9). Another clinical study of the effect of albumin given during cardiopulmonary bypass showed lower intraoperative hematocrit in patients receiving albumin. Patients who received no albumin had greater net water balance than those who did. The study showed that large amounts of albumin (up to 175 gm) would

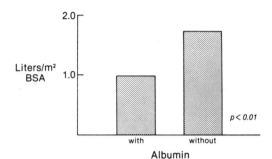

Figure 3.7. Fluid accumulation during cardiopulmonary bypass. Comparison of fluid accumulation in patients with and without 50 gm albumin in the priming solution shows a significant decrease in fluid accumulation with albumin.

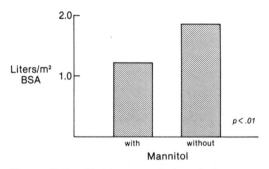

Figure 3.8. Fluid accumulation during cardiopulmonary bypass. The addition of 12.5 gm mannitol to the priming solution during cardiopulmonary bypass significantly decreases fluid accumulation.

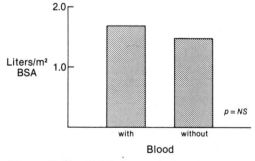

Figure 3.9. Fluid accumulation during cardiopulmonary bypass. The use of blood in priming the pump oxygenator was not associated with significant differences in fluid accumulation during cardiopulmonary bypass.

not completely eliminate the accumulation of fluid during cardiopulmonary bypass.[58] Studies of hemodilution cardiopulmonary bypass in the pig with varying levels of albumin replacement show that the amount of fluid accumulation is inversely proportional to the level of plasma albumin.[59]

Other studies have failed to demonstrate a return of plasma colloidal oncotic pressure to normal with albumin administration during cardiopulmonary bypass. No effect on postoperative alveolar-arterial oxygen gradient could be demonstrated with albumin administration.[60]

The effect of albumin in the priming solution may be less important that the total albumin kinetics during cardiopulmonary bypass. Normally one-third of the exchangeable albumin is intravascular, and two-thirds is in the extravascular spaces. This extravascular exchangeable albumin exists in two components based on rates of exchange. The slowly exchangeable albumin is mainly in skin and muscle.[61] The factors determining distribution of rapidly exchangeable albumin are not known. Part of the changes in plasma colloidal oncotic pressure during cardiopulmonary bypass may be related to the influx of albumin from the extravascular stores. Approximately 40% of the extravascular rapidly exchangeable albumin may be transferred to the intravascular space during cardiopulmonary bypass.[11, 12, 62]

A study of water accumulation in various organs at different albumin levels showed that fluid retention was significantly correlated with plasma colloidal oncotic pressure and albumin level in all tissues except liver. The relationship was strongest in intestine, muscle, myocardium, and skin and less strong in kidney, lung, and fat. The authors noted an adverse effect on renal function with the addition of albumin.[63] The study concluded that the optimal level of plasma colloidal oncotic pressure was 16 mm Hg and that of serum protein concentration was 4.2 gm%.

Diminished levels of plasma albumin increase glomerular filtration and diminish the reabsorption of filtrate from the proximal renal tubule[62]; thus, restoring the albumin concentration in the hemodiluted patient may have a deleterious effect on renal function. Diminished sludging of red cells has been observed with albumin added to the priming solution.[62, 64]

Studies of dextran as a volume expander in extracorporeal circulation showed that cellular oxygenation was diminished by dextran. Dextran is readily filtered at the glomerulus and may act as an osmotic diuretic. Blood volume was better maintained during cardiopulmonary bypass with low molecular weight dextran.[65] Blood volume actually increased at the onset of bypass with low molecular weight dextran in the priming solution. Urine flow was less with dextran in the perfusate than with mannitol or with saline alone. Thus, dextran may have an effect similar to albumin in decreasing urine output while diminishing interstitial fluid accumulation.[66] The studies of hydroxyethyl starch and gelatin have not evaluated their effect on fluid retention.[67]

MYOCARDIAL EDEMA

Although the edema that develops in the myocardium is not a significant volume of fluid compared to the interstitial edema which accumulates throughout the body, myocardial edema is an important factor in perioperative myocardial dysfunction.[68] Hemodilution alone may cause significant myocardial water accumulation. Lowering hematocrit by plasmapheresis preserving the concentration of plasma proteins does not lead to myocardial edema.[69] Cardiopulmonary bypass with whole blood or colloid prime did not produce significant myocardial edema (wet:dry weight increase approximately 5%), whereas crystalloid prime caused a much greater increase in water content. The accumulation of water observed by gravimetric technique was confirmed by double indicator dilution techniques with tritiated water and Evans blue. The indicator techniques measured about 85% of the water determined by gravimetric methods. Histologic and electron microscopy showed the edema in the crystalloid group to be interstitial. Ultrastructural studies showed swollen sarcoplasmic reticulum and mitochondrial cristae and clearing of the mitochondrial matrix.[64]

Among the other factors which may increase myocardial edema are high coronary perfusion pressure, ventricular distention, multiple defibrillations, and perfusion with bubble oxygenator.[68]

The distribution of water content within the heart may be altered by the onset of edema with various surgical interventions. Normally the water content is greater in the subendocardial region. This relation is maintained with up to 3 hours of hemodilution cardiopulmonary bypass in the fibrillating heart. If hypercalcemia is induced during ventricular fibrillation, the volume of the left ventricle diminishes and the water content of the subendocardial region increases more than the subepicardial region.[68] Increased subendocardial water content may be related to regional increases in capillary permeability.[70] The small, firmly contracting fibrillating left ventricle causes subendocardial vascular distortion and venous obstruction in the subendocardium.[71]

Ventricular fibrillation during cardiopulmonary bypass is accompanied by a fall in lymph flow from the heart. After 2 hours of fibrillation the flow of lymph returns to previous levels.[72] Increased myocardial contractility may increase cardial lymph flow. Thus, the flow of lymph with normal systolic contraction is diminished during ventricular fibrillation similar to the effect of diminished muscle contraction in the flow of lymph in the extremities. Total body lymph flow is increased during cardiopulmonary bypass.[73]

"Reperfusion" edema of the myocardium after periods of myocardial ischemia is a common cause of perioperative cardiac dysfunction. Hypothermic potassium cardioplegia protects against reperfusion edema. High perfusion pressures during reperfusion may contribute to edema. Osmotic agents including mannitol may protect against cell swelling during reperfusion.[74]

Reperfusion following normothermic ischemia is accompanied by higher rates of flow than following hypothermic ischemia. The increased flow and edema following normothermic perfusion is greater in the epicardium.[75] Increased capillary permeability following ischemic arrest undoubtedly contributes to reperfusion myocardial edema. These capillary changes were not demonstrable unless the ischemia had been greater than 20 minutes. The changes included irregular cytoplasmic expansion, vacuoles, and swelling of the endothelium.[76]

References

1. Litwak RS, Slonim R, Kiem Iris, Gadboys HL: Alterations in blood volume during "normovolemic" total body perfusion. J Thorac Cardiovasc Surg 42:477, 1961.
2. Kaplan S, Edwards FK, Helmsworth JA, Clark LC: Blood volume during and after total extracorporeal circulation. Arch Surg 80:31, 1960.
3. McClenahan JB, Yamauchi H, Roe BB: Blood-volume studies in cardiac-surgery patients. JAMA 195:112, 1966.
4. Neville WE, Thomason RD, Hirsch DM: Postperfusion hypervolemia after hemodilution cardiopulmonary bypass. Arch Surg 93:715, 1966.
5. Carr EA, Sloan HE, Tovar E: The clinical importance of erythrocyte and plasma volume determinations before and after open-heart surgery. J Nucl Med 1:165, 1960.
6. Utley JR, Stephens DB: Unpublished data.
7. Flanagan JP, Steinmetz GP, Crawford EW, Merendino KA: Observations on blood volume with special attention to loss and replacement in cardiac surgery. Surgery 56:925, 1964.
8. Breckenridge IM, Digerness SB, Kirklin JW: Increased extracellular fluid after open intracardiac operation. Surg Gynecol Obstet 131:53, 1970.
9. Cleland J, Pluth JR, Tauxe WN, Kirklin JW: Blood volume and body fluid compartment changes soon after closed and open intracardiac surgery. J Thorac Cardiovasc Surg 52:698, 1966.
10. Berger RL, Boyd TF, Marcus PS: A pattern of blood-volume response to open-heart surgery. N Engl J Med 271:59, 1964.
11. Beattie HW, Evans G, Garnett ES, Webber CE: Sustained hypovolemia and extracellular fluid volume expansion following cardiopulmonary bypass. Surgery 71:891, 1972.
12. Beattie HW, Evans G, Garnett ES, Regoeczi E, Webber CE, Wong KL: Albumin and water fluxes during cardiopulmonary bypass. J Thorac Cardiovasc Surg 67:926, 1974.
13. Reid DJ, Digerness S, Kirklin JW: Intracellular fluid volume in surgical patients measured by the simultaneous determination of total body water and extracellular fluid. Surg Forum 18:29, 1967.
14. Beall AC, Johnson PC, Shirkey AL, Crosthwait RW, Cooley DA, DeBakey ME: Effects of temporary cardiopulmonary bypass on extracellular fluid volume and total body water in man. Circulation 29 (Suppl.):59, 1964.
15. Lilleaasen P, Stokke, O: Moderate and extreme hemodilution in open-heart surgery: Fluid balance and acid-base studies. Ann Thorac Surg 25:127, 1978.
16. Pluth JR, Cleland J, Tauxe WN, Kirklin JW: Late changes in body fluid and blood volume after

intracardiac surgery. J Thorac Cardiovasc Surg 56:108, 1968.

17. Sturtz GS, Kirklin JW, Burke EC, Power MH: Water metabolism after cardiac operations involving a Gibbon-type pump oxygenator. Circulation 16:1000, 1957.

18. Dordoni L, Oddi N, Schiavello R, Magalini SI, Bondoli A: Biochemical changes in extracorporeal circulation in patients. Resuscitation 5:111, 1976.

19. Pacifico AD, Digerness S, Kirklin JW: Sodium-excreting ability before and after intracardiac surgery. Circulation 2 (Suppl.):142, 1970.

20. Pacifico AD, Digerness S, Kirklin JW: Regression of body compositional abnormalities of heart failure after intracardiac operations. Circulation 42:999, 1970.

21. Pacifico AD, Digerness S, Kirklin JW: Acute alterations of body composition after open intracardiac operations. Circulation 41:331, 1970.

22. Kirklin, JW, Pacifico AD: Effect of intracardiac operations upon congestive heart failure and body composition. Am J Cardiol 22:183, 1968.

23. Cohn LH, Klovekorn P, Moore FD, Collins JJ: Intrinsic plasma volume deficits in patients with coronary artery disease. Arch Surg 108:57, 1974.

24. Wigboldus AH, Urzua J, Viljoen JF: The "empty heart" phenomenon. J Thorac Cardiovasc Surg 66:807, 1973.

25. Utley JR, Moores WY, Stephens DB: Blood conservation techniques. Ann Thorac Surg 31:482, 1981.

26. Vertrees RA, Stark M, Auvil J, Rohrer C, Rousou JH, Engelman RM: Weight gain and cardiopulmonary bypass. J Extra-Corporeal Technol 12:74, 1980.

27. Utley JR, Wachtel C, Cain RB, Spaw EA, Collins JC, Stephens DB: Effect of hypothermia, hemodilution and pump oxygenation on organ water content, blood flow and oxygen delivery, and renal function. Ann Thorac Surg 31:121, 1981.

28. Webber CE, Garnett ES: The relationship between colloid osmotic pressure and plasma proteins during and after cardiopulmonary bypass. J Thorac Cardiovasc Surg 65:234, 1973.

29. English TA, Digerness S, Kirklin JW: Changes in colloid osmotic pressure during and shortly after open intracardiac operation. J Thorac Cardiovasc Surg 61:338, 1971.

30. Gollub S, Schechter DC, Schaefer C, Svigals R, Bailey CP: Absolute hemodilution cardiopulmonary bypass: Free water distribution and protein mobilization in body compartments. Am Heart J 78:626, 1969.

31. Roe BB, Swenson EE, Hepps SA, Bruns DL: Total body perfusion in cardiac operations. Arch Surg 88:128, 1964.

32. Neville WE, Faber LP, Peacock H: Total prime of the disc oxygenator with Ringer's and Ringer's lactate solution for cardiopulmonary bypass. Dis Chest 45:320, 1964.

33. Cooley DA, Beall AC, Grondin P: Open heart operations with disposable oxygenators, 5 per cent dextrose prime, and normothermia. Surgery 52:713, 1962.

34. Gordon RJ, Ravin M, Rawitscher RE, Daicoff GR: Changes in arterial pressure, viscosity, and resist-ance during cardiopulmonary bypass. J Thorac Cardiovasc Surg 69:552, 1975.

35. Gordon RJ, Ravin M, Daicoff GR, Rawitsher RE: Effects of hemodilution on hypotension during cardiopulmonary bypass. Anesth Analg (Cleve) 54:482, 1975.

36. Eiseman B, Spencer FC: Effect of hypothermia on the flow characteristics of blood. Surgery 52:532, 1962.

37. Fedor EJ, Fisher B: Simultaneous determination of blood volume with Cr^{51} and T-1824 during hypothermia and rewarming. Am J Physiol 196:703, 1959.

38. Oz M, Kameya S, Neville W, Clowes GHA: The relationship of blood volume, systemic peripheral resistance, and flow rate during profound hypothermia. Trans Soc Artif Intern Org 6:204, 1960.

39. Lofstrom B: Changes in blood volume in induced hypothermia. Acta Anaesthesiol Scand 1:1, 1957.

40. Kanter GS: Hypothermic hemoconcentration. Am J Physiol 214:856, 1968.

41. Chang CB, Shoemaker WC: Effect of hypothermia on red cell volumes. J Thorac Cardiovasc Surg 46:117, 1963.

42. Svanes K, Zweifach BW, Intaglietta M: Effect of hypothermia on transcapillary fluid exchange. Am J Physiol 218:981, 1970.

43. Kahler RL, Goldblatt A, Braunwald E: Circulatory effects of profound hypothermia during extracorporeal circulation. Am J Physiol 202:523, 1962.

44. Yeh TJ, Ellison LT, Ellison RG: Hemodynamic and metabolic responses of the whole body and individual organs to cardiopulmonary bypass with profound hypothermia. J Thorac Cardiovasc Surg 42:782, 1961.

45. Lopez-Belio M, Tasaki G, Balagot R, Sanchez L, Gomez F, Julian OC: Effect of hypothermia during cardiopulmonary bypass on peripheral resistance. Arch Surg 81:283, 1960.

46. Clasen RA, Pandolfi S, Hass GM: Interrupted hypothermia in experimental cerebral edema. Neurology 20:2779, 1970.

47. Fenstermacher JD, LI C-L, Levin VA: Extracellular space of the cerebral cortex of normothermic and hypothermic cats. Exp Neurol 27:101, 1970.

48. Lee WH, Krumhaar D, Fondalsrud EW, Schjeide OA, Maloney JV: Denaturation of plasma proteins as a cause of morbidity and death after intracardiac operations. Surgery 50:29, 1961.

49. Parker DJ, Cantrell JW, Karp RB, Stroud RM, Digerness SB: Changes in serum complement and immunoglobins following cardiopulmonary bypass. Surgery 71:824, 1972.

50. Cook WA, Webb WR: Pump oxygenators and hypothermia. Ann Thorac Surg 1:466, 1965.

51. Guyton AC: Interstitial fluid pressure: II. Pressure-volume curves of interstitial space. Circ Res 16:452, 1965.

52. Menninger FJ III, Rosenkranz ER, Utley JR, Dembitsky WP, Hargens AR, Peters RM: Interstitial hydrostatic pressure in patients undergoing CABG and valve replacement. J Thorac Cardiovasc Surg 79:181, 1980.

53. Rosenkranz ER, Utley JR, Menninger FJ, Dembitsky WP, Hargens AR, Peters RM: Interstitial fluid pres-

sure changes during cardiopulmonary bypass. Ann Thorac Surg 30:538, 1980.

54. Larmi TKI, Karkola P: Plasma protein electrophoresis during a three hour cardiopulmonary bypass in dogs. Scand J Thorac Cardiovasc Surg 8:162, 1974.

55. Wisselink P, Feola M, Alfrey CP, Suzuki M, Ross JN, Kennedy JH: Prolonged partial cardiopulmonary bypass and the integrity of small blood vessels. J Thorac Cardiovasc Surg 60:789, 1970.

56. Martin DS, DelCastillo J, Martinex M, Pickens J, Hudson PJ: Beneficial influence of a serotonin-histamine antagonist on perfusion sequelae. Surgery 56:1064, 1964.

57. Parker DJ, Cook S, Turner-Warwick M: Serum complement studies during and following cardiopulmonary bypass. In *Lung Metabolism*, edited by AF Junod and R de Haller. New York, Academic Press, 1975.

58. Hallowell P, Bland JHL, Dalton BC, Erdmann AJ, Lappas DG, Laver MB, Philbin D, Thomas S, Lowenstein E: The effect of hemodilution with albumin or Ringer's lactate on water balance and blood use in open heart surgery. Ann Thorac Surg 25:22, 1978.

59. Lilleaasen P, Stokke O, Thoresen O, Aasen A, Engesaeter L, Froysaker T: Effects of different nonhaemic fluids in open-heart surgery. Scand J Thorac Cardiovasc Surg 13:233, 1979.

60. Marty AT, Prather J, Matloff JM, Schauble J: Oncotic effects of dilutional bypass, albumin, and diuretics. Arch Surg 107:21, 1973.

61. Rothschild MA, Oratz M, Schreiber SS: Extravascular albumin. N Engl J Med 301:497, 1979.

62. Utley Jr, Stephens DB, Wachtel C, Cain RB, Collins JC, Spaw EA, Moores WY: Effect of albumin and mannitol on organ blood flow, oxygen delivery, water content and renal function during hypothermic hemodilution cardiopulmonary bypass. Ann Thorac Surg 33:250, 1982.

63. Schupbach P, Pappova E, Schilt W, Kollar J, Kollar M, Sipos P, Vucic D: Perfusate oncotic pressure during cardiopulmonary bypass: Optimum level as determined by metabolic acidosis, tissue edema and renal function. Vox Sang 35:332, 1978.

64. Laks H, Standeven J, Blair O, Hahn J, Jellinek M, Willman VL: The effects of cardiopulmonary bypass with crystaloid and colloid hemodilution on myocardial extravascular water. J Thorac Cardio-

vasc Surg 73:129, 1977.

65. Hymes AC, Safavian MH, Arbulu A, Baute P: A comparison of Pluronic F-68, low molecular weight dextran, mannitol, and saline as priming agents in the heart-lung apparatus. J Thorac Cardiovasc Surg 56:16, 1968.

66. Albrechtsen OK, Althaus U, Berg E, Jeyasingham K, Kim CH, Silberschmid M: Haemodilution techniques in canine extracorporeal circulation using bubble and disc oxygenators. Scand J Thorac Cardiovasc Surg 6:178, 1972.

67. Merikallio E: Haemodilution in cardiopulmonary bypass using a gelatine derivative for priming. Ann Chir Gynaecol Fenn 65:138, 1976.

68. Utley JR, Michalsky GB, Bryant LR, Mobin-Uddin K, McKean HE: Determinants of myocardial water content during cardiopulmonary bypass. J Thorac Cardiovasc Surg 68:8, 1974.

69. Lowenstein E, Cooper JD, Erdman AJ, Geffin G, Laver MB, Yoshikawa H: Lung and heart water accumulation associated with hemodilution. Bibl Haematol 41:190, 1975.

70. Anversa P, Giacomelli F, Wiener J: Regional variation in capillary permeability of ventricular myocardium. Microvasc Res 6:273, 1973.

71. Utley JR, Michalsky GB, Mobin-Uddin K, Bryant LR: Subendocardial vascular distortion at small ventricular volumes. J Surg Res 17:114, 1974.

72. Taira A, Yamashita M, Arikawa K, Hamada Y, Toyohira H, Akita H: Cardiac lymph in electrical ventricular fibrillation: An experimental study. Ann Thorac Surg 27:144, 1978.

73. Pasqui U, Cedrangolo L, Parmeggiani U, Molea G, Barbarisi A, Procaccini E, Gentile A, DeSiena M: Drenaggio linfatico in corso di circolazione extracorporea ed arresto circolatoria ipotermico nel cane. Arch Chir Thorac Cardiovasc 33:69, 1976.

74. Engelman RM: Myocardial edema, a complication of ischemic arrest during cardiopulmonary bypass. Am Heart J 95:128, 1978.

75. Todd EP, Utley JR, Collins JC, Wachtel CC: Normothermic vs. hypothermic ischemia. Effects on coronary flow, myocardial water content and systemic vascular resistance. Surg Forum 26:232, 1975.

76. DeGasperis C, Gonzales-Lavin L, Pellegrini A, Ross DN: Ultrastructural aspects of human myocardial capillaries during open heart surgery. Cardiology 56:333, 1971.

CHAPTER 4

DEEP HYPOTHERMIA AND CIRCULATORY ARREST IN THE ADULT

BENSON B. ROE, M.D.

HISTORY AND BACKGROUND

Clinical experience with hypothermia dates back to antiquity. The medical literature documents several cases of uncomplicated survival from accidental hypothermia to body temperatures from 25°C to below 20°C[1,2]. And the hemodynamics of profound hypothermia have been extensively studied.[3–6]

Although circulatory arrest under deep hypothermia has recently proven to be a useful and widely accepted adjunct in neonatal cardiac surgery,[7,8] it is interesting to recall that this modality was introduced clinically for intracardiac operations before the advent of cardiopulmonary bypass.[9,10] Mild hypothermia—just above the arrhythmia level—was successfully used to permit quite safe inflow occlusion for periods of 6 to 8 minutes during which we were able to carry out a few simple intracardiac procedures.[11] Later we successfully closed aortopulmonary (Potts) shunts through the pulmonary artery during a brief period of suspended machine perfusion prior to repairing a tetralogy of Fallot. And cerebral aneurysms were successfully repaired under prolonged circulatory arrest during deep hypothermia induced with extracorporeal circulation (via femoro-femoral bypass).[12–14]

Despite this background of favorable experience with hypothermia and despite minimal evidence to demonstrate any harmful effects of hypothermia (other than causing cardiac arrhythmias and respiratory arrest) clinicians have long feared or imagined detrimental consequences from hypothermia and were reluctant to use the modality except when it was necessary. Abundant experimental evidence has verified the protective effect of hypothermia against ischemic damage.[15–17] On the other hand, the alternative of perfusion from cardiopulmonary bypass is known to produce organ damage and physiological changes that are still not completely understood. Despite this knowledge, most cardiac surgeons routinely employ high flow extracorporeal circulation for adult heart surgery in preference to diminished or suspended flows at low body tempereatures. Is it possible that we are missing something?

CIRCULATORY ARREST WITHOUT HYPOTHERMIA

We are so imbued with the vital importance of maintaining circulation—as the very symbol of life—that we sometimes fail to recognize the potential alternatives. When the circulation itself provides a serious threat to survival, such as in exsanguinating hemorrhage, it may be life-saving to arrest it briefly—even at normothermia, thus preserving critical intravascular volume

Table 4.1
Deliberate Circulatory Arrest to Treat Massive Hemorrhage

Episode	Age	Period of Arrest (Minutes)	Outcome
Left atrial tear during forced avulsion of free-floating myxoma	55	6	No sequelae
Traction tear at junction of left pulmonary vein and left atrium during closed mitral commissurotomy	52	14	No sequelae
Traumatic 4-cm tear in right atrium with pericardial tamponade	22	11	No sequelae
Rent in soft left ventricle during implanting of epicardial pacemaker electrode	83	5½	No sequelae
Clamp slipped off during coarctation repair	9	4	No sequelae
Pulmonary artery tie slipped off during pneumonectomy	57	6	No sequelae
Aortic valve replacement with bleeding from posterior suture line (perfusion cannulae removed)	62	2½	Low output syndrome with recovery
Aortic valve replacement with bleeding from posterior suture line (perfusion cannulae removed)	53	4	Low output syndrome with recovery
Disruption of friable aortic suture line during division of adult patent ductus arteriosus	37	7	No sequelae
Uncontrollable bleeding from right ventricular cannulation site after left thoracotomy cardiopulmonary bypass	56	4	No sequelae

and providing visual access to the bleeding source. We have deliberately induced ventricular fibrillation in a series of circumstances where major bleeding had not been readily controllable and were thus able to stem the tide before exsanguination occurred and then to massage and defibrillate before ischemic brain damage occurred. The significant risk of deliberately arresting the circulation is a favorable trade-off against the combined effects of gradual exsanguination, impaired access to surgical control of bleeding, and relatively slow volume replacement with donor blood. These experiences convinced me that the advertized limits of circulatory arrest were excessively restrictive and that we should remain aware of the potential benefits of that modality. That contention is documented by our own results which were substantiated in Table 4.1.[18,19]

HYPOTHERMIA PHYSIOLOGY

The principles and limitations of decelerating bacterial growth and biochemical action by refrigeration are well established and are directly transposable to the living organism. Even as some foods spoil more rapidly than others so are some tissues more susceptible to ischemic damage than others. As we all know it is the central nervous system that is least tolerant of anoxia, followed by the kidneys, liver, and heart. The spectrum of ischemic tolerance (at normothermia) spreads from 5 to 6 minutes for brain cells to many hours for fat and skin. Hypothermia roughly doubles this tolerance time for each 5°C of cooling, thus the brain (and, of course, other tissues) are almost completely protected from ischemic damage for 6 to 9 minutes at 32°C, for 40 minutes at 23°C, and for 100 minutes at 12°C.

Much remains to be learned about the metabolic and enzymatic consequences of hypothermia. Significant changes in pH occur during hypothermia, and correction of the acidosis has been recommended by some on the basis of elevated pH in hybernating animals and some improvement of post hypothermia cardiac function in experimental animals whose pH was artificially raised during the cooling phase.[20] From a practical standpoint, however, the metabolic aberrations of hypothermia appear to correct themselves spontaneously on rewarming and do not have residual effect.

PITFALLS AND FAILURES

It is true that damage to the brain and other organs has been encountered after both experimental and clinical use of hypothermic arrest. However, these reports are sporadic and should not be the basis for inferring hazards of the fundamental concept. Instead, it is more likely that the method of application is faulty either by failing to provide the objective or by introducing other hazards. The protective effect of hypothermia may be diminished or obliterated by various mechanisms which may be obscure to the surgeon: (1) Cooling may not be homogeneous, so that the temperature measurement does not reflect that some of the ischemic tissue is warmer and thus susceptible to damage. (2) When hypothermia and rewarming are induced by extracorporeal perfusion the inherent embolic hazards of that system can insidiously cause tissue damage. (3) Circulatory arrest can create a gravitational vacuum in the vascular compartment so that air can be aspirated from the operative field and later embolized to cause infarction. (4) When surface cooling with ice is used to induce hypothermia it is possible to damage tissue by freezing and crystalization.

The safe lower limits of hypothermia are still in dispute. Studies have shown impaired ventricular function after temperatures of 10°C, but others have demonstrated no damage after temperatures below 0°C. For all practical purposes, however, we can consider hypothermia itself to be a harmless modality over a broad range so long as measures are provided to protect against its arrhythmogenic, respiratory, and perhaps metabolic effects.

UTILITY OF CIRCULATORY ARREST

There are a number of circumstances in operations on the heart or great vessels when it is either unsafe, technically difficult or even impossible to work effectively while the extracorporeal circulation is maintained. Among those circumstances are: (1) over-developed bronchial circulation causing massive extracardiac shunting from the pump-supported systemic circulation into the pulmonary circulation and thence to flood the left heart; (2) aortopulmonary surgical shunt (Potts-Smith) which cannot easily and safely be surgically controlled prior to initiating cardiopulmonary bypass and which cannot be visualized with systemic blood flowing through it; (3) saccular aneurysms of the thoracic aorta whose size or location precludes or complicates control of the adjacent aorta; (4) fusiform aneurysms of the thoracic aorta which extend either proximally into the mediastinum or distally to the diaphragm where clamping the aorta beyond them is difficult or dangerous; (5) aneurysms of the ascending aorta which extend into the transverse arch and therefore require clamping of the innominate or carotid artery so as to endanger the cerebral circulation; (6) aneurysms of the (transverse) aortic arch.

There are alternative approaches to these lesions which require difficult dissection and/or they employ separate additional cannulation and perfusion of the arch vessels. While these techniques have been used successfully, they introduce distinct hazards which I believe to be significantly greater than those of circulatory arrest under appropriate conditions. An additional benefit of circulatory arrest is that blood damage associated with the extracorporeal circuit is diminished while it is shut off.

COMPLICATIONS OF CIRCULATORY ARREST

When the extracorporeal circulation is interrupted the intravascular pressure drops to zero so that air will enter an open semi-rigid vessel (such as the aorta) to replace the blood which spills or is aspirated from it. This air may not easily be evacuated at the end of the procedure, and on reinstituting the perfusion it can easily be forced into the cerebral circulation (particularly if the arterial perfusion enters the femoral artery). To avoid this serious and potentially fatal complication we have introduced carbon dioxide into the (clamped) perfusion line just as the aorta is to be opened. The blood is thus forced into the operative field from within and is displaced by a transparent gas which is later rapidly absorbed into the blood and diffused in the oxygenator without remaining in the circulation as embolic bubbles. This mechanism prevents nitrogenous air from entering the circulation and prevents its embolization.[21] This innovation was prompted by a disastrous experience with air embolism following the simple closure of a large saccular intramediastinal aortic aneurysm from within the sac during a very brief circulatory arrest at 25°C. Measures to evacuate intraaortic air were unsuccessful and unrecognized because it gravitated distally when the patient was put in Trendelberg position to keep the head vessels filled and then was driven up the aorta when the femoral artery perfusion was resumed. Our first use of intravascular CO_2 was followed by the usual maneuvers to evacuate the gas, but these efforts were subsequently abandoned as we appreciated how harmless it was. All patients have awakened immediately after the operation completely free of neurological deficit.

SUMMARY

Deep hypothermia has proven to be a safe and effective mechanism to protect even the most sensitive tissues from ischemic damage when the circulation is arrested. The extent of this protection is great enough to justify the utilization of circulatory arrest during a variety of operative procedures that are impaired by maintaining the circulation. Experience from its use under these circumstances suggests that broader application may be indicated, particularly when balanced against the hazards of prolonged extracorporeal circulation.

References

1. Wickerstron P, Ruiz E, Lilja GP, Hinterkopf JP, Haglin JJ: Accidental hypothermia: Core rewarming with partial bypas. Am J Surg 131:622, 1976.
2. Truscott DG, Firor WB, Clein LJ: Accidental profound hypothermia: Successful resuscitation by core rewarming and assisted circulation. Arch Surg 106:216, 1973.
3. Zarins CK, Skinner DB: Hemodynamics and blood flow distribution following prolonged circulation at 5°C. Am J Physiol 229:275, 1975.
4. Aoyagi M, Flasterskin AH, Barnette J, et al: Cerebral effects of profound hypothermia (18°C) and circulatory arrest. Circulation 49, 50:60, 1974.
5. Edmunds LH, Folkman J, Snodgrass AB, Brown RB: Prevention of brain damage during profound hypothermia and circulatory arrest. Ann Surg 157:637, 1963.
6. Egerton N, Egerton WS, Kay JH: Neurologic changes following profound hypothermia. Ann Surg 157:366, 1963.
7. Barratt-Boyes BG, Simpson M, Neutze JM: Intracardiac surgery in neonates and infants using deep hypothermia with surface cooling and limited cardiopulmonary bypass. Circulation 43:25, 1971.
8. Drew CE: Profound hypothermia in cardiac surgery. Lond Clin Med J 7:15, 1966.
9. Swan H, Zeavin I, Blount SG Jr, Virtue RW: Surgery by direct vision in the open heart during hypothermia. JAMA 153:1081, 1953.
10. Swan H, Virtue RW, Blount SG, Kircher LT: Hypothermia in surgery: Analysis of 100 clinical cases. Ann Surg 142:382, 1955.
11. Lewis FJ, Taufic M: Closure of atrial septal defects with aid of hypothermia: Experimental accomplishments and report of one successful case. Surgery 33:52, 1953.
12. St. Ville JM, Tobias E: Intracranial surgery: Profound hypothermia and cardiac arrest. Arch Surg 92:573, 1966.
13. Patterson RH, Ray BS: Profound hypothermia for intracranial surgery. Ann Surg 156:377, 1962.
14. Rehder K, Kirklin JW, MacCarthy CS, Theye RA: Physiologic studies following profound hypothermia and circulatory arrest for treatment of intracranial aneurysm. Ann Surg 156:882, 1962.
15. Swan H: Clinical hypothermia: A lady with a past and some promise for the future. Surgery 73:736, 1973.
16. Perna AM, Gardner TJ, Tabaddor K, et al: Cerebral metabolism and blood flow after circulatory arrest during deep hypothermia. Ann Surg 178:95, 1973.
17. Connolly JE, Harris EJ, Bruns DL, Smith JW, Guernsey J, Boyd R: An experimental study of the techniques and effects of selective brain cooling. Surg Forum 11:405, 1960.
18. Roe BB, Zanger LC, Behnke JC: Induced ventricular fibrillation to control massive hemorrhage during closed cardiac surgery. Surgery 51:112–120, 1962.
19. Roe BB: Induced ventricular fibrillation to control cardiac surgical emergencies. Dis Chest 42:422–424, 1962.
20. Becker H, et al: Myocardial damage caused by keeping pH 7.40 during systemic deep hypothermia. J Thorac Cardiovasc Surg 82:810–820, 1981.
21. Roe BB: Prevention of air embolism with intravascular carbon dioxide washout. J Thorac Cardiovasc Surg 71:628, 1976.

CHAPTER 5

CARBON DIOXIDE TRANSPORT AND ACID-BASE BALANCE DURING HYPOTHERMIA*

FRED N. WHITE, Ph.D.
YITZHAK WEINSTEIN, Ph.D.

A major goal of the cardiac surgeon and the perfusionist is the establishment of blood flow rates and blood gas and acid-base conditions which assure the welfare of tissues during hypothermic procedures. Hemodilution is commonly employed, a practice which has the advantage of reducing blood viscosity and hemolysis. The gas phase of pump oxygenators is typified by high partial pressures of oxygen and carbon dioxide tensions of approximately 40 torr. A common objective is to establish an arterial pH of approximately 7.4 at low temperature. This criterion is based upon the general assumption that this pH, characterizing as it does a normal arterial blood at 37°C, should represent the most propitious level at lower temperatures.

TEMPERATURE-pH RELATIONSHIPS OF BLOOD AT CONSTANT CO$_2$ CONTENT

A sample of arterial blood exhibiting a P_{CO_2} of 40 torr and pH of 7.4 at 37°C will exhibit a progressively higher pH and a lower P_{CO_2} as temperature is reduced. The pH will exhibit $\Delta pH/°C \cong -0.015$ so long as the sample is maintained tight from the atmosphere, i.e., maintained at constant to-tal CO$_2$ content. This relationship, described by Rosenthal,[1] allows the calculation of the pH of blood at low temperature when pH electrodes are thermostated at the usual 37°C level: $pH_{22°C} = pH_{37°C} + (37 - 22)$ (0.015). The slope of pH on temperature ($\Delta pH/°C \cong -0.015$) is remarkable in its similarity to the slope of the neutral pH of water. Pure water exhibits pH = 7 at 25° C. At all other temperatures, owing to the temperature-dependent dissociation constant, the neutral pH of water follows the relationship: $\Delta pH/°C = -0.017$. Thus, at 37°C, the neutral pH of H$_2$O = 6.8, while at 15°C it is 7.17. Albery and Lloyd[2] predicted that the buffer system responsible for the relationship of blood pH and temperature would exhibit a pK of 7 and heat of enthalpy of 7 kcal/mole. If in sufficient concentration in the blood, such a buffer would allow its pK to change in parallel with that of water. It is now known that the imidazole moiety of protein-bound histidine supplies this property and is present in sufficient quantity to account for the pH-temperature relationships observed in vitro.[3]

The relationship of blood pH to temperature is usefully placed in perspective when we consider man as thermally heterogeneous. Exercising man, or man in the cold, exhibits a range of tissue temperatures. Exercising muscle temperatures may exceed

* Supported in part by NSF Grant PCM 79-05052.

that of the core, while the temperature of the skin may be several degrees below core values. Because of the behavior of blood, at constant CO_2 content, we come to appreciate that cool skin exhibits pH values higher than warmer tissues.[4] The particular pH will depend upon the thermal state of the pre-capillary blood as it equilibrates with tissue temperatures. It thus seems important to realize that as we indulge, periodically, in varying degrees of hyper- and hypothermia in our daily lives, the arterial pH is heterogeneous in nature.

PATTERNS OF ACID-BASE HOMEOSTASIS IN ANIMALS

The vast majority of animals exhibit body temperatures which are dictated by their thermal environment. Many of these ectothermic creatures are subject to a wide range of body temperatures as a result of daily or seasonal cycles in temperatures. It is instructive to examine the patterns of acid-base regulation of ectotherms, especially since biochemical pathways may be quite sensitive to changes in hydrogen ion concentration.

Examination of the arterial blood of various ectothermic animals (reptiles, amphibians, fishes, crabs, etc.) has revealed a general pattern in the pH-temperature relationship: pH is inversely related to temperature (Fig. 5.1). The relationship, $\Delta pH/°C \cong -0.015$, shown by these organisms, is essentially that described for *in vitro* blood at constant CO_2 content. The *in vivo* slope of pH on temperature is very nearly parallel to the curve for the neutral pH of water. It can also be shown that the pOH^- follows a similar slope. Thus, over the wide range of temperatures experienced by ectotherms, the ratio $[OH^-]/[H^+]$ remains essentially constant, and the arterial blood exhibits constant alkalinity relative to the pH of neutral water. Studies on the intracellular compartment have demonstrated a similar relationship to temperature with pH_i for various tissues. This curve is to the acid side of the extracellular fluid and generally approximates the curve of pH for neutral water (recent reviews in refs. 5 and 6).

The behavior of the blood of these lower

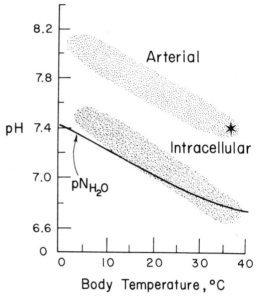

Figure 5.1. Arterial and intracellular pH as a function of body temperature in ectothermic animals. Arterial pH values for fishes, amphibians, reptiles, and crabs fall within the stippled area. Intracellular pHs for liver, smooth, skeletal, and cardiac muscle for a turtle fall to the acid side of arterial values and near the neutral $pH(pN_{H_2O})$ of water. Arterial pH of man indicated by *asterisk*.

vertebrates would find its sole explanation in the buffer properties of blood (as in a closed syringe) were it not that animals are *open* systems exchanging gases with the environment. We are challenged to explain how animals can mimic the *in vitro* behavior of blood while transporting carbon dioxide to the environment. The problem takes on new definition when we consider the buffering properties of the blood, which are summarized in the Henderson-Hasselbalch relationship: $pH = pK + \log [HCO_3^-]/S \cdot P_{CO_2}$.

As described by Severinghaus,[7,8] there are important temperature influences on two of the variables of this equation. First, pK is a function of both temperature and pH. S, the solubility factor, varies inversely with temperature. The nomogram[7] and table of S values[8] produced by Severinghaus are useful in making these corrections. In an open system, such as a reptile experiencing temperature changes, the maintenance of arterial blood at constant carbon dioxide content could be achieved *either* by reducing $[HCO_3^-]$ or elevating P_{CO_2} as a function of temperature. Examination of the arterial blood proves that $[HCO_3^-]$ remains essentially constant while P_{CO_2} varies directly with body temperature. The result is constant total CO_2 of the blood, and consequently the pH resembles the behavior of blood *in vitro*.

The primary system responsible for regulating arterial P_{CO_2} is, of course, the respiratory system. It can be seen that the condition of arterial blood observed at various temperatures can be explained if it is shown that the ratio of ventilation to CO_2 production is in a precise inverse relationship to body temperature. This condition is met by

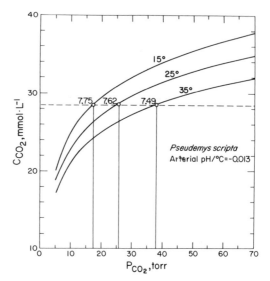

Figure 5.3. Carbon dioxide dissociation curves of oxygenated blood of the turtle, *Pseudemys scripta*, at three temperatures. Arterial pH and associated Pa_{CO_2} values observed in intact animals are shown. Note that the total CO_2 content of blood is maintained at a constant level. (Based on reference 10 and dissociation curves derived by Y. Weinstein, R. A. Ackerman, and F. N. White.)

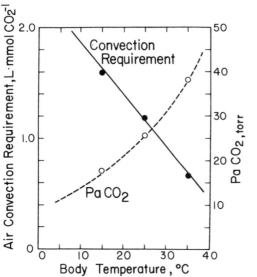

Figure 5.2. Relationships of body temperature to air convection requirement and arterial P_{CO_2} in a turtle. The direct relationship between body temperature and Pa_{CO_2} is the result of the fall in convection requirement (liters of gas ventilated per unit of carbon dioxide produced). The regulation of arterial Pa_{CO_2} at the values shown is required to maintain total CO_2 content of blood at a constant level and $\Delta pH/°C \cong -0.015$. (Based on reference 10.)

experimental observations on a number of ectothermic lung breathers. The pattern exhibited by the turtle is rather typical,[9, 10] although the precise values for the ratio of ventilation to CO_2 production, and thus the arterial P_{CO_2} values, are highly influenced by the $[HCO_3^-]$ values typifying given species (Fig. 5.2).

The temperature-specific arterial P_{CO_2}s, when related to corresponding CO_2 dissociation curves, dramatically illustrate that the respiratory poise is so regulated that a constant CO_2 content of arterial blood is achieved at various temperatures (Fig. 5.3). The nature of the sensory systems which achieve this precise modulation of alveolar and arterial P_{CO_2} levels as temperature *and* the CO_2 dissociation curve are altered is not understood. The achievement, however, is quite clear: maintenance of a $\Delta pH/°C \cong -0.015$, constant CO_2 content of blood and $[OH^-]/[H^+]$. The system behaves like *in vi-*

tro blood in a closed system, although the *in vivo* organism is obviously an open system exchanging gases with the atmosphere.

It was stated above that intracellular compartments follow a pH-temperature slope similar to that of blood, the slope being displaced to the acid side of blood in the zone of the neutral pH of water. This condition has important implications for enzymic functions.

The principal intracellular buffers appear to be proteins. Of the amino acids forming proteins, only histidine is titratable over the range of intracellular pH values, a characteristic which must be ascribed to the imidazole moiety of histidine. Because the change in pK of imidazole with temperature (dpK_{im}/dT) is similar to that of H_2O, the dominance of this component of intracellular buffering maintains the net protein charge state protected, *i.e.*, protons are neither taken up nor given off by imidazole groups, and the carbonic acid buffer system will not be titrated. The necessity of maintaining total CO_2 content constant is achieved at the respiratory level.

The state of protonization (charge state) of imidazole is expressed as a variable (alpha) equal to the ratio of deprotonated to total imidazole groups. Maintenance of a constant alpha, referred to as *alpha-stat* behavior, occurs *in vivo* when carbon dioxide partial pressure is appropriately regulated by ventilation, such as to control carbonic acid titration of imidazole. This regulated interplay between these principal buffer systems may be expected to set the stage for enzyme systems which utilize histidine imidazole groups as binding sites. An instructive example is lactic acid dehydrogenase.[11] The activity of this enzyme is dependent on the charge state of the imidazole active site which must maintain alpha at around 0.5. Protonization of the imidazole group favors pyruvate binding, while deprotonization favors lactate binding. Regulation of the charge state is thus necessary in order to allow catalysis of these reactions in both directions. It is alpha-stat regulation which preserves this property with changing temperature, a feature requiring that pH compensates in such a manner as to conserve the K_m values (affinity constants) for substrates. Similar behaviors requiring alpha-stat regulation have been described for ribonuclease, phosphofructokinase, and sodium-potassium ATP-ase.[6] As emphasized by Rahn and Reeves,[12] the entire strategy behind the regulation of constant CO_2 content through respiratory control of the P_{CO_2} may be rationalized in terms of alpha-stat control. The consequence of this regulation is the stabilization of biochemical reactions fundamental to the metabolic welfare of organisms in a heterogeneous thermal world.

An additional effect of alpha-stat regulation is the stabilization of Donnan ratios as demonstrated by Reeves.[13] Not only is the Donnan ratio maintained constant but cell volume as well. Regulation to the acid-side of the alpha-stat regime will promote an increase in Donnan ratio and cell volume.

There is a fascinating departure from patterns of acid-base regulation exhibited by ectothermic animals. Hibernating mammals maintain arterial pH values at essentially constant levels, and recent observations indicate that this is true for intracellular values as well.[14] By ecothermic standards they are quite acidotic at hibernating temperatures. It is of interest that these animals do not exhibit metabolic acidosis at low temperature, while this is a common complication in human hypothermia where normothermic pH values are maintained. The extent to which isoenzymes with differing pH optima may contribute to the metabolic pathways of hibernation is unknown.

ACID-BASE STUDIES IN HYPOTHERMIC MAMMALS AND MAN

The rationale underlying current acid-base management in hypothermic patients appears to reside primarily on the general concept that pH values normal to 37°C are, *post hoc ergo propter hoc*, appropriate to lower temperatures. Consideration of alternative acid-base regimes is a serious matter, considering the impressive results obtained by current surgical methods. Yet, complications involving acid-base disorders and electrical and conductive abnormalities of the heart still remain major management problems. Alpha-stat regulation offers a rationale and potential method of improving the welfare of the tissues of hypothermic subjects. Recent experimental and clinical studies bear on this question.

An early attempt to evaluate alpha-stat regulation during hypothermia focused on canine cardiac functions.[15] It was shown that, at 28°C, the maintenance of an arterial pH of 7.7 resulted in significant elevations in coronary blood flow, left ventricular oxygen consumption, and lactate consumption by comparison to pH 7.4. There was also a significant increase in peak ventricular pressure when a standard load was applied. Subsequent studies[16] report that during surface cooling hypothermia, the maintenance of pH 7.4 (CO_2 management) was associated with marked arterial hypotension, low cardiac output, systemic lactic acidosis, and declines in cerebral and renal blood flows. There was a net production in lactic acid by the heart. Management of arterial pH by lowering P_{CO_2} to achieve an "ectothermic" pH resulted in improvement in arterial pressure, a doubling of cerebral blood flow, net extraction of lactic acid by the heart, and normal systemic lactate metabolism.

Hypothermic isolated, perfused papillary muscle exhibits greater contractility when the pH of the perfusate is to the alkaline side of pH 7.4.[17] Furthermore, when pH was reduced by increasing perfusate P_{CO_2}, the resulting acidosis was associated with a rapid fall in myocardial tension development and an inhibition of the efflux of slow exchanging $^{45}Ca^{2+}$ and uptake of $^{47}Ca^{2+}$.[18]

Recently Swain[19] has demonstrated that alpha-stat regulation in hypothermic dogs results in stabilization of the electrical threshold for cardiac fibrillation, while maintenance of pH 7.4 lowered the threshold.

The central nervous susceptibility to the damaging effects of circulatory arrest or perfusion with anoxic blood has been evaluated in regard to the influence of perfusate pH prior to the period of insult in the hypothermic (20°C) dog. Arterial pHs to the alkaline side of pH 7.4, while not preventing lesions, clearly ameliorated their extent and magnitude. Acidic perfusate enhanced the extent of lesions.[20]

A goal of hypothermic perfusional preservation of the kidney is the choice of a perfusion fluid which will best preserve function and survival on transplantation to a recipient. Experimental studies of kidney function following cold preservation and retransplantation of rabbit and canine kidneys show a positive correlation between function and preservation pHs at low temperature to the alkaline side of pH 7.4.[21,22] There is associated with pHs to the alkaline side of pH 7.4, during cold perfusion, a reduction in vascular resistance and reduced lysosomal enzyme release.[23]

Detailed studies of the application of alpha-stat regulation in humans are few. Prakash et al.[24] maintained 29 hypothermic infants at their normal 35°C ventilation rate throughout open chest operations for cardiac repair. Due to the fall in metabolic rate, this procedure resulted in an increase in air convection requirement, a fall in arterial P_{CO_2}, and a rise in pH. The result was a $\Delta pH/°C$ which closely resembled that of ectothermic animals, or blood held *in vitro*, at constant CO_2 content. While these workers interpreted this circumstance as "respiratory alkalosis," it is clearly an example of alpha-stat regulation and respiratory management of blood at constant CO_2 content. No neurological damage was observed, and it was concluded that there is no need for added CO_2 to inhaled gas to avoid cerebral damage and that the method is safe.

Blayo et al.[25] reported results on 11 hypothermic adults on cardiopulmonary bypass in which the P_{CO_2} of the gas mixture was adjusted downward from 40 torr, such that normal values of pH and P_{CO_2} for arterial blood were obtained when measured at 37°C. When chilled blood returns to normal values at normothermic temperatures it can only indicate that alpha-stat regulation pertained in the hypothermic state. It was found that this procedure resulted in stabilization of [HCO_3^-] and total CO_2 content of arterial and mixed venous blood during both hypothermia and rewarming. No metabolic acidosis was observed under these conditions.

ALPHA-STAT REGULATION AND THE CO_2 DISSOCIATION CURVE

Reference to Figure 5.3 provides guidelines, from an example of alpha-stat regulation by an ectothermic animal, governing the necessary alterations in Pa_{CO_2} to assure the maintenance of constant carbon dioxide content of the blood as temperature is altered. In the case illustrated, the *inverse* relationship between air convection requirement and body temperature assures the *direct* relationship between alveolar and arterial P_{CO_2} which is required for constant CO_2 content of the blood. As previously discussed, this is a necessary condition for alpha-stat regulation and a $\Delta pH/°C \cong -0.015$.

The strategy for such regulation during hypothermic cardiopulmonary bypass procedures would appear quite straightforward when blood of normal composition is used. It is only required during cooling, that the P_{CO_2} of the gas phase be reduced to a level at which the normothermic Pa_{CO_2} and pH values are achieved by a blood gas instrument thermostated at 37°C. This is the procedure utilized in hypothermic man by Blayo et al.[25] However, it is important to realize that the particular P_{CO_2} necessary to achieve this result will vary, depending upon blood compositional influences on the CO_2 dissociation curve. A common compositional change is that introduced by hemodilution.

Carbon dioxide dissociation curves, derived by the Van Slyke manometric technique, are presented in Figure 5.4. These curves are useful in assessing the influence of temperature, hemodilution, and P_{CO_2} on the CO_2 transport properties of the blood. The usual practice of gassing the blood to achieve a Pa_{CO_2} of 40 torr results in the progression of points connected by the vertical line emanating at the P_{CO_2} 40 torr point on the horizontal axis. While at each point, an essentially common pH is attained, it is important to note that both low temperature and hemodilution are associated with increasing CO_2 content at any given P_{CO_2}. If alpha-stat regulation is desired ($\Delta pH/°C \cong -0.015$), the points represented by pH 7.54

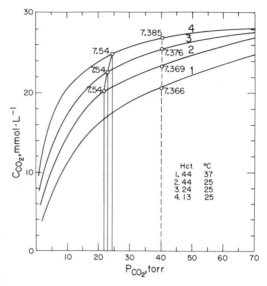

Figure 5.4. Carbon dioxide dissociation curves for oxygenated human blood under normothermic and hypothermic conditions at two levels of hemodilution. Vertical lines indicate P_{CO_2}s and associated pH values. Alpha-stat regulation ($\Delta pH/°C \cong -0.015$) will prevail at the pH 7.54 value. Curves were derived by the Van Slyke manometric technique.

can be achieved at the arterial P_{CO_2}s indicated on the graph. In contrasting the differences which emerge from constant pH and alpha-stat regulation, it is apparent that total CO_2 content of blood is more closely conserved under alpha-stat control. Furthermore, the slope of the dissociation curve is higher at the more alkaline pH point. The instantaneous slope of the CO_2 dissociation curve is equivalent to the capacitance coefficient, β (mmole $\cdot$ liter$^{-1} \cdot$ torr^{-1}) and, as we will see below, β is an important determinant of venous-arterial partial pressure gradients when CO_2 production is in balance with delivery to the gas phase.

In evaluating the influence of these alternative acid-base schemes, it is useful to view them from the perspective of gas exchange equations deriving from the Fick principle. Symbols used are: M, transfer rate of gas, mmole $\cdot$ min^{-1}; C, concentration of gas, mmole $\cdot$ liter $^{-1}$; P, partial pressure of gas, torr = mm Hg; β, capacitance coefficient. The increment in concentration per incremental in partial pressure, $\Delta C / \Delta P$, mmole $\cdot$ liter^{-1} $\cdot$ torr^{-1}; $\dot{V}_b$, flow rate of blood, liter $\cdot$ min^{-1}; $\dot{V}_b / M$, blood convection requirement, liters $\cdot$ mmole^{-1}; G_{perf}, perfusive conductance: $\dot{V}_b \cdot \beta$, mmole $\cdot$ min^{-1} $\cdot$ torr^{-1}.

The Fick equation, $\dot{M}_{CO_2} = \dot{V}_b \cdot (C_{\bar{v}} - C_a)_{CO_2}$, allows the calculation of venous and arterial content difference when the other variables are known. Knowledge of $(C_a)_{CO_2}$ is known from the CO_2 dissociation curve when Pa_{CO_2} is specified (Fig. 5.4) and $(C_{\bar{v}})_{CO_2}$ can be easily calculated.

We can usefully alter the form of the Fick equation:[26] $\dot{M}_{CO_2} = \dot{V}_b \cdot \beta \cdot (P_{\bar{v}} - P_a)_{CO_2}$. This allows calculation of the partial pressure difference between venous and arterial blood. β derived from the CO_2 dissociation curve at any stated $P_{CO_2} \cdot (\dot{V}_b \cdot \beta)$ has the meaning of perfusive conductance, G_{perf}. Here the *slope* of the CO_2 dissociation curve at any specified point is seen as equipotent with $\dot{V}_b$ as a determinant of gas exchange.

Table 5.1 presents calculations which emphasize the qualitative differences which are expected in consequence of constant pH or alpha-stat regulation of the arterial blood. Data for a 59-kg normothermic man[27] are used to derive metabolic data at 25°C and are based on the assumptions: $\dot{V}_b / \dot{M}_{CO_2}$ and RQ are constants; metabolic production of CO_2 is matched by delivery to the gas ex-

changer; and, there is a twofold alteration in metabolism per 10°C, i.e., $Q_{10} = 2$. The calculations apply to blood at 25°C, Hct 23 (Fig. 5.4), and reveal several important contrasts between constant pH and alpha-stat regulation. Because of the alteration in the CO_2 dissociation curve due to hemodilution and low temperature, maintenance of a Pa_{CO_2} of 40 torr imposes a rather large increment in total CO_2, whereas in alpha-stat management the incremental is modest. This is reflected in elevation of $C_{\bar{v}CO_2}$ to 27 mmole $\cdot$ L^{-1}, a value which must reflect the equilibrium between interstitial fluid and venous blood. From the $[HCO_3^-] - pH$ curve (Fig. 5.5), a venous pH of around 7.3 prevails. It must be concluded that maintenance of Pa_{CO_2} at 40 torr during hypothermia may lead to respiratory acidosis and that total body CO_2 stores are apt to be significantly elevated under these conditions. Table 5.2 makes the point that the capacitance coefficient, being of a low value at Pa_{CO_2} 40 torr, imposes a requirement for a large venous-arterial partial pressure gradient (20 torr), a circumstance where $P_{\bar{v}CO_2}$ must be massively elevated in order to maintain a flux of CO_2 equivalent to production rate. By contrast, alpha-stat regulation is characterized by large G_{perf} owing to high β. Consequently, the venous-arterial partial pressure gradient (7.3 torr) resembles healthy normothermic man. These calcula-

Table 5.1
Alphastat Regulation Contrasted with Constant pH Regulation

°C	RQ	$\dot{V}b/\dot{M}_{O_2}$ (liter $\cdot$ mmole^{-1})	$\dot{M}_{O_2}$ (mmole $\cdot$ min^{-1})	$\dot{M}_{CO_2}$ (mmole $\cdot$ min^{-1})	$\dot{V}b/\dot{M}_{CO_2}$ (liter $\cdot$ mmole^{-1})	$\dot{V}b$ (liter $\cdot$ min^{-1})	Q_{10}	Hct (%)
37	0.8	0.50	11.20	8.96	0.62	5.60	—	44
25	0.8	0.50	5.04	4.03	0.62	2.50	2	23

Constant pH$_a$
25°C, Hct 23, $Pa_{CO_2} = 40$, $pH_a = 7.38$, $Ca_{CO_2} = 25.4$:
$\dot{M}_{CO_2} = \dot{V}_b \cdot (C_{\bar{v}} - C_a)_{CO_2}$; $(C_{\bar{v}} - C_a)_{CO_2} = 1.6$
$(C_{\bar{v}})_{CO_2} = 27^*$; from dissociation curve, $P_{\bar{v}CO_2} \cong 60$ torr
$pH_{\bar{v}} = 7.33$ (calculated from $[HCO_3^-] - pH$ curve)
$\Delta pH/°C = -0.015$
25°C, Hct 23, $Pa_{CO_2} = 22.7$, $pH_a = 7.54$, $Ca_{CO_2} = 22.4$:
$\dot{M}_{CO_2} = \dot{V}_b \cdot (C_{\bar{v}} - C_a)_{CO_2}$; $(C_{\bar{v}} - C_a)_{CO_2} = 1.6$
$(C_{\bar{v}})_{CO_2} = 24^*$; from dissociation curve, $P_{CO_2} \cong 30$ torr
$pH_{\bar{v}} = 7.50$

* Note difference in $(C_{\bar{v}})_{CO_2}$ which reflects excess tissue stores at $pH_a = 7.38$.

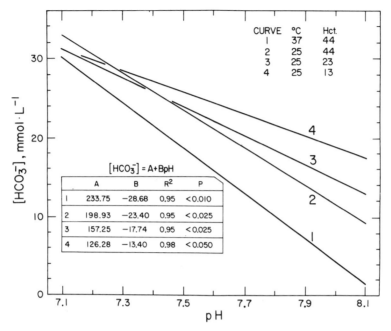

Figure 5.5. Plasma pH-[HCO_3^-] curves as a function of temperature and hemodilution. These data pertain to the CO_2 dissociation curves presented in Figure 5.4.

Table 5.2

Role of Capacitance Coefficient, β, as a Determinant of Arterial-Venous P_{CO_2} Difference

From: $\dot{M}_{CO_2} = \dot{V}_b \cdot (C_{\bar{v}} - C_a)_{CO_2}$ we derive:

$\quad \dot{M}_{CO_2} = \dot{V}_b \cdot \beta \cdot (P_{\bar{v}} - P_a)_{CO_2}$

For Hct 23, 25°C, $Pa_{CO_2} = 40$ torr:

$\quad \beta = 0.08$ mmole $\cdot$ liter$^{-1} \cdot$ torr^{-1}

$\quad \dot{V}_b \cdot \beta = G_{perf} = 0.2$ mmole $\cdot$ min$^{-1} \cdot$ torr^{-1}

$\quad (P_{\bar{v}} - P_a)_{CO_2} = 20$ torr; $P_{\bar{v}CO_2} = 60$ torr

For Hct 23, 25°C, $Pa_{CO_2} = 22.7$ torr

$\quad \beta = 0.22$ mmol $\cdot$ liter$^{-1} \cdot$ torr^{-1}

$\quad \dot{V}_b \cdot \beta = G_{perf} = 0.55$ mmole $\cdot$ min$^{-1} \cdot$ torr^{-1}

$\quad (P_{\bar{v}} - P_a)_{CO_2} = 7.3$ torr; $P_{\bar{v}CO_2} = 30$ torr

tions are meant to illustrate directional trends which suggest that the common practice of regulating P_{CO_2} to achieve an invariant arterial pH is likely to impose respiratory acidosis during hypothermia and that the resultant excess body stores of CO_2 will be manifest, on warming, as a potential acid-base management problem. These risks should be minimized by regulating the CO_2 content of the blood such that $\Delta pH/°C \cong -0.015$ prevails at all temperatures. This can

be achieved by adjusting Pa_{CO_2} at the gas exchanger such that arterial pH is 7.4 when evaluated with electrodes thermostated to 37°C.

Indeed, Blayo et al.[25] report that blood [HCO_3^-] remains at a constant level during hypothermia and postoperatively in man when alpha-stat control is utilized. Alpha-stat regulation also appears to avoid metabolic acidosis and hyperpnea on rewarming.[25] These features, coupled with stabilization of Donnan ratio, improved blood flow and electrical stability of the heart, higher cerebral perfusion and optimization of enzyme activities, suggest that alpha-stat regulation, as exhibited by ecothermic vertebrates, represents a useful alternative to current acid-base practices during hypothermia.

References

1. Rosenthal TB: The effect of temperature on the pH of blood and plasma *in vitro*. J Biol Chem 173:25, 1948.
2. Albery WJ, Lloyd BB: Variation of chemical potential with temperature. In *Development of the Lung*, edited by AVS deReuck and R Porter. London, Churchill, 1967, p. 30.

3. Reeves RB: An imidazole alpha-stat hypothesis for vertebrate acid-base regulation: Tissue carbon dioxide content and body temperature in bullfrogs. Respir Physiol 14:219, 1972.

4. Rahn H: Body temperature and acid-base regulation. Pneumonologie 151:87, 1974.

5. White FN: A comparative physiological approach to hyperthermia. J Thorac Cardiovasc Surg 82:821, 1981.

6. White FN, Somero G: Acid-base regulation and phospholipid adaptations to temperature: Time courses and physiological significance of modifying the milieu for protein function. Physiol Rev 62:40, 1982.

7. Severinghaus JW, Stupfel M, Bradley AF: Variation of serum carbonic acid pK' with pH and temperature. J Appl Physiol 9:197, 1956a.

8. Severinghaus JW, Stupfel M, Bradley AF: Accuracy of blood pH and P_{CO_2} determinations. J Appl Physiol 9:189, 1956b.

9. Jackson DC: Respiratory control in air-breathing ectotherms. In *Regulation of Ventilation and Gas Exchange*, edited by DG Davies and CD Barnes. New York, Academic Press, 1978, p. 93.

10. Kinney JL, Matsuura DT, White FN: Cardiorespiratory effects of temperature in the turtle, *Pseudemys floridana*. Respir Physiol 31:309, 1977.

11. Yancey PH, Somero GN: Temperature dependence of intracellular pH: Its role in the conservation of pyruvate apparent Km values of vertebrate lactate dehydrogenase. J Comp Physiol 125:129, 1978.

12. Rahn H, Reeves RB: *Protons, proteins and Claude Bernard's "Fixite du Milieu Interieur."* Colloque Claude Bernard (Foundation Singer-Polignac), edited by ED Robin. Paris, Masson et Cie, 1980, p. 263.

13. Reeves RB: Temperature-induced changes in blood acid-base status. Donnan R_{cl} and red cell volume. J Appl Physiol 40:762, 1976.

14. Lyman CP, Hastings AB: Total CO_2, plasma pH and pCO_2 of hamsters and ground squirrels during hibernation. Am J Physiol 167:633, 1951.

15. McConnel DH, White FN, Nelson RL, Goldstein SM, Maloney JV, DeLand EC, Buckberg GD: Importance of "alkalosis" in maintainence of ideal blood pH during hypothermia. Surg Forum 26:263, 1975.

16. Becker H, Vinten-Johansen J, Buckberg GD, Robertson JM, Leaf JD, Lazer HL, Manganaro AJ: Myocardial damage caused by keeping pH 7.40 during systemic deep hypothermia. J Thorac Cardiovasc Surg 82:810, 1982.

17. Poole-Wilson PA, Langer GA: Effect of pH on ionic exchange and function in rat and rabbit myocardium. Am J Physiol 229:570, 1975.

18. Poole-Wilson PA, Langer GA: Effects of acidosis on mechanical function and Ca^{2+} exchange in rabbit myocardium. Am J Physiol 236:H525, 1979.

19. Swain JA, White FN, Peters RM, Bickler P, Boyle M, Utley JR: Effect of pH on hypothermic ventricular fibrillation. Samson Thor Surg Soc, 1982.

20. Norwood WI, Norwood CR, Castaneda AR: Cerebral anoxia. Effect of deep hypothermia and pH. Surgery 86:203, 1979.

21. Halasz NA, Collins GM, White FN: The right pH for preservation? *Organ Preservation III*, edited by D Pegg. London, Churchill-Livingstone, 1979, p. 259.

22. Carter JN, White FN, Collins GM, Halasz NA: Studies of the ideal [H⁺] for perfusional preservation. Transplantation 30:409, 1980.

23. Romolo JL, Ariyan S, Halasz NA: Evaluation of perfusion techniques in renal perfusion. Cryobiology 8:407, 1971.

24. Prakash O, Jonson G, Bos E, Simon M, Hugenholtz PG, Hekman W: Cardiorespiratory and metabolic effects of profound hypothermia. Crit Care Med 6:340, 1978.

25. Blayo MC, Lecompte Y, Pocidalo JJ: Control of acid-base status during hypothermia in man. Respir Physiol 42:287, 1980.

26. Piiper J, Scheid P: Comparative physiology of respiration: Functional analysis of gas exchange organs in vertebrates. In *International Review of Physiology: Respiratory Physiology II*, edited by JG Widdicombe, Vol. 14. Baltimore, University Park Press, 1977, p. 219.

27. Dejours P: *Principles of Comparative Respiratory Physiology.* Amsterdam, Elsevier/North-Holland Biomedical Press, 1981, p. 120.

CHAPTER 6

COMPLEMENT ACTIVATION DURING CARDIOPULMONARY BYPASS*

DENNIS E. CHENOWETH, Ph.D., M.D.

Cardiopulmonary bypass is employed tens of thousands of times each year. Even though the procedures that utilize extracorporeal circulation might be expected to have a high incidence of mortality and morbidity, the typical patient tolerates cardiac surgery and cardiopulmonary bypass very well. However, in roughly 3 to 5% of cases, significant alterations that lead to prolonged postoperative recovery are observed. While these situations seem to be sporadic in nature, certain risk factors have been identified. For example, extremely young or elderly patients tend to have an increased risk of postoperative sequellae after open heart surgery. Another risk factor is prolongation of cardiopulmonary bypass. Although problems related to any organ system are encountered postoperatively, the surgeon may recognize a pattern composed of a vague systemic toxicity, increased susceptibility to infection, pulmonary impairment, renal insufficiency, or central nervous system manifestations of a global or focal nature. One of the central issues facing the cardiovascular surgical team today is to define the pathophysiological mechanisms that are re-

sponsible for these varied sequellae. Once the causes of these problems have been delineated, it should be possible to modify either surgical techniques and/or equipment, and thus reduce the risks associated with open heart surgery.

Our attempts to understand the causes of these syndromes have been predicated upon the following hypotheses. First, since these phenomena are unique to open heart surgery, we assumed that components or mechanical properties of the pump oxygenator circuit itself were directly responsible for the observed postoperative sequellae. Second, it seemed likely that the "toxins" or bioactive factors that were being formed in the extracorporeal circuit were derived from plasma precursors that normally circulated in an inactive form. Biological systems that fulfilled these criteria would include the coagulation cascade, the closely related, kinin-generating system, and/or human complement.

We have chosen to focus on the complement system as potentially causative of these syndromes for a number of reasons. Human complement is known to be converted from an inactive to active form in extracorporeal circuits, i.e., those utilized for either hemodialysis for nylon fiber leukapheresis. More importantly, activation of complement results in the formation of potent inflammatory mediators, known as the

* Supported by a grant from the National Institutes of Health administered through the University of Alabama (UAB 81-16). Portions of this work were completed during Dr. Chenoweth's tenure as an Established Investigator of the American Heart Association.

49

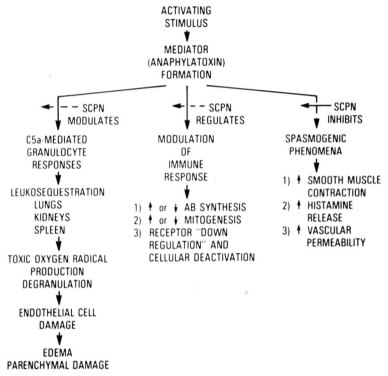

Figure 6.1. Schematic diagram representing the proposed consequences of intravascular complement activation.

anaphylatoxins (Fig. 6.1). These low molecular weight split products possess diverse biological activities that possibly could account for the phenomena observed in patients after cardiopulmonary bypass. For example, these factors potentially could alter vascular permeability or modulate the host's immune responsiveness. Furthermore, one particular anaphylatoxin, C5a, could play an especially significant role as a mediator of postoperative syndromes. Human C5a is known to interact with granulocytes and promote leukosequestration in the microvasculature where these activated cells may induce local tissue injury. Thus, in theory, activation of complement during cardiopulmonary bypass could result in the production of inflammatory mediators whose systemic manifestations might include edema, increased susceptibility to infection, and diffuse tissue damage that is most apparent in very vascular organs, such as the lungs, kidneys, and central nervous system. These

phenomena, which may be predicted from the known biological activities of the anaphylatoxins, so closely resemble the problems encountered with certain open heart surgical patients that it seemed logical to examine the effects of cardiopulmonary bypass on the human complement system. Before describing the results of these studies, it is worthwhile to briefly review what is currently known about the human anaphylatoxins.

COMPLEMENT ACTIVATION: FORMATION OF THE HUMAN ANAPHYLATOXINS

The human complement system is composed of more than 20 plasma proteins that act together in a concerted fashion to promote host defense mechanisms.[1] Conceptually, complement is analogous to the coagulation system, i.e., an initiating stimulus triggers a cascade-like series of regulated enzymatic reactions that terminate in the formation of a macromolecular membrane attack complex which facilitates cell lysis. Functionally, complement is an integral part of the humoral immune system. Current evidence favors the hypothesis that complement serves to bridge the gap between acute and chronic inflammatory events. For example, certain of the cleavage products formed during complement activation, such as the anaphylatoxins, act as acute inflammatory mediators, while other complement split products enhance opsonization or alter lymphocyte and/or macrophage function.

Much as blood clotting may proceed through either intrinsic or extrinsic pathways, complement may be activated by either of two independent mechanisms, termed the classical and alternative pathways. In general, antibody-dependent activation of complement by either immunoglobulins bound to cell surface antigens or by immune complexes proceeds via the classical pathway route. In contrast, "foreign" materials, such as bacterial cell wall determinants or biopolymers found in devices

utilized for extracorporeal circulation, tend to promote activation through alternative pathway mechanisms. As depicted in Figure 6.2, the active enzymes of both the classical and alternative pathways converge to promote enzymatic conversion and activation of the pivotal protein C3. The enzymatically active form of C3 in turn initiates a sequence of events that comprise the final common pathway of complement activation, assembly of the membrane attach complex.

Three different low molecular weight polypeptides or glycopolypeptides known as anaphylatoxins are formed and released into the fluid phase as a result of complement activation (Fig. 6.2). One anaphylatoxin, C4a, is specifically produced when complement is activated only through the classical pathway. The other two anaphylatoxins, C3a and C5a, are cleaved from their respective precursors, C3 and C5, following activation by either classical or alternative pathway mechanisms. Thus, detection of elevated plasma levels of C4a specifically implies classical pathway activation processes, while the appearance of either

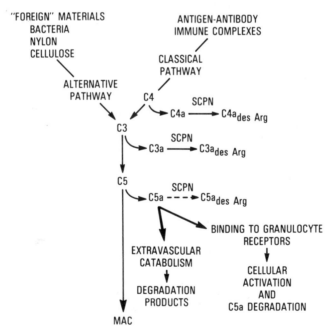

Figure 6.2. Schematic diagram outlining the complement system and emphasis on the formation and catabolism of the human anaphylatoxins C4a, C3a, and C5a.

C3a or C5a in circulation indicates complement activation without defining the responsible pathway.

All three of the human anaphylatoxins are chemically similar.[2-4] The polypeptide chains of each molecule contain 74 to 77 amino acid residues. As a result, the molecular weights of C3a and C4a are about 9,000 daltons. The molecular weight of the polypeptide portion of C5a is 8,300, but this anaphylatoxin has a complex oligosaccharide moiety (MW ca. 3000) attached to the asparigine residue in position 64. Thus, the molecular weight of the human C5a glycopolypeptide is approximately 12,000. All three anaphylatoxins contain 3 intrachain disulfide bonds; thus they are chemically stable and resist denaturation at extremely low pH or elevated temperature. The former property, acid stability, has been exploited in development of radioimmunoassay procedures that permit quantitation of the plasma levels of C3a, C4a and C5a.

BIOLOGICAL ACTIVITIES OF THE ANAPHYLATOXINS

In addition to being chemically similar, human C3a, C4a, and C5a share certain common biological properties.[5] Each of the anaphylatoxins possesses spasmogenic activity, being capable of promoting contraction of guinea pig ileal smooth muscle. Other tissue changes induced by the anaphylatoxins include: vascular (arteriolar) constriction, increased vascular permeability, wheal and erythema formation, and induction of histamine release from mast cells. Quantitative comparisons demonstrate that C5a is a more potent spasmogen than C3a, which is in turn considerably more active than C4a. These observations suggest that the anaphylatoxins may perform as inflammatory mediators, acting to alter vascular permiability and blood flow at localized sites of inflammation.

Human C5a differs from both C3a and C4a in that it has a unique ability to trigger cellular responses in granulocytes, including mast cells,[6] basophils,[7] eosinophils,[8] monocytes,[9] macrophages,[10, 11] and peripheral blood neutrophils.[12-16] The C5a-mediated responses of neutrophils have received the greatest attention and are summarized in Table 6.1. According to current concepts, C5a functions as a potent acute inflammatory mediator by initially causing circulating granulocytes to adhere to the endothelium and then stimulating directed migration (chemotaxis) of these cells, thus promoting their accumulation in inflammatory foci. Once present as exudate cells, the C5a-stimulated granulocyte functions to protect the host by releasing its lysosomal enzymes and producing toxic oxygen species that are injurious to invading organisms. When these processes take place within carefully regulated limits in a delineated locale, they play an invaluable role in host defense. However, if unregulated intravascular formation of C5a occurs, the systemic manifestations of C5a-mediated granulocyte responses may be injurious to the host. For example, it is known that intravenous infusion of C5a produces immediate and profound neutropenia.[15-17] The C5a-activated cells aggregate and disappear from circulation as they become sequesterred in the pulmonary microvasculature. While the activated granulocytes are in contact with the endothelial cell they may either release their lytic enzymes or produce toxic oxygen radicals that induce significant parenchymal damage.[18] Thus,

Table 6.1
Human C5a-Mediated Responses of Granulocytes

Cell movement
  Chemotaxis
  Chemokinesis
Release of lysosomal enzymes (degranulation) from
  Adherent cells
  Cells treated with cytochalasin B
Production of toxic oxygen species
Enhanced arachidonic acid metabolism
Increased adherence and/or autoaggregation
In vivo responses to infused C5a
  Neutropenia
  Vascular leukosequestration in
    Lungs
    Kidneys
    Spleen

there is great interest in the role of C5a as an indirect mediator of pulmonary injury and dysfunction following cardiopulmonary bypass,[19] hemodialysis,[20] or nylon fiber leukapheresis,[21] and during the initial phases of adult respiratory distress syndrome.[22]

Human C5a exerts its leukocyte-related biological activities by binding to specific receptors that are present on the granulocyte plasma membrane. Each human peripheral blood neutrophil has about 200,000 C5a receptors, and each of these has an apparent affinity of approximately 1 nm.[23] In practical terms, these observations imply that C5a is such an extremely potent effector of neutrophil function that significant cellular responses will result when as little as 1% of the available plasma C5 is converted to C5a. Clearly, extracorporeal events that promote even modest complement activation may result in profound neutrophil stimulation by C5a.

Once bound to the neutrophil receptors, C5a is rapidly internalized and degraded to its constituent amino acids which are subsequently released from the intact cell.[24] These events not only trigger cellular responses by as yet undefined mechanisms, but also inactivate both C5a and its target cell as well. In the first case, C5a is inactivated in two steps. Cellular internalization effectively clears the ligand from circulation, and then proteolytic degradation ensures that the active factor will not reappear in blood. In the second case, cellular deactivation results, at least in part, from a phenomenon termed receptor "down regulation." Thus, we observe that neutrophils that have been allowed to internalize C5a have very few residual C5a receptors left on their surface and consequently fail to respond when challenged with a second exposure to the ligand.

CONTROL MECHANISMS

The biological activities and circulating concentrations of the anaphylatoxins are regulated by both enzymatic and physiological mechanisms.

When the anaphylatoxins are formed in human serum or plasma, they are rapidly acted upon by carboxypeptidase N, an enzyme that selectively removes only the carboxyl terminal arginyl residue from each molecule to yield its respective des Arg derivative (Figs. 6.2 and 6.5). These des Arg derivatives possess less than 0.01% of the spasmogenic activity of their parent molecules. Thus, rapid enzymatic inactivation tends to limit the systemic vasoactive effects of C3a, C4a, and C5a. However, the leukocyte-directed activity of C5a is only partially abrogated by this enzymatic control mechanism. Human C5a$_{des\ Arg}$ still retains a considerable ability to promote granulocyte responses, being only 20 to 50-fold less active than C5a.[12]

Because C3a and C4a, as well as their respective des Arg derivatives, are not bound to circulating leukocytes, these molecules appear free in circulation until they equilibrate with the extravascular fluid compartment and/or are excreted intact in the urine.

Human C5a and C5a$_{des\ Arg}$ are catabolized in a somewhat different fashion.[17] Experiments conducted in rabbits have demonstrated that both C5a and C5a$_{des\ Arg}$ are almost completely cleared from circulation within 5 minutes after intravenous infusion. The extremely rapid clearance of C5a is regulated by at least two factors. First, C5a binds to and is internalized by peripheral blood neutrophils. These C5a activated cells in turn aggregate and/or adhere and become trapped in the microcirculation of the lungs, kidneys, and spleen. A second phenomenon accounts for the clearance of nearly 80% of the C5a injected into rabbits. Specific organs, including the liver, kidneys, muscle, and the skin, bind and actively remove C5a directly from blood. White blood cells are not required for this clearance phenomenon, but instead cellular elements associated with the vascular bed seem to be responsible. Once C5a is bound to either leukocytes or vascular elements within target organs, it is degraded to amino acids or low molecular weight peptides that are excreted in the urine. The net effect of these *in vivo* catabolic events is to limit circulating quantities of C5a to low levels until both leukocyte and extravascular binding sites have become saturated.

RADIOIMMUNOASSAY QUANTITATION OF THE ANAPHYLATOXINS

The ability to detect traces of the complement-derived anaphylatoxins in human plasma provides a precise and extremely sensitive measure of *in vivo* complement activation. As mentioned previously, elevated levels of plasma C4a provide evidence of classical pathway activation events, while increased amounts of either C3a or C5a signify complement activation without defining the pathway involved. Because C4a and C3a, or their des Arg derivatives, do not bind to leukocytes, they tend to remain in circulation for a longer period of time than does the leukocyte-bound C5a molecule. Thus, the appearance of C4a or C3a in circulation affords a more sensitive means of detecting complement activation than the quantitation of plasma C5a levels. Facile detection of C3a, but not C5a, is also favored by the fact that the absolute concentration of the C3a precursor, C3, is 10 to 15 times greater than that of the C5a parent molecule (C5).

All three of the anaphylatoxins may be quantitated in human plasma or other biological fluids by standard radioimmunoassay (RIA) procedures.[25] Specific antibodies directed against unique antigenic determinants on each of the human anaphylatoxins have been elicited in rabbits. Therefore, it is possible to identify and quantitate each of the anaphylatoxins, or their des Arg analogs, even though they exist as a mixture in the clinical sample. The major technical obstacle encountered in the anaphylatoxin RIA procedure is the fact that each of the antibodies utilized cross-reacts with the anaphylatoxin precursor, *i.e.*, anti-C3a cross-reacts with C3. Therefore, special techniques have been developed to denature and remove C3, C4, and C5 from plasma samples prior to performing the RIA quantitation of the corresponding anaphylatoxin.

While complement activation may be detected with classical hemolytic or immuno-logical assays, these types of assays tend to be relatively insensitive when compared to the anaphylatoxin RIA procedures. For example, C3 radial immunodiffusion and nephlometric techniques have a lower limit of detection of about 5% conversion of the molecule. In contrast, the C3a RIA possesses sufficient sensitivity to detect as little as 0.1% conversion of C3. Therefore, the RIA procedures are preferred for detection of low level complement activation in certain clinical settings.

COMPLEMENT ACTIVATION DURING CARDIOPULMONARY BYPASS

To investigate our hypothesis that human complement might be activated during cardiopulmonary bypass procedures, we utilized RIA procedures to quantitate the plasma levels of C3a and C5a in 15 adults undergoing elective saphenous vein coronary artery bypass grafting.[19]

As shown in Figure 6.3, the plasma levels of C3a detected preoperatively (baseline) and following sternotomy and heparinizatin (prebypass) were not different, suggesting that routine surgical procedures and medi-

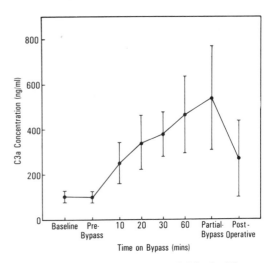

Figure 6.3. Plasma levels of C3a in 15 patients undergoing cardiopulmonary bypass. Levels were unaffected by routine surgical procedures (*Pre-Bypass*) but displayed a time-dependent elevation during bypass.

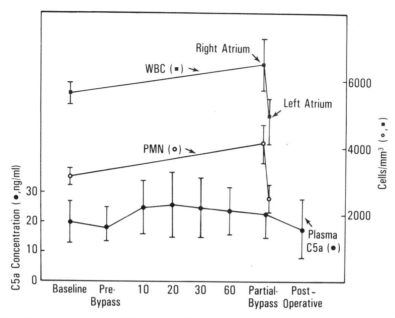

Figure 6.4. Plasma levels of C5a and white blood cell counts in 15 patients undergoing cardiopulmonary bypass. Levels of C5a did not change significantly during bypass. Instead, an increase in white cells (*WBC, solid squares*) due to neutrophilia (*PMN, open circles*) was observed, and when pulmonary circulation was re-established at partial bypass, transpulmonary leukosequestration and neutropenia were demonstrable.

cations did not promote complement activation. In marked contrast, within 10 minutes after institution of bypass with an extracorporeal circuit consisting of a Sarns roller pump, a Bentley BOS-10 bubble oxygenator, and Swank cardiotomy filters, the plasma C3a levels were significantly elevated. Continued activation of complement in the extracorporeal circuit was demonstrated by the fact that plasma C3a levels continued to increase in a time-dependent fashion throughout the duration of bypass. In fact, statistical analysis demonstrated that the plasma level of the C3a split product was directly dependent on the duration of cardiopulmonary bypass. These observations provided confirmation of our original hypotheses. We could clearly demonstrate activation of the human complement system during open heart surgery. Furthermore, the extracorporeal circuit appeared to be primarily responsible for these events.

When we evaluated the plasma C5a levels in this same group of patients, no significant changes from preoperative values were noted (Fig. 6.4). If complement was being activated during bypass, why couldn't we observe an increase in the C5a levels that paralleled the appearance of free C3a? The explanation for this apparent discrepancy was that C5a was being bound to granulocytes and catabolized more rapidly than was C3a. Activation of granulocytes by the C5a produced during cardiopulmonary bypass was demonstrated by comparing the white blood cell counts proximal and distal to the pulmonary circulation at termination of bypass, *i.e.*, at a time when the pulmonary vascular bed is effectively returned to circulation (Table 6.2). We observed a significant ($p = 0.0002$) trapping of neutrophils in the pulmonary circulation at this time. These findings not only suggested that C5a was indeed produced during cardiopulmonary bypass but provided direct evidence of vascular trapping of the activated granulocyte at completion of the surgical procedure.

Because certain components of the extra-

Table 6.2
White Blood Cell Counts Proximal and Distal to the Pulmonary Circulation at Termination of Cardiopulmonary Bypass

Cell Type	Right Atrium at Partial Bypass*	Left Atrium at Partial Bypass*	Difference†	p Value‡
Total white cells	6500 ± 760	4800 ± 680	−1700 ± 710	0.03
Segmented neutrophils	4200 ± 530	2500 ± 410	−1700 ± 330	0.0002
Lymphocytes	1900 ± 240	2000 ± 310	100 ± 340	0.8
Monocytes	120 ± 32	54 ± 18	−66 ± 39	0.11
Eosinophils	54 ± 18	49 ± 12	−5 ± 21	0.8
Basophils	11 ± 6	14 ± 12	3 ± 14	0.8
Band neutrophils	230 ± 47	200 ± 38	−30 ± 55	0.6

* Mean ± SEM.
† Left atrium at partial bypass − right atrium at partial bypass.
‡ Determined from paired t-test with data from 15 operations.

corporeal circuit so clearly seemed to cause complement activation, we were interested in attempting to identify the possible sources of anaphylatoxin production. One suggestion was that all oxygenators possessed some type of oxygen-blood interface, and therefore, the complement-related effects of vigorous oxygenation of blood ought to be explored. When we evaluated this possibility in vitro, a small but measurable time-dependent increase in plasma C3a levels was produced by vigorous oxygenation of whole blood. Therefore, the requisite blood-gas interface of bubble oxygenators could by itself be partially responsible for the complement activation we observed. However, an alternative source of anaphylatoxin formation was also found in the extracorporeal circuit, and it seems likely to play a much greater role in activating complement than does simply oxygenating blood.

Other investigators had shown that nylon fiber leukapheresis devices produced significant complement activation when employed in clinical settings.[21] When we found that a nylon tricot mesh linear was employed to defoam the oxygenated blood in bubble oxygenators, we immediately suspected that this biomaterial might be one of the potential sources of complement activation. This hypothesis was dramatically confirmed by in vitro experimentation (Fig. 6.5). Incubation of either heparinized whole blood or serum with nylon produced immediate formation of C3a which continued for the next 60 minutes. After this time, the plasma levels of C3a had risen to 8 μg/ml or nearly 80 times baseline levels. Comparisons of oxygen- and nylon-mediated complement conversion indicated that nylon was capable of producing 15 to 20 times more C3a than the oxygenation procedure. Therefore, we feel that biopolymers, such as nylon, probably play a major role in facilitating formation of the complement-derived inflammatory mediators during cardiopulmonary bypass.

PRELIMINARY OBSERVATIONS AND SPECULATIONS

Our clinical and experimental observations to date demonstrate the validity of our original hypotheses. Complement activation during cardiopulmonary bypass seems to be a universal phenomenon observed in all of the patients that we have examined so far. The activation phenomenon is promoted by components of the extracorporeal circuit and is observed with both bubble and membrane type oxygenators.[26] Formation of the anaphylatoxins, especially C5a, can promote significant physiological perturbations, such as pulmonary vascular leukosequestration. Are any of these observations important to cardiovascular surgeons or their colleagues who are involved with pa-

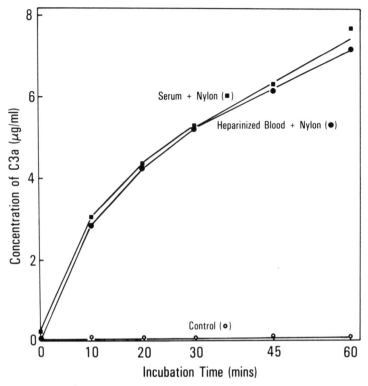

Figure 6.5. Human C3a in serum (*solid squares*) or in heparinized whole blood (*solid circles*) when incubated with a nylon tricot mesh liner from a bubble-type oxgenator. Control samples of serum or whole blood (*open circles*) were incubated in the absence of nylon, and these samples showed no C3a formation.

tient care during open heart procedures? We don't know yet. Presently, we can only speculate about their significance. Therefore, I would like to outline briefly some of our current areas of investigation, whose major objectives are to provide a better understanding of the clinical significance of our initial observations.

First, we would like to know if the amount of complement activation that occurs during bypass may be related directly to the eventual development of postoperative complications. To answer this question, we determined the intraoperative plasma levels of C3a in 140 consecutive patients undergoing all types of open heart surgery at the University of Alabama, Birmingham. The values obtained are currently being correlated with intraoperative, postoperative, and clinical parameters in an attempt to determine if we can identify a link between comple-

ment activation and unusual postoperative sequellae of cardiopulmonary bypass. Because it is extremely difficult to define clearly cause and effect relationships in such a complex clinical setting and the computer-assisted data analysis represents such a massive undertaking, it may be some time yet before we can provide definitive answers to these important questions.

A second area of interest seems more amenable to investigation. We have reasoned that since the complement activation processes consist of a series of temperature-dependent enzymatic reactions, hypothermic conditions should retard anaphylatoxin formation. Preliminary studies tend to confirm this hypothesis. We have observed that the rate of formation of C3a is slowed during the hypothermic phase of cardiopulmonary bypass. These findings imply that the clinically apparent benefits of hypothermia may in part be related to the fact that complement activation is significantly slowed during this phase of the operative procedure. On the other hand, the rate of C3a production appears to be significantly enhanced during the rewarming phase of bypass. Thus, as might be predicted from biochemical principles, what is gained by lowering the body temperature is in turn partially lost during the essential return to normothermia. Clearly, we need to compare complement activation phenomena in groups of patients undergoing hypothermic and normothermic bypass procedures to determine if the beneficial effects of hypothermia are indeed related to limitation of inflammatory mediator formation.

Another interesting area of investigation has been suggested and should be explored. Many surgeons feel that open heart patients have a greater susceptibility to postoperative infection than other types of surgical patients. Could this observation be explained by our findings? We don't know yet, but certain facts suggest that complement activation during cardiopulmonary bypass could predispose the open heart patient to infection. First, we know that exposure of granulocytes to C5a not only transiently activates these cells, but subsequently "deactivates" them, i.e., they fail to respond when challenged with a second exposure to the ligand. Thus one possible explanation for the observation that neutrophils isolated from the blood of patients after open heart surgery display impaired chemotactic responsiveness[27] is that the cells have been exposed to C5a in vivo and are effectively "deactivated." Second, in vitro studies have demonstrated that both C3a and C5a may alter macrophage and/or lymphocyte responses. Additional complement split products also may play a role in regulating the immune response or modulating phagocytosis. Clearly, the complex interplay that exists between these varied complement-derived mediators of granulocyte and immune function needs to be more completely defined in vivo, but it isn't unreasonable to suspect that these factors could account, at least in part, for the relative susceptibility to infection in open heart patients.

Less speculation is required to answer another question that has been posed. Other investigations had previously shown that heparin-protamine sulfate complexes promote in vitro activation of complement by classical pathway mechanisms.[28] Could the same phenomena be demonstrated in open heart patients after completion of bypass? To investigate this possibility, we determined the plasma levels of C4a (a classicial pathway marker), C3a, and C5a in open heart patients prior to and at 5-minute intervals after neutralization of heparin with protamine sulfate. Our findings clearly demonstrated that administration of protamine sulfate produced an immediate and prolonged (30 to 35 minutes) generation of C4a, C3a, and C5a. We have concluded that heparin-protamine sulfate complexes activate the classical pathway of complement in vivo as well as in vitro. Additionally, we now appreciate that postoperative intervention can trigger a second wave of complement activation. Obviously, the clinical consequences of these events and their potential relationship to problems encountered after protamine sulfate administration remain to be defined. However, this specific phenomenon might prove to be a fruitful area for future investigations.

Finally, we are especially interested in applying basic biomedical research to clinical problems. I feel that we now have an excellent opportunity to do just that. Our studies to date clearly suggest that the anaphylatoxin RIA methods may be directly applied to assess the complement-activating potential of both cardiopulmonary bypass devices and biomaterials employed in their manufacturer. We have already shown that nylon acts as a source of complement activation. Therefore, we anticipate that it will be possible to screen alternative biomaterials and identify a suitable substitute for nylon that can be used to promote oxygenators and filters with a much lower propensity to activate complement. Realistic application of this approach should permit redesign of extracorporeal circuit components with greatly reduced complement-activating potential. If complement-derived mediators provoke significant systemic or organ dysfunction, these design changes may play an important role in reducing the mortality and morbidity of open heart surgery.

In conclusion, we now know that complement-derived inflammatory mediators are formed in the extracorporeal circuit during cardiopulmonary bypass. These bioactive polypeptides may induce systemic changes in the open heart patient when they are returned to circulation. One particular mediator, C5a, plays an important role in promoting granulocyte adherence and sequestration in the microvasculature. These C5a-activated cells in turn may initiate parenchymal injury. While this much is known, we must still define the clinical relevance of these phenomena. However, it seems reasonable to assume that reducing complement activation during cardiopulmonary bypass could limit some of the diffuse tissue injury that is clinically manifest in about 3 to 5% of open heart surgery patients. If this concept proves to be true, we can directly apply our knowledge of biochemical and immunological phenomena to provide improved patient care following these commonly performed surgical procedures.

Acknowledgment. These studies would not have been possible without the close scientific and personal cooperation of the members of the Department of Surgery at the University of Alabama, Birmingham: Eugene Blackstone, Robert Stewart, Steven Westaby, and John Kirklin. Collaborators in La Jolla included: Tony Hugli, Steven Cooper, and Carol Soderberg.

References

1. Müller-Eberhard HJ: Complement. Annu Rev Biochem 44:697, 1975.
2. Fernandez HN, Hugli TE: Primary structural analysis of the polypeptide portion of human C5a anaphylatoxin. Polypeptide sequence determination and assignment of the oligosaccharide attachment site in C5a. J Biol Chem 253:6955, 1978.
3. Hugli TE: Human anaphylatoxin (C3a) from the third component of complement. J Biol Chem 250:8293, 1975.
4. Moon KE, Gorski JP, Hugli TE: Complete primary structure of human C4a anaphylatoxin. J Biol Chem 256:8685, 1981.
5. Hugli TE, Müller-Eberhard HJ: Anaphylatoxins: C3a and C5a. Adv Immunol 26:1, 1978.
6. Johnson AR, Hugli TE, Müller-Eberhard HJ: Release of histamine from rat mast cells by the complement peptides C3a and C5a. Immunology 28:1067, 1975.
7. Grant JA, Dupree E, Goldman AS, Schultz DR, Jackson AL: Complement-mediated release of histamine from human leukocytes. J Immunol 114:1101, 1975.
8. Kay AB, Shin HS, Austen KF: Selective attraction of eosinophil chemotactic factor of anaphylaxis (ECF-A) and a fragment cleaved from the fifth component of complement (C5a). Immunology 24:969, 1973.
9. Nelson RD, Quie PG, Simmons RL: Chemotaxis under agarose: A new and simple method for measuring chemotaxis and spontaneous migration of human polymorphonuclear leukocytes and monocytes. J Immunol 115:1650, 1975.
10. Synderman, R., Shin HS, Hausman MS: A chemotactic factor for mononuclear leukocytes. Proc Soc Exp Biol Med 138:387, 1971.
11. Synderman R, Pike MC, McCarley D, Lang L: Quantification of mouse macrophage chemotaxis *in vitro*: Role of C5 for the production of chemotactic activity. Infect Immun 11:488, 1975.
12. Chenoweth DE, Hugli TE: Human C5a and C5a analogs as probes of the neutrophil C5a receptor. Mol Immunol 17:151, 1980.
13. Webster RO, Hong SR, Johnston RB, Jr, Henson PM: Biological effects of the human complement fragments C5a and C5a$_{des\ Arg}$ on neutrophil function. Immunopharmacology 2:201, 1980.
14. Craddock PR, Hammerschmidt D, White JG, Dalmasso AP, Jacob HS: Complement (C5a)-induced granulocyte aggregation *in vitro*. A possible mechanism of complement-mediated leukostasis and leukopenia. J Clin Invest 60:260, 1977.
15. O'Flaherty J, Showell HJ, Ward PA: Neutropenia induced by systemic infusion of chemotactic factors. J Immunol 118:1586, 1977.
16. Goetzl EJ, Derian CK, Owens CJ, Valone FH: Modulation of the PMN leukocyte component of hypersensitivity reactions by lipoxygenase products of arachadonic acid. In *Advances in Immunopharmacology*, edited by J Hadden, L Chedid, P Mullen and F Spreafico. New York, Pergamon Press, 1981, pp. 343–351.
17. Chenoweth DE, Nitsche JF, Curd JG: Catabolism of human C5a in the rabbit. I. Roles of neutrophils and extravascular sites. J Immunol, in press, 1983.
18. Sacks T, Moldow CF, Craddock PR, Bowers TK, Jacob HS: Oxygen radicals mediate endothelial cell damage by complement-stimulated granulocytes. An *in vitro* model of immune vascular damage. J Clin Invest 61:1161, 1978.
19. Chenoweth DE, Cooper SW, Hugli TE, Stewart RW, Blackstone EH, Kirklin JW: Complement activation during cardiopulmonary bypass. Evidence for generation of C3a and C5a anaphylatoxins. N Engl J Med 304:497, 1981.
20. Craddock PR, Fehr J, Brigham KL, Kronenberg RS, Jacob HS: Complement and leukocyte-mediated

pulmonary dysfunction in hemodialysis. N Engl J Med 296:769, 1977.

21. Hammerschmidt DE, Craddock PR, McCullough J, Kronenberg RS, Dalmasso AP, Jacob HS: Complement activation and pulmonary leukostasis during nylon fiber filtration leukapheresis. Blood 51:721, 1978.

22. Hammerschmidt DE, Weaver LJ, Hudson LD, Craddock PR, Jacob HS: Association of complement activation and elevated plasma C5a with adult respiratory distress syndrome. Lancet I:947, 1980.

23. Chenoweth DE, Hugli TE: Demonstration of specific C5a receptor on intact human polymorphonuclear leukocytes. Proc Natl Acad Sci USA 75:3943, 1978.

24. Chenoweth DE, Hugli TE: Binding internalization and degradation of human C5a by human neutrophils. Fed Proc 39:1049, 1980.

25. Hugli TE, Chenoweth DE: Biologically active peptides of complement: Techniques and significance of C3a and C5a measurements. In *Future Perspectives in Clinical Laboratory Immunoassays*, edited by RM Nakamura, WR Dito, and ES Tucker III. New York, Alan R Liss, 1981, pp. 443–460.

26. Hammerschmidt DE, Stroncek DF, Bowers TK, Lammi-Keefe CJ, Kurth DM, Ozalins A, Nicoloff DM, Lillehei RC, Craddock PR, Jacob HS: Complement activation and neutropenia occurring during cardiopulmonary bypass. J Thorac Cardiovasc Surg 81:370, 1981.

27. Mayer JE, McCullough J, Weiblen BJ, Kaplan EL, Lindsay WG, Nicoloff DM: Effects of cardiopulmonary bypass on neutrophil chemotaxis. Surg Forum 27:285, 1976.

28. Rent R, Ertel N, Eisenstein R, Gewurz H: Complement activation by interactions of polyanious and polycations: Heparin-protamine induced consumption of complement. J Immunol 114:120, 1975.

CHAPTER 7

CARDIOPULMONARY BYPASS IN NONCARDIAC DISEASE

JULIE A. SWAIN, M.D.

Cardiopulmonary bypass is becoming more commonly used in hospitals because of the increasing number of cardiac surgery operations. Because of this increased familiarity, the use of cardiopulmonary bypass has been extended to other disease states where temporary circulatory support or extracorporeal oxygenation is needed. This chapter will summarize the indications for use, technical considerations, and specific applications of cardiopulmonary bypass for noncardiac conditions.

Cardiopulmonary bypass has four main areas of use: (1) when circulatory arrest and deep hypothermia is needed for a dry field, such as during vascular and neurosurgery; (2) for oxygenation in tracheal or pulmonary surgery, or for temporary oxygenation during acute respiratory insufficiency; (3) for circulatory support while specific medical conditions are being treated, such as hypothermia and drug overdose; and (4) for blood filtration and extracorporeal treatment of blood.

The concept of "suspended animation" has intrigued people for years. In 1953, with the first use of cardiopulmonary bypass by Gibbon,[1] the possibility of suspending the circulation became a reality. In the late 1950s, as bypass was more frequently used for cardiac surgery, Drs. Seely and Woodall at Duke combined cardiopulmonary bypass with neurosurgical procedures.[2] This was followed in 1961 by Woods' use of bypass for oxygenation during a resection of a re-

current tracheal cylindroma.[3] Since that time, an increasing number of surgeons have elected to employ cardiopulmonary bypass as an adjunct to other surgical procedures and as a treatment of various medical conditions.

BYPASS CIRCUITS

There are several options available for bypass circuitry; venoarterial bypass, venovenous bypass, arteriovenous bypass, and a mixture of these. Unlike cardiac surgery where the venoarterial route is used exclusively, other circuits may be more advantageous. One may design the extracorporeal circuit after considering concurrent operations, specific physiologic factors requiring altered blood flow, and other special situations.

With venoarterial perfusion, blood is drained from the venous system to the oxygenator and returned to the arterial system. The inferior and superior vena cava commonly are drained and blood returned to the aorta or femoral artery. Another variation of venoarterial perfusion includes femoral vein drainage and axillary artery return. The advantages of this type of perfusion are that it decompresses the pulmonary artery, right and left ventricular work are decreased, circulatory support is provided, and if the arterial return is to the aorta or axillary artery, there is increased cerebral oxygen delivery.

The disadvantage of venoarterial perfusion is that if a peripheral artery, such as the femoral artery, is cannulated there can be an uneven distribution of oxygenated blood through the upper and lower half of the body, which would inhibit oxygen delivery and warming and cooling of the upper half of the body. Other disadvantages include the occurrence of systemic emboli because of the return of blood to the arterial circulation, and cannulation of the arterial side of the circulation is technically more complex than venous cannulation.

Venovenous perfusion utilizes drainage from the inferior vena cava or femoral vein with oxygenator return to the jugular vein. The advantages of this form of perfusion are that: (1) there is a physiological distribution of oxygenated blood because blood is pumped in the normal distribution from the left ventricle; (2) the mixed venous blood is preoxygenated before presentation to the lungs so that if there is an increased shunt fraction (ventilation-perfusion imbalance), the effect of this is lessened, therefore increasing systemic oxygen tension; (3) the lungs trap all particulate matter, and there is no possibility for systemic emboli. The disadvantages of this perfusion system are that no circulatory support is provided, there is no pulmonary artery decompression, left or right ventricular failure may be aggravated, and generally lower flows are obtainable.

Arteriovenous perfusion is less commonly used. In the past it has been utilized for respiratory support of neonates. The advantages are that high flows are obtainable, there is a physiological distribution of oxygenated blood because of passage from the left ventricle to the aorta, the lungs trap emboli, and as with venovenous perfusion, there is an increased mixed venous oxygen tension and a lessening of the effect of high shunt fractions on systemic oxygenation. The disadvantage of this route of perfusion is that it does not provide circulatory support, there is no pulmonary artery decompression, and because of the large arterial to venous shunt, there is increased right and left ventricular work.

Several complex perfusion circuits have been designed to employ venoarterial and venovenous perfusion. By varying the ratio of blood being pumped back to the superior vena cava *vs.* blood returned to the femoral artery, the pulmonary arterial circulation can be decompressed while circulatory support is being maintained during partial cardiopulmonary bypass.

PERIPHERAL CANNULATION

Median sternotomy or thoracotomy for cardiopulmonary bypass cannulation during heart surgery is standard procedure. However, when bypass is being instituted for noncardiac and nonthoracic conditions, avoiding a median sternotomy or thoracotomy is advantageous. In the past it had been thought that cannulation of the heart directly was necessary for adequate venous drainage and the prevention of overdistension of the heart. Left ventricular venting and prevention of overdistension of the left ventricle and left atrium is essential during cardiopulmonary bypass, especially when the heart becomes ineffective due to hypothermia or fibrillation. In early experiments utilizing peripheral cannulation of the femoral artery and vein, death occurred from pulmonary edema. In 1959, Woodall et al.[2] were among the first to perform hypothermic bypass successfully without thoracotomy. This was in conjunction with a neurological procedure for the excision of a brain tumor. In 1962, the experimental basis for the safe performance of bypass was provided by Patterson and Ray,[4] who showed that with jugular and femoral vein cannulation for venous drainage and return to the femoral artery, the heart could be adequately decompressed, thus demonstrating that by maintaining a low CVP with excellent venous drainage, the left heart could be decompressed (Fig. 7.1). It was theorized that venous suction would keep the pulmonary valve incompetent, thereby decompressing the pulmonary artery and preventing left atrial distension. This was confirmed experimentally, showing an excellent correlation between low CVP and low left atrial pressure. In the 20 years since Patterson's experiments, several other

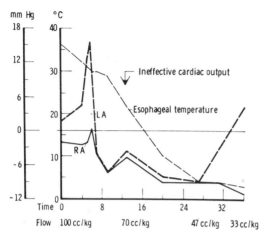

Figure 7.1. A demonstration that the left atrium can be decompressed by peripheral cannulation if the right atrial pressure remains low. (Reproduced with permission from R. H. Patterson and B. S. Ray.[4])

measures have been shown to be important for decompressing the left atrium. The central venous pressure must be kept low when the heart becomes ineffective, and gradual cooling should be performed to delay ventricular fibrillation as long as possible. Early defibrillation should be performed during warming to restore effective contraction of the heart, and careful attention should be paid to the acid-base status of the hypothermic patient. This last point is assuming increasing importance because of the work of McConnell *et al.*,[5] which demonstrated that the widely used pH scheme of keeping the pH 7.4 at all temperatures may not be optimum for the hypothermic patient. Our laboratory has recently shown that the electrical stability of the heart can be increased markedly by allowing the pH to vary with the temperature of the patient.

NEUROSURGERY

The most exciting use of cardiopulmonary bypass as an adjunct to other surgical procedures has occurred in the field of neurosurgery. Hypothermic cardiopulmonary bypass with circulatory arrest has been used during surgery for the correction of arteriovenous malformations, cerebral tumors, and

giant cerebral aneurysms, which account for 3 to 5% of all intracranial aneurysms.[2,4,6–12] Prior to utilizing bypass and circulatory arrest, many of these aneurysms were felt to be unresectable, and when resection was attempted the mortality was 30 to 50%.

By utilizing cardiopulmonary bypass, deep hypothermia, and circulatory arrest, the aneurysm can be decompressed and the neck exposed, which allows for a clear assessment of anatomy. With the neck of the aneurysm exposed, clipping or aneurysmorrhaphy can be accomplished. In 1959, Woodall et al.[2] demonstrated that circulatory arrest could be used for resection of intracranial aneurysms, and in 1963, Uihlein et al.[10] reported 15 patients at Mayo Clinic undergoing circulatory arrest and neurosurgical procedures with generally good results. However, in 1963 Drake et al.[8] presented 10 patients with poor results because of complications of the hypothermic bypass method. Because of this, the interest in combining cardiopulmonary bypass and neurosurgical procedures waned. The method was largely abandoned because of blood clotting abnormalities, temperature drift, and local problems occurring because surface hypothermia was used which entailed packing the patients in ice, which was a very time-consuming and technically complex method. Also, median sternotomy was still being performed by most surgeons for cannulation for bypass. For all of these reasons, the technique came into disuse. The modern era of use began in 1971, when Sundt et al.[9] at the Mayo Clinic had success with this technique using modern bypass methods. The largest series currently is by Silverberg et al.,[7] who has reported nine patients with excellent results using peripheral cannulation and core cooling (Fig. 7.2). Several technical points are important when utilizing bypass for neurosurgical procedures. It is important to measure brain temperature, because there can be a 10°C difference between esophageal core temperature and brain temperature (Fig. 7.3). Either a direct brain temperature probe or a tympanic membrane probe is necessary. At a brain temperature of 10°C, oxygen consumption is only 6% of normal, which

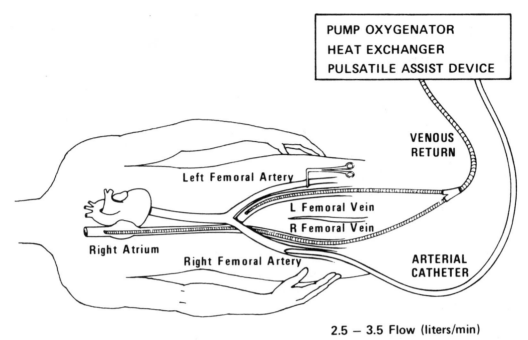

2.5 – 3.5 Flow (liters/min)

Figure 7.2. A method of venoarterial perfusion that provides excellent left and right heart decompression. (Reproduced with permission from G. D. Silverberg et al.[7])

would theoretically permit 60 to 80 minutes of circulatory arrest at 10°C. However, previous work has shown that at 40 minutes of 10°C circulatory arrest the oxygen tension is zero in cerebrospinal fluid.[13] This would indicate that the arrest should be limited to 20 or 30 minutes, with reperfusion in between if additional circulatory arrest time is necessary. The cannulation technique is important with neurosurgical procedures. Jugular cannulation should be avoided because, in addition to crowding the operative field, intracranial pressure is increased when the jugular vein is obstructed, which leads to increased bleeding and cerebral edema. During circulatory arrest the blood can be drained back into the oxygenator which decompresses the cerebral circulation and stops intracranial bleeding. Absolute hemostasis is necessary for the neurosurgical procedure, and coagulation defects should be aggressively corrected at the completion of bypass.

VASCULAR SURGERY

Circulatory arrest can be very valuable as an adjunct to the surgical correction of com-plex vascular lesions. Griffin et al.[14] first reported the use of hypothermic cardiopulmonary bypass and circulatory arrest in the treatment of a traumatic renal arteriovenous fistula. Other uses have included operations on traumatic vertebral artery aneurysms, traumatic iliac artery arteriovenous fistulas, and resection of complex facial arteriovenous malformations.[15-20] The indications for bypass in vascular surgery include large fistulas where standard operative procedures are dangerous or impossible because of distended vessels in the area, such as occurs with chronic arteriovenous fistulas.

TRACHEAL SURGERY

There are occasional rare complex tracheal tumors that are unresectable by conventional means because of the inability to provide oxygenation during the resection. In 1961, Woods et al.[3] resected a recurrent tracheal cylindroma of the carina. Multiple other surgical teams have reported use of cardiopulmonary bypass to provide oxygenation during tracheal surgery for tumor, stenosis, or disruption.[21-24] Bypass has generally been used only as an emergency procedure when imminent hypoxic arrest had led to rapid cardiopulmonary deterioration. By instituting bypass the situation could be stabilized and the resection completed. It is to be emphasized that these are extremely rare lesions, and routine use of bypass is not indicated. In 1965, Neville et al.[22] performed cardiopulmonary bypass as an adjunct to elective pulmonary resections in 11 patients. The operative mortality was 73% in this series and represents a questionable use of this method. In the future, high frequency ventilation may prove to be feasible, which will decrease the indications for bypass for oxygenation.

PULMONARY LAVAGE

Alveolar proteinosis is a disease which produces an accumulation of proteinaceous material in the alveoli with subsequent hy-poxia and suffocation. Whole lung pulmonary lavage, which involves placing a double-lumen endotracheal tube and ventilating one lung while saline lavage is accomplished repeatedly in the other lung, has been found to be a satisfactory treatment for this condition. Because of the small size of the trachea of children, adequate double-lumen endotracheal tubes are not available and lavage cannot be performed by the standard method.[25] Seard et al.[26] first successfully performed pulmonary lavage in two children utilizing cardiopulmonary bypass for oxygenation. This technique has also been used in adults whose pulmonary status was so precarious that ventilation of one lung was not adequate to sustain oxygenation.[27–29] By instituting bypass to provide oxygenation, pulmonary lavage can be accomplished in these extremely sick patients. Because there is transient worsening

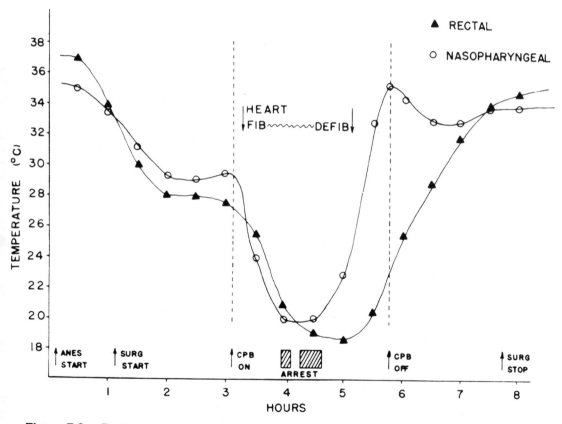

Figure 7.3. Brain temperature may not be proportional to rectal temperature. For maximum cerebral protection, an accurate brain temperature must be obtained. (Reproduced with permission from G. D. Silverberg et al.[12])

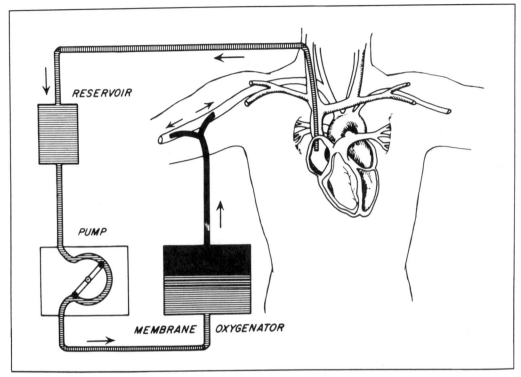

Figure 7.4. By cannulating the axillary artery for arterial return, increased arterial blood saturation can be provided for perfusion of the cerebral vessels (Reproduced with permission from M. D. Altose *et al.*[29] Copyright 1976, American Medical Association.)

of hypoxia after pulmonary lavage due to the increased shunt fraction, the patient often requires extracorporeal oxygenation during and for a short time after the lavage.

In the two children reported by Seard et al.,[26] severe hypoxemia occurred during the lavage with PO_2 levels of 25 to 30 mm Hg on bypass.[26] Because they were children and were acclimated to chronic hypoxemia, there were no untoward results. However, a PO_2 this low in adults would produce severe cerebral hypoxia. During femoral artery perfusion, with low flows during partial bypass, very little change in radial artery oxygen saturation can be detected.[29] For this reason, other bypass techniques may be more appropriate during pulmonary lavage. Venoarterial perfusion can be performed with axillary artery cannulation (Fig. 7.4). This allows highly saturated arterial blood to be delivered to the arch vessels with increased upper body oxygenation.

When the circulatory status permits, venovenous bypass is advantageous because it provides increased mixed venous oxygenation, which decreases the significance of the pulmonary shunt by preoxygenating the pulmonary blood. However, many of these patients may have pulmonary hypertension and incipient right ventricular failure which would preclude the use of this technique.

OXYGENATION

In the late 1960s and early 1970s it was postulated that long-term extracorporeal membrane oxygenation (ECMO) might be useful in treating the respiratory distress syndrome. It was postulated that by sustaining oxygenation, the disease process in the lungs could be allowed to heal with subsequent return of lung function. A multicenter trial was accomplished wherein 233 cases from 90 teams were reported.[30] Significant questions were raised about the reversibility of the lung disease in many of the patients. Because of these poor results, the use of ECMO for respiratory failure was largely abandoned. The advantages of ECMO during respiratory failure are that it prevents hypoxic damage of other organs, such as the myocardium, brain, and kidneys, and that pulmonary toilet for control of secretions is facilitated. With extracorporeal oxygenation one avoids direct oxygen toxicity to the lungs and may also prevent barotrauma secondary to mechanical ventilation. The disadvantages of ECMO are that: (1) it requires heparinization with the attendant bleeding complications; (2) it leads to widespread systemic endocrine alterations that occur with long-term nonpulsatile bypass; (3) the immunocompetence of the host is decreased and infections are facilitated; (4) mechanical blood vessel damage may occur at the cannulation sites; (5) red blood cell destruction occurs with decreased production and decreased red blood cell survival; and (6) proteins are denatured with destruction of clotting factors. Despite these disadvantages, a few patients were salvaged. It was found that patients with respiratory failure that was secondary to trauma and was present for less than 3 weeks did better than those with longer term failure due to infection.[31]

A recent report by an Italian group reports on the treatment of three patients who were provided with extracorporeal membrane oxygenation from 1½ to 13 days.[32] Venovenous bypass was used with peripheral cannulation. Oxygen diffusion to the lung was provided by mechanical ventilation of only 3 breaths/min and by a tracheal catheter with a continuous oxygen flow, with extracorporeal circulation being used for carbon dioxide removal. It was postulated that by avoiding pulmonary barotrauma secondary to mechanical ventilation the lungs were allowed to heal. The entry criteria to this group were the same as with the multicenter ECMO trial, but the criteria for weaning from ECMO were different. Aside from looking at oxygenation and PCO_2, lung compliance was measured. Until there was evidence of lung healing by decreased com-

pliance, ECMO was continued. All three of these patients were weaned successfully from ECMO and had excellent clinical results. By using more selective criteria for initiation of ECMO and more sophisticated treatment and evaluation protocols, there may be a limited place for a long-term ECMO in the treatment of respiratory failure.

CIRCULATORY SUPPORT

Cardiopulmonary bypass can provide oxygenation, carbon dioxide removal, circulatory support and perfusion, correction of metabolic acidosis, and whole body warming or cooling, which can be useful in the treatment of such conditions as hypothermia, malignant hyperthermia, drug overdose, electric shock, traumatic injuries, and massive pulmonary emboli.[33-38]

The first report of the use of cardiopulmonary bypass for rewarming and circulatory stabilization during hypothermia was in 1967.[37] Circulatory support is especially useful in accidental hypothermia where the patient is biochemically and physiologically unprepared for the hypothermic event. Multiple studies have shown that rapid rewarming is essential for salvage of the hypothermic patient and, by rewarming the central organs first with core rewarming, the organs are ready for the increased metabolic demands placed upon them by the peripheral tissues. One of the most common causes of death in hypothermic patients occurs secondary to intractable ventricular fibrillation in the hypothermic heart. Because of the hypoperfusion of peripheral tissues during hypothermia, metabolic acidosis is common and can lead to ventricular arrhythmias. Again, it is important to emphasize the control of the acid-base status in the hypothermic patient. The concept of maintaining a pH at 7.4 at all temperatures has to be reevaluated in light of recent evidence that a more physiological variation of pH with temperature produces increased hemodynamic and electrical stability of the heart.[39]

Again, it is important to emphasize the control of the acid-base status in the hypothermic patient. The concept of maintaining a pH at 7.4 at all temperatures has to be reevaluated in light of recent evidence that a more physiological variation of pH with temperature produces increased hemodynamic and electrical stability of the heart.[39]

Recently, an unsuccessful attempt was made at our institution to resuscitate a patient who developed cardiac arrest and circulatory decompensation because of malignant hyperthermia secondary to an anesthetic. Reports of resuscitation using cardiopulmonary bypass in the treatment of drug overdose and traumatic injuries have appeared.[34, 35]

OTHER CONDITIONS

In the past, multiple other conditions have been treated with the use of cardiopulmonary bypass, including endotoxic shock, psoriasis, and schistosomiasis.[40–44] None of these uses have found widespread application.

SUMMARY

Cardiopulmonary bypass can be a useful adjunct to other operative procedures, such as surgery for intracranial aneurysms, complex vascular fistulas during pulmonary lavage for alveolar proteinosis, and in the treatment of various medical conditions, including respiratory distress syndrome, hypothermia, malignant hyperthermia, and drug overdose.

Median sternotomy or thoracotomy can usually be avoided because peripheral cannulation for bypass can be accomplished with good ventricular decompression. It is essential to design the perfusion circuits with the specific physiological situation and the needs of the patient in mind.

References

1. Gibbon JH Jr: Development of the artificial heart and lung extracorporeal blood circuit. JAMA 206:1983, 1968.
2. Woodhall B, Sealy WC, Hall KD, Floyd WL: Craniotomy under conditions of quinidine-protected cardioplegia and profound hypothermia. Ann Surg 152:37, 1960.
3. Woods FM, Neptune WB, Palatchi A: Resection of the carina and main-stem bronchi with the use of

4. Patterson RH, Ray BS: Profound hypothermia for intracranial surgery: Laboratory and clinical experiences with extracorporeal circulation by peripheral cannulation. Ann Surg 156:377, 1962.
5. McConnell DH, White FN, Nelson RL, et al.: Importance of alkalosis in maintenance of "ideal" blood pH during hypothermia. Surg Forum 26:263, 1975.
6. Michenfelder JD, Kirklin JW, Uihlein A, Svien HJ, MacCarthy CS: Clinical experience with a closed-chest method of producing profound hyothermia and total circulatory arrest in neurosurgery. Ann Surg 159:125, 1964.
7. Silverberg GD, Reitz BA, Ream AK: Hypothermia and cardiac arrest in the treatment of giant aneurysms of the cerebral circulation and hemangioblastoma of the medulla. J Neurosurg 55:337, 1981.
8. Drake CG, Barr HWK, Coles JC, Gergely NF: The use of extracorporeal circulation and profound hypothermia in the treatment of ruptured intracranial aneurysm. J Neurosurg 21:575, 1964.
9. Sundt TM, Pluth JR, Gronert GA: Excision of giant basilar aneurysm under profound hypothermia. Mayo Clin Proc 47:631, 1972.
10. Uihlein A, Theye RA, Dawson B, Terry HR, McGoon DC, Daw EF, Kirklin JW: The use of profound hypothermia, extracorporeal circulation and total circulatory arrest for an intracranial aneurysm. Staff Meet Mayo Clin 35:567, 1960.
11. McMurtry JG, Housepian EM, Bowman FO, Matteo RS: Surgical treatment of basilar artery aneurysms. J Neurosurg 40:486, 1974.
12. Silverberg GD, Reitz BA, Ream AK, Taylor G, Enzmann DR: Operative treatment of a giant cerebral artery aneurysm with hypothermia and circulatory arrest: Report of a case. Neurosurgery 6:301, 1980.
13. Neville WE, Thomason RD, Peacock H, Colby C: Cardiopulmonary bypass during noncardiac surgery. Arch Surg 92:576, 1966.
14. Griffin LH Jr, Fishback ME, Galloway RF, Shearer GL: Traumatic aortorenal vein fistula: Repair using total circulatory arrest. Surgery 81:480, 1977.
15. Little KET, Cywes S, Davies MRQ, Louw JH: Complicated giant hemangioma: Excision using cardiopulmonary bypass and deep hypothermia. J Pediatr Surg 11:533, 1976.
16. Zannini G, Spampinato N, Cuocolo R: Partial cardiopulmonary bypass in peripheral vascular surgery. J Cardiovasc Surg 16:308, 1975.
17. Mulliken JB, Murray JE, Castaneda AR, Kaban LB: Management of a vascular malformation of the face using total circulatory arrest. Surg Gynecol Obstet 146:168, 1978.
18. Brickman RD, Yates AJ, Crisler C, Schwentker E, Bron K, Bahnson HT: Circulatory arrest during profound hypothermia. Arch Surg 103:259, 1971.
19. Schwentker EP, Bahnson HT: Total circulatory arrest for treatment of advanced arteriovenous fistula. Ann Surg 175:70, 1972.
20. Neville WE: Cardiopulmonary bypass for noncardiac surgery. Surg Gynecol Obstet 124:592, 1967.

extracorporeal circulation. N Engl J Med 264:492, 1961.

21. Hall KD, Friedman M: Extracorporeal oxygenation for induction of anesthesia in a patient with an intrathoracic tumor. Anesthesiology 42:493, 1975.
22. Neville WE, Langston HT, Correll N, Maben H: Cardiopulmonary bypass during pulmonary surgery. J Thorac Cardiovasc Surg 50:266, 1965.
23. Sadony V, Schramm G, Doetsch N: Management of extensive lesions of the lower trachea using emergency cardiopulmonary bypass. Thorac Cardiovasc Surg 27:195, 1979.
24. Adkins PC, Izawa EM: Resection of tracheal cylindroma using cardiopulmonary bypass. Arch Surg 88:405, 1964.
25. Lippmann M, Mok MS, Wasserman K: Anaesthetic management for children with alveolar proteinosis using extracorporeal circulation. Br J Anaesth 49:173, 1977.
26. Seard C, Wasserman K, Benfield J, Cleveland R, Costley DO, Heimlich EM: Simultaneous bilateral lung lavage (alveolar washing) using partial cardiopulmonary bypass. Am Rev Respir Dis 101:877, 1970.
27. Gille JP, Schrijen F, Horsky P, Cabezon-Cepedes A, Foliguet B: Medical extracorporeal circulation supporting experimental pulmonary lavage. Trans Am Soc Artif Intern Organs 24:638, 1978.
28. Cooper JD, Duffin J, Glynn MFX, Nelems JM, Teasdale S, Scott AA: Combination of membrane oxygenator support and pulmonary lavage for acute respiratory failure. J Thorac Cardiovasc Surg 71:304, 1976.
29. Altose MD, Hicks RE, Edwards MW: Extracorporeal membrane oxygenation during bronchopulmonary lavage. Arch Surg 111:1148, 1976.
30. Zapol WM, Snider MT, Hill JD, et al.: Extracorporeal membrane oxygenation in severe acute respiratory failure. A randomized prospective study. JAMA 242:2193, 1979.
31. Newland PE: Extracorporeal membrane oxygenation in the treatment of respiratory failure—a review. Anaesth Intensive Care 5:99, 1977.
32. Gattinoni L, Pesenti A, Rossi GP, et al.: Treatment of acute respiratory failure with low-frequency positive-pressure ventilation and extracorporeal removal of CO_2. Lancet 2:292, 1980.
33. Tschirkov A, Krause E, Elert O, Satter P: Surgical management of massive pulmonary embolism. J Thorac Cardiovasc Surg 75:730, 1977.
34. Mattox KL, Beall AC: Application of portable cardiopulmonary bypass to emergency instrumentation. Med Instrum 11:347, 1977.
35. Mattox KL, Beall AC: Resuscitation of the moribund patient using portable cardiopulmonary bypass. Ann Thorac Surg 22:436, 1976.
36. Truscott DG, Firor WB, Clein LJ: Accidental profound hypothermia. Arch Surg 106:216, 1973.
37. Kugelberg J, Schuller H, Berg B, Kallum B: Treatment of accidental hypothermia. Scand J Thorac Cardiovasc Surg 1:142, 1967.
38. Davies DM, Millar EJ, Miller IA: Accidental hypothermia treated by extracorporeal blood-warming. Lancet 1:1036, 1967.
39. White FN: A comparative physiological approach to hypothermia. J Thorac Cardiovasc Surg 82:821, 1981.
40. Buselmeier TJ, Cantieri JS, Dahl MV, Nelson RS, Bsumgaertner JC, Bentley CR, Goltz RW: Clearing of psoriasis after cardiac surgery requiring cardiopulmonary bypass oxygenation: A corollary to clearance after dialysis? Br J Dermatol 100:311, 1979.
41. Goldsmith EI, Carvalho Luz FF, Prata A, Kean BH: Surgical recovery of schistosomes from the portal blood. JAMA 199:83, 1967.
42. Kean BH, Goldsmith EI: Schistosomiasis Japonica. Treatment by extracorporeal hemofiltration. Am J Med 47:546, 1969.
43. Goldsmith EI, Kean BH: Surgical treatment of schistosomiasis by extracorporeal hemofiltration in baboons and in man: S. mansoni and S. haematobium. Ann NY Acad Sci 162:453, 1969.
44. Ito Y, Wakabayashi A, Guilmette JE, Connolly JE: Temporary cardiopulmonary bypass for the treatment of endotoxic shock. Am J Surg 136:80, 1978.

CHAPTER 8

HYPOTHERMIA AND CARDIOCIRCULATORY ARREST FOR NEUROSURGICAL INTERVENTIONS

RICARDO J. MORENO-CABRAL, M.D.
BRUCE A. REITZ, M.D.
ALLEN K. REAM, M.D.
GERALD D. SILVERBERG, M.D.

The fascinating method of hypothermia and circulatory arrest as an aid to intracranial aneurysm surgery was initially used in the early 1960s.[1,2,3] This method provided a safe period of circulatory arrest which allowed neurosurgeons to approach otherwise inoperable brain lesions.

The method gradually fell into disuse due to its complexity and to new developments in conventional neurosurgical techniques. Some lesions of the brain, however, remain a technical challenge to neurosurgeons. These include giant aneurysms and hemangioblastomas of the medulla.

In recent years we have seen patients who underwent unsuccessful neurosurgical interventions due to the size and location of the lesions: these lesions were subsequently approached with success with the aid of cardiopulmonary bypass, deep hypothermia, and circulatory arrest.

We will discuss in this chapter the technical aspects of our current method to achieve *deep hypothermia by core cooling in the adult*. This technique has evolved from the time-consuming method of *immersion surface cooling*, applied for resection of aortic arch aneurysms at Stanford in earlier years.[4] A detailed discussion of the neurosurgical indications and techniques at our institution and the physiological aspects of hypothermia have been published elsewhere.[5,6]

PREOPERATIVE PREPARATION

Due to the complexity of the procedure and the large number of personnel involved, all requirements for special equipment are arranged in advance. A written protocol is circulated prior to the scheduled date of surgery.

Preoperative medication is restricted to short acting narcotics, such as fentanyl. Unnecessary sedation is avoided due to its lingering effects following hypothermia. Antibiotic coverage with a cephalosporin (Mandol, 1 to 2 gm i.v.) is provided prior to induction of anesthesia.

A hypothermia blanket is placed on the operating table and activated once the patient is anesthetized. Monitoring lines include both radial arteries, central venous and pulmonary artery by means of a Swan Ganz catheter. Other monitored variables

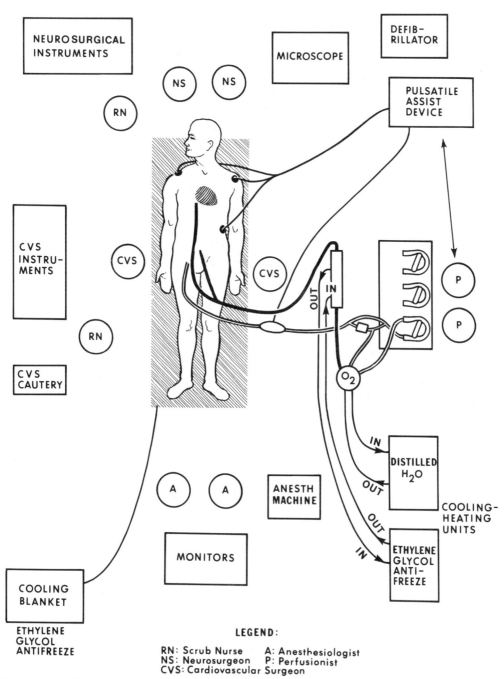

Figure 8.1. Personnel and equipment for hypothermia and circulatory arrest in neurosurgery.

include urine output, nasopharyngeal and rectal temperatures, EKG, O_2 and end-tidal CO_2.

The cardiopulmonary bypass circuit used in this series is illustrated in Figures 8.1 and 8.2. It includes a Harvey H-1000 oxygenator, a Harvey H-500 cardiotomy reservoir and a Harvey H-600 filter, which is re-

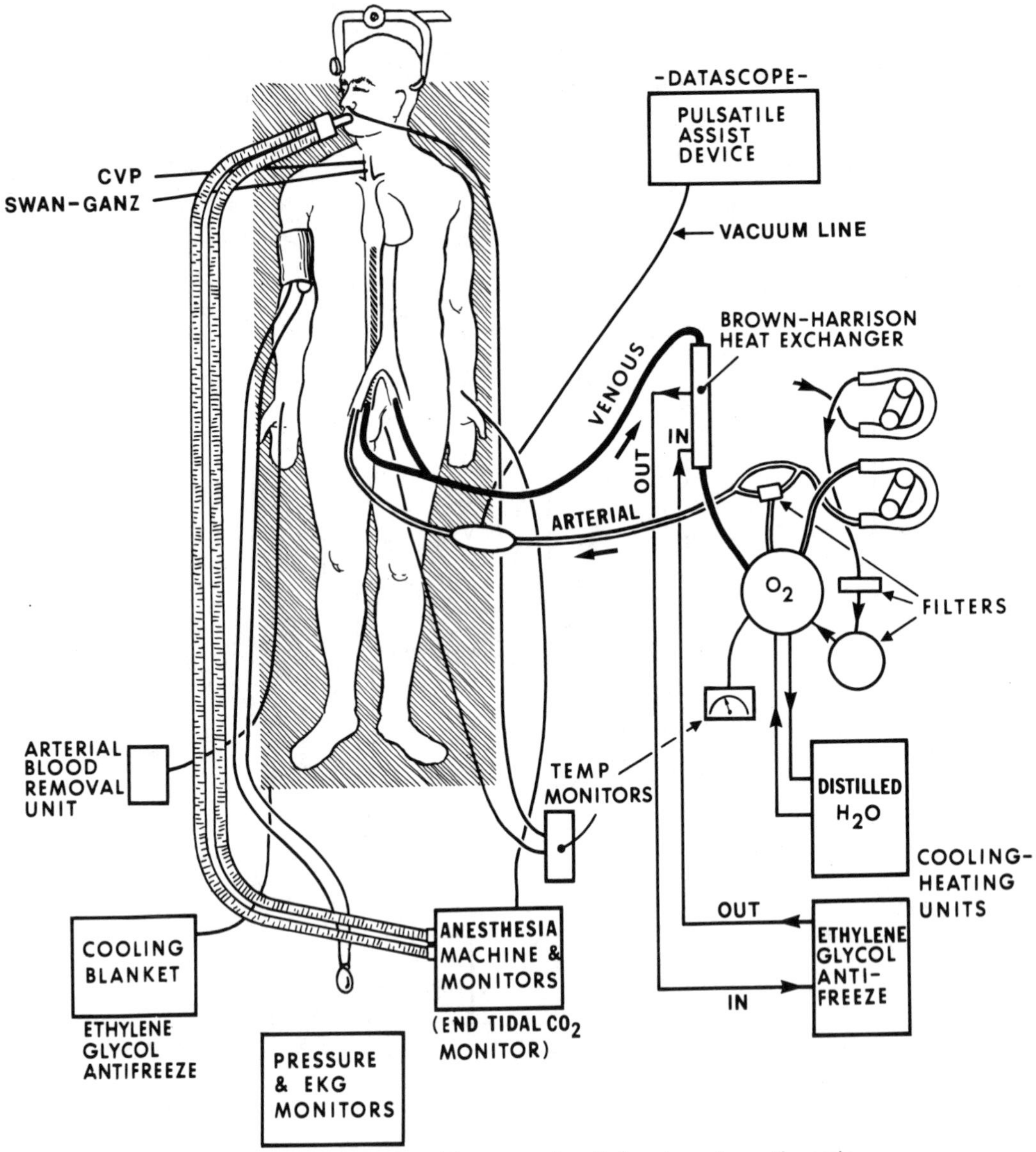

Figure 8.2. Details of bypass circuit for deep hypothermia.

moved from the circuit after the prime has been filtered, a Bentley bypass blood filter, a Brown-Harrison heat exchanger set in the venous line in countercurrent mode, a Pall arterial line filter, and three Blanketrol (Blanketrol Cincinnati Subzero Products, Inc., Cincinnati, Ohio) cooling-heating units, one with distilled water for the oxygenator and two with ethylene glycol antifreeze for the hypothermia blanket and the Brown-Harrison heat exchanger. All venous and arterial tubing is ⅜ inch (internal diameter) except for ⅝-inch silastic tube in the arterial pump head. The prime composition is shown in Table 8.1.

INDUCTION, ANESTHESIA, AND PREBYPASS COOLING

Anesthesia is induced with Demerol (3 to 9 mg/kg) or fentanyl (6 µg/kg) and pancuronium (1.3 mg/kg), and maintained with

Table 8.1
Prime for Hypothermia and Circulatory Arrest (Adult)

Lactated ringers	2000 ml
Packed red blood cells	1 unit
Sodium bicarbonate	100 mEq
Heparin	8,800 IU
Mannitol	12.5 gm
Potassium chloride	20 mEq

nitrous oxide; halothane is used electively to potentiate vasodilating agents. Thiopental (30 mg/kg i.v. drip, 30 to 90 min) is given for its presumed protective effect in brain ischemia.

After induction of anesthesia, the hypothermia blanket is activated and perfused with 4°C fluid. Gentle vasodilation is effected with intravenous sodium nitroprusside (0.5 to 2 μg/kg/min) to improve perfusion. Small doses of chlorpromazine (1 mg/dose · maximum 10 mg) enhance this effect and prevent shivering as temperature falls.

Blood is drawn through one of the radial arterial lines (3 units in a 70-kg patient)* and replaced with normal saline at 4°C (1 liter + 4 to 8 mEq Cal per unit of blood removed). Crystalloid infusion is targeted to maintain a stable central venous pressure and a prebypass hematocrit of 25 to 30%. Serum potassium levels are monitored and adjusted as needed. All fluids administered after induction should be chilled to 4°C to assist cooling. For the same reason the patient is ventilated using high gas flows (open circuit).

As the patient's P_{CO_2} decreases approximately 40% per 10°C cooling, end-tidal CO_2 is monitored and correlated with arterial blood gas values. End-tidal values are typically 3 to 5 torr higher than arterial values. In earlier cases CO_2 (1 to 2%) was added to keep arterial P_{CO_2} above 27 torr when the temperature fell below 30°C. Currently we accept arterial P_{CO_2} between 26

---

* Method of calculating estimated blood volume to remove. Blood volume estimate $(BV_1) = 0.07 \times$ weight (kg); initial RBC mass $(RBC_1) = PCV_1 \times BV_1$; RBC bypass mass $= 0.30 \times (1500 \text{ cc} + BV_1)$; estimated blood to remove: V remove $= RBC_1 - RBC$ bypass$/PVC_1$.

and 33 torr, and CO_2 is rarely added to the inspired gas. It must be remembered that a low CO_2 tension may precipitate arrhythmias and cardiac arrest and that intractable fibrillation may occur if the CO_2 tension is too high. Drug administration, including an additional dose of muscle relaxant (pancuronium, 0.04 mg/kg), is completed prior to circulatory arrest, since no medications can be given during this interval. With the combination of these interventions the patient's temperature usually reaches 30°C prior to bypass. The blood removed is stored in citrate phosphate dextrose (CPD) bags at room temperature and reinfused at the end of the operation.

CARDIOPULMONARY BYPASS

The operative field must include sterile preparation and draping of the entire chest to allow access for an anterolateral thoracotomy or median sternotomy if necessary. During the time spent by the neurosurgeons to gain surgical exposure, both common femoral arteries and veins are dissected free and prepared for cannulation. When the neurosurgical dissection is complete, the patient is heparinized (300 units/kg i.v.) and cannulation carried out.

We typically cannulate the common right femoral artery first, using a large (no. 22 or 24 French) Bardic cannula. The cannula is tied to the artery with tapes, secured to the skin by sutures, and the arterial line is secured to the drapes with clamps. The distal femoral artery is occluded by tourniquets or soft (Fogarty) vascular clamps. In recent cases we have placed a pulsatile assist device (Datascope) in the arterial line.

A long venous cannula (no. 32 French) is then inserted via the right common femoral vein; its length is estimated prior to insertion in order to position its tip at the right atrial level. The left common femoral artery is then clamped to avoid leg distention and the left common femoral vein cannulated. This cannula is short; its tip is ideally placed at the level of the left common iliac vein as it enters the inferior vena cava. This completes the bypass circuit. Except for collateral flow, the lower extremities are practically excluded from the circulation.

Perfusion is initiated, and flow rates are kept between 2.5 and 3.5 liters/min (~50 cc/kg/min). The gas flow consists of a mixture of 95% O_2 and 5% CO_2 at 2 liters/min and 100% O_2 at 1 liter/min. The gas flow is corrected after each blood gas result. Since the prime is cooled at 12 to 14°C by recirculation prior to bypass, the patient's temperature rapidly falls and within minutes the heart fibrillates; at this point the pulsatile assist device is activated. With pulsatile flow, a rectal temperature of 18 to 20°C is reached within 30 minutes in the average patient. During bypass, careful attention is paid to perfusion and central pressures, blood gas, activated clotting time (ACT), and K^+ levels. Bypass hematocrit is kept at 18 to 20%. Of particular concern is the possibility of left ventricular damage by distention in patients with any degree of aortic valve incompetence. An undue elevation of pulmonary wedge pressure as indicated by Swan Ganz catheter monitoring dictates the use of left ventricular venting by an anterior thoracotomy.

After initiation of bypass, the coolant temperatures are lowered to 5°C for distilled water and 0°C for antifreeze-water mixture of the countercurrent heat exchanger. The prime temperature is lowered to 8 to 10°C, and as the patient's nasopharyngeal temperature approaches the desired level, the coolants are gradually warmed to prevent further temperature drift. The hypothermia blanket is disconnected and warming of the bath begun. The heart lung machine is stopped when the targeted temperature is reached (17 to 20°C nasopharyngeal). The venous line is left open and the patient exsanguinated into the oxygenator reservoir. This further facilitates the neurosurgical procedure by providing a bloodless field, reducing brain bulk, and collapsing the aneurysm or vascular tumor.

The safe limits of continuous circulatory arrest under deep hypothermia in the adult are not firmly established. We have limited its duration to less than 30 minutes at 20°C. If the operation cannot be completed in this time, we use short periods of reperfusion alternating with periods of arrest and take advantage during reperfusion to achieve hemostasis in brain vessels not seen during circulatory arrest.

REWARMING

The hypothermia blanket is reconnected, set at 10°C warmer than the patient's core temperature (maximum 40°C), and pulsatile perfusion restarted; the heat exchanger circulation is kept 10 to 12°C warmer than the perfusate to a maximum of 41°C. Any higher temperature gradient increases the risk of gas embolism and thermal damage. For this reason, the additional heat exchanger unit (Brown-Harrison) is placed in the venous side so that any bubbles are trapped in the oxygenator. Rectal and nasopharyngeal temperatures are recorded every degree centigrade or 5 minutes; arterial and venous blood gases are drawn every 5 minutes; ACT is measured every 30 minutes or 5°C. Mannitol, 12.5 gm, is added every hour on bypass, and additional heparin is given according to ACT results to keep it >450 seconds. Potassium supplement is given as necessary after 1 hour on bypass. Calcium chloride, 1 gm, is given as nasopharyngeal temperature approaches 25°C.

Spontaneous cardiac defibrillation may occur when the heart reaches a temperature of 27 to 28°C; otherwise electrical defibrillation is accomplished by external countershock of 100 to 300 W-seconds when coarse ventricular fibrillation is observed. As the heart rewarms faster with perfusion than the nasopharynx or rectum, defibrillation may be accomplished at nasopharyngeal temperatures of 23 to 25°C. Five minutes after defibrillation, blood is gradually returned to the patient from the oxygenator reservoir. When cardiac ejection is effective, the pulsatile assist device is stopped. Once the nasopharyngeal temperature reaches 34 to 36°C, perfusion is discontinued. Further rewarming is assured by the continued use of thermal blankets. Typically, it takes 45 to 60 minutes of perfusion to rewarm.

Vasodilators are used to improve perfusion, increase cardiac output, and thereby facilitate rewarming. During the rewarming phase it may be necessary to add carbon dioxide to the ventilation gases to normalize PCO_2.

POSTPERFUSION PERIOD

The heparin effect is neutralized with protamine. The initial protamine dose is 1½ times the total heparin dose in milliliters (15 mg of protamine for 1000 units heparin). Further doses of protamine are given according to ACT results. Decannulation is carried out expeditiously, since the cannulae should not stay in place after administration of protamine. The left cannula is removed first, the venotomy repaired with continuous 6.0 monofilament suture, and the left femoral artery unclamped. This is followed by removal of the right femoral vein cannula, venotomy repair, removal of the arterial perfusion line, and repair of the right common femoral artery. As there may be transient periods of hypotension upon reperfusion of the lower extremities, appropriate precautions are taken by the anesthesiologist for rapid volume replacement.

Excessive bleeding is a potential, lethal complication of perfusion hypothermia; we routinely use infusion of platelets (6 units), fresh frozen plasma (4 units), the patient's own blood, and frequently factor IX concentrate (Proplex 2 units), and cryoprecipitate. Further blood component therapy is tailored according to coagulation studies in the postoperative period. Although we have not routinely used aminocaproic acid (Amicar), this may also be useful since fibrinolysis may be increased with hypothermia.[7] The rapid administration of blood and blood component therapy can result in myocardial depression; this usually responds to infusion of 500 to 2000 mg of calcium chloride.

Urine output is stimulated if necessary with small doses of furosemide (5 to 10 mg). A urine output of more than 100 cc/hr is expected in a normal patient within 30 minutes from the time a pulsatile flow and physiologic pressures are reestablished. Both lower extremities are wrapped with elastic bandages in order to decrease venous stasis, and the patient is completely covered with warm blankets. Rewarming is continued in the intensive care unit with thermal blankets; usually within 3 to 5 hours after arrival in the ICU the temperature stabilizes at 37°C.

Epidural intracranial pressure and hemodynamics are monitored postoperatively. Extubation is carried out on the evening of surgery if possible.

CLINICAL EXPERIENCE

Our first patient had a history of two previous craniotomies at another institution for a giant aneurysm of the left middle cerebral artery. During the first operation the aneurysm was invested with gauze. As symptoms progressed and the aneurysm enlarged a second craniotomy was performed, but the surgeon was forced to abandon the procedure due to the size of the aneurysm and its dense adhesions to surrounding dominant temporal and frontal lobes. A third craniotomy was performed on November 2, 1978; this time the aneurysm was successfully resected with the aid of hypothermia and circulatory arrest.

Table 8.2 summarizes a 2-year clinical experience. The first nine patients listed were operated on at Stanford University Medical Center and the last patient at the Palo Alto Veterans Administration Hospital. This last patient also had a history of an unsuccessful previous attempt at surgical resection with conventional technique. The tumor was successfully resected under cardiac arrest and low flow (2500 to 3500 cc/min) low pressure (25 to 30 mm Hg) cardiopulmonary bypass.

Of particular interest is case 3, a 38-year-old female with bilateral giant aneurysms who underwent craniotomies under hypothermia and circulatory arrest 2 months apart. The first operation was accomplished with nonpulsatile perfusion and the second with pulsatile flow. We noticed a significant reduction in cooling and rewarming times with the use of pulsatile flow. (Total perfusion time 2 hours, 21 minutes *vs.* 1 hour, 6 minutes). We have used pulsatile flow in most subsequent cases.

The total arrest times have ranged from 7 to 51 minutes. However, on the three patients with the longest recorded times (29, 36, and 51 minutes), there were several brief periods of reperfusion. On the patient with the longest arrest time (51 minutes), this

Table 8.2
Hypothermia and Circulatory Arrest in Neurosurgery

Case	Age-Sex	Diagnosis*	Perfusion Time	Circulatory Arrest Time	Lowest Core Temperature
1	46 M	Giant MCAA	2 hr 30 min	29 min	22°C
2	29 M	Hemangioblastoma of medulla	1 hr 27 min	9 min	16°C
3	38 F†	Giant (R) MCAA	2 hr 21 min	23 min	19°C
4	38 F†	Giant (L) MCAA	1 hr 6 min	7 min	19°C
5	44 M	Giant basilar A	1 hr 35 min	27 min	19°C
6	57 M	Giant MCAA	2 hr 41 min	36 min	18°C
7	59 F	Giant basilar A	4 hr 42 min	51 min	16°C
8	48 F	Giant MCAA	2 hr 16 min	20 min	18.5°C
9	62 F	Giant ICAA	1 hr 51 min	21 min	18°C
10	29 M	Hemangioblastoma of medulla	3 hr 15 min	0‡	11.5°C

* Abbreviations used are: MCAA, middle cerebral artery aneurysm; ICAA, internal carotid artery aneurysm.
† Same patient underwent bilateral craniotomies, 2 months apart.
‡ Procedure completed under cardiac arrest and low flow. Low pressure cardiopulmonary bypass.

was accumulated by five periods of arrest of 11, 9, 14, 11, and 6 minutes. Therefore, the continuous arrest time did not reach 30 minutes in this series.

There was no difficulty in resuscitation of the heart. In some patients, sinus rhythm returned spontaneously upon rewarming; others required external defibrillation by electric countershock.

One patient required brain reexploration for excessive postoperative bleeding, and two patients had small pulmonary emboli 1 and 3 months postoperatively which responded well to anticoagulation therapy.

All patients survived without neurologic complications attributable to hypothermia and circulatory arrest.

APPLICABILITY OF TECHNIQUE

Initial enthusiasm for the application of deep hypothermia and circulatory arrest in brain surgery was tempered by its technical complexity and by improvement in neurosurgical techniques, including hypotensive anesthesia, the operating microscope, microvascular anastomosis, etc. Only occasional reports on the clinical application of hypothermia in neurosurgery have appeared in the recent literature.[8]

With technological advances and wide application of cardiopulmonary bypass during the last decade, we have simplified our technique and made perfusions safer. A great amount of knowledge has been acquired by the extensive application of deep hypothermia by surface cooling and limited cardiopulmonary bypass in pediatric cardiac surgery.[9-11] Sophisticated research techniques have further enhanced our knowledge in the physiologic aspects of deep hypothermia.[12,13]

Several factors have improved the safety of perfusion hypothermia. These include: hemodilution, smaller prime volumes, more efficient heat exchangers and oxygenation, pulsatile flow, better intraoperative monitoring and availability of blood components to correct the clotting abnormalities associated with perfusion hypothermia. Complications associated with deep hypothermia, such as thermal damage, acid base disturbances, arrhythmias, and gas embolism can be minimized by careful attention to detail.

Our method of peripheral cannulation without thoracotomy simplifies the operative approach by keeping all lines away from the neurosurgeons and markedly reduces the operative trauma and thus morbidity. Venous drainage in all cases has been excellent. Only in one instance the arterial line had to be taken out of the pump housing and drained to the oxygenator because of failure to decompress a giant aneurysm after exsanguination by opening the venous lines.

The possibility of left ventricular distention during cardiac arrest has been mentioned. We have not experienced difficulty resuscitating the hearts. Central pressure monitoring, including pulmonary artery wedge pressure, has shown no undue elevations. However, we would not hesitate to insert an apical left ventricular vent through a thoracotomy if the pulmonary wedge pressure rose over 35 mm Hg. A pulmonary artery vent through the same approach would be useful to improve venous drainage and reduce the possibility of left ventricular distention.

Experimentally, it has been shown that maximal gravity drainage of the right atrium may act as a vent to the pulmonary circuit during perfusion.[1] However, if the pulmonary and mitral valves were competent in an arrested heart, retrograde drainage would not be possible. Other experiments have shown improved survival from 40 to 100% by routine venting of the left ventricle in dogs cooled to 4°C.[14]

The techniqual advantages and protection provided by perfusion hypothermia and the results obtained in this initial series of complex neurosurgical cases have stimulated us to continue its clinical application. The results suggest that the technique should be more widely applied in the future for cases not amendable to standard procedures.

References

1. Patterson RN, Ray BS: Profound hypothermia for intracranial surgery: Laboratory and clinical experiences with extracorporeal circulation by peripheral cannulation. Ann Surg 156:377, 1962.
2. Michenfelder JD, Kirklin JW, Vihlein A, et al: Clinical experience with a closed chest method of producing profound hypothermia and total circulatory arrest in neurosurgery. Ann Surg 159:125, 1964.
3. Vihlein A, MacCarty CS, Michenfelder JD, et al: Deep hypothermia and surgical treatment of intracranial aneurysms. JAMA 195:639, 1966.
4. Griepp RB, Stinson EB, Hollingsworth JF, et al: Prosthetic replacement of the aortic arch. J Thorac Cardiovasc Surg 70:1051, 1975.
5. Silverberg GD, Reitz BA, Ream AK: Hypothermia and cardiac arrest in the treatment of giant aneurysms of the cerebral circulation and hemangioblastoma of the medulla. J Neurosurg 55:337, 1981.
6. Reitz BA, Ream AK: Uses of hypothermia in cardiovascular surgery. In *Acute Cardiovascular Management. Anesthesia and Intensive Care*, edited by AK Ream and RP Fogdall. Philadelphia, Lippincott, 1982.
7. Barnard CN, Terblanche J, Ozinski J: Profound hypothermia and the helix reservoir bubble oxygenator. S Afr Med J 35:107, 1961.
8. Sundt TM, Pluth JR, Gronert GA: Excision of giant basilar aneurysm under profound hypothermia. Report of a case. Mayo Clin Proc 47:631, 1972.
9. Barrat-Boyes BG, Simpson M, Neutze JJ: Intracardiac surgery in neonates and infants using deep hypothermia with surface cooling and limited cardiopulmonary bypass. Circulation 43(Suppl. 1):25, 1971.
10. Rittenhouse EA, Mohri H, Dillard DH, Merendino AK: Deep hypothermia in cardiovascular surgery. Ann Thorac Surg 17:63, 1974.
11. Lamberti JJ, Lin CHY, Cutilleta A, et al: Surface cooling (20°C) and circulatory arrest in infants undergoing cardiac surgery. Results in ventricular septal defect, complete atrioventricular canal and total anomalous pulmonary venous connection. Arch Surg 113:822, 1978.
12. Popovic V, Popovic P: Hypothermia in biology and medicine. New York, Grune & Stratton, 1974.
13. Black PR, Van Devanter S, Cohn L: Effects of hypothermia on systemic organ system metabolism and function. J Surg Res 20:49, 1976.
14. Popovic V, Kostolny I, Pass K, et al: Survival of extracorporeally cooled dogs after one hour circulatory arrest. Cryobiology 8:390, 1971.

CHAPTER 9

AIR EMBOLUS DURING CARDIOPULMONARY BYPASS

JOE R. UTLEY, M.D.
D. BARTON STEPHENS, C.C.P.

Air embolus is an important cause of morbidity and mortality during cardiopulmonary bypass. The pump oxygenator is a potential source of air emboli. Systemic air emboli from intracardiac sources are possible when the left side of the heart is opened. Air in any cardiac chamber may embolize to the systemic arteries in the presence of an atrial or ventricular septal defect. Entry of blood into the aorta, left ventricle, left atrium, or pulmonary veins is affected by the site of venting, by cardiac chamber which is opened, and by the presence of septal defects, valve incompetence, or valve stenosis.

The techniques to prevent air entry into left-sided cardiac chambers as well as the techniques necessary for removal of air depends on the presence of valve abnormalities, septal defects, and the chamber containing air. There is evidence that pulmonary artery air emboli following cardiopulmonary bypass are a cause of increased pulmonary vascular resistance or lung dysfunction.

It was known before the era of cardiac surgery that the greatest risk of systemic air emboli was related to entry of air into the coronary or cerebral circulation.[1] The deleterious effect of air in the systemic circulation is related to the volume of air injected and the injection site. Air entering the heart without cardiopulmonary bypass may be a cause of immediate death due to asystole,

ventricular fibrillation or tachycardia, or ischemic myocardial depression.[2] Air that enters the cerebral circulation causes morbidity or death from stroke-like syndromes. Much larger amounts of air are tolerated without mortality when injected directly into the cerebral circulation, thus avoiding the coronary circulation.[1]

In 1967 Nicks[3, 4] reported air embolus in 6 of 127 patients following atrial septal defect repair, 6 of 36 after ventricular septal defect repair, 7 of 42 after mitral valve replacement, and 14 of 155 after aortic valve replacement. The current incidence of air embolism is undoubtedly less. The incidence of cerebral air embolism has diminished with improved techniques of air evacuation.

PATHOPHYSIOLOGY OF INTRAVASCULAR AIR

The surface tension at the gas-blood interface is a critical factor in the consequence of gas emboli. The size of bubbles, the solubility of the gas, and the alteration of surface tension by surface-active agents may be important in the consequences of gas emboli. Air emboli are less harmful than oxygen emboli.[5] Carbon dioxide is the most benign gas embolus because of its high solubility. Occlusion of arteries by gas emboli may be followed immediately by a neurovascular response characterized by spasm followed in hours by hyperemia. Perivascular hemorrhages have been observed experimentally.[6] The interaction at the surface of the bubble includes adhesion and consumption of platelets and damage to endothelium[7] (Fig. 9.1).

Air bubbles are often dispersed as they arrive at small arteries and cause an immediate but temporary block. The immediate occlusion is followed by vasodilatation of arteries, capillaries, venules, and collateral vessels. The vascular dilatation is followed by congestion, hyperemia, stasis, and perivascular hemorrhage. The bubbles are gradually pushed through the capillary bed. The hyperemic phase may last from 1 to 48 hours in experimental studies. The increased flow is greatly in excess of that necessary to repay oxygen debt. Payback of 30 times the oxygen debt has been observed. Denervation does not alter the response. The response follows emboli from virtually any gas including air, oxygen, nitrous oxide, cyclopropane, carbon dioxide, and helium. This suggests that the response is due to direct vascular injury by the gas emboli.[8]

Cerebral Air Emboli

Experimentally, cerebral air embolism is followed very quickly by cessation of flow with restoration of flow to normal within 3 minutes. The electroencephalogram may show depression or silence within 30 seconds of the embolism. The EEG may also

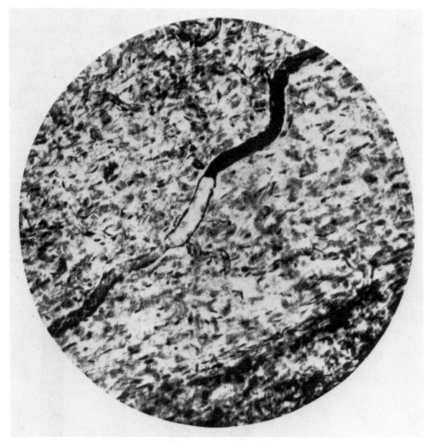

Figure 9.1. The photo shows an air embolus in an arteriole of the mesentery of the rabbit. The segment of the artery with the air embolus is dilated. The red cells are conglutinated proximal to the air embolus. The mass of red cells is less dense distal to the air embolus. (Reproduced with permission from W. H. Chase.[6])

show few changes despite prominent changes in blood flow. Despite prompt return of blood flow, the EEG may show delay in its return to normal. The magnitude of EEG and blood flow changes were roughly proportional. Ischemic lesions are most prominent in the end arteries of border zones between arterial territories.[9]

The distribution of gas emboli may be affected by hypothermia, hematocrit, radius of bubble, and velocity of flow.[10] In experimental animals, survival and risk of neurologic deficit is a function of the volume of air embolized[2] (Fig. 9.2).

Experimental studies have shown no advantage to the use of heparin, low molecular weight dextran, or hyperbaric oxygen following cerebral embolism.[11] The clinical course of cerebral air embolism is usually that of progressive, although often not complete, recovery.[12]

Coronary Air Emboli

There is wide variability in the myocardial response to air injected into the left ventricle.[13] This is probably related to the variable amount which may reach the coronary circulation and to the variation in the part of the coronary circulation embolized. Ventricular fibrillation, ventricular tachyarrhythmia, bradycardia, A-V dissociation, widening of the QRS complex, as well as ST and T wave changes may be observed following coronary air embolism.[14, 15] While coronary air emboli are often fatal without cardiopulmonary bypass, they are rarely fatal if cardiopulmonary bypass is available to support the circulation. Thus, the surgeon may choose to keep the cardiopulmonary bypass cannulae in place for a time after discontinuing cardiopulmonary bypass if there seems to be a risk of delayed emboli[16] (Fig. 9.3). Fornaro et al.[17] was unable to show that cardiopulmonary bypass reduced the degree of left ventricular injury following air emboli. He concluded that the main effect of cardiopulmonary bypass was to support the circulation until the acute effects of the embolism were passed.

Both right and left ventricles have significant decreases in function following coronary emboli.[18] The effect of coronary air embolism is additive, and even though recovery may be complete after a single episode, subsequent episodes of equal magnitude are followed by successive decreases in myocardial function[19] (Fig. 9.4).

Carbon dioxide emboli are much better tolerated by the coronary circulation than

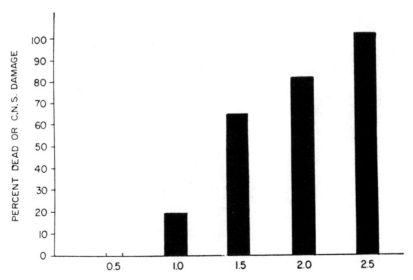

Figure 9.2. The risk of death and neurologic deficit increases with the volume of air injected in experimental animals. (Reproduced with permission from R. B. Benjamin et al.[2])

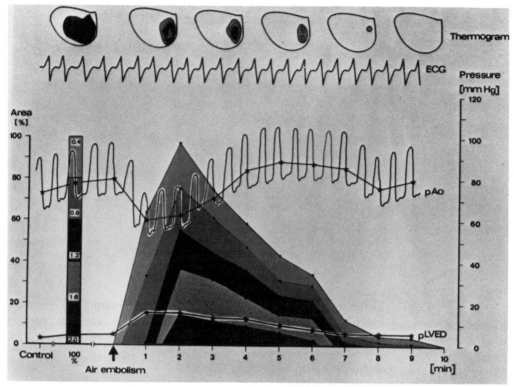

Figure 9.3. This diagram depicts the events following a single episode of coronary air embolus in an experimental animal. The aortic pressure falls with a simultaneous rise in ventricular end-diastolic pressure. The degree of regional ischemia is depicted as a function of the change in regional temperature (0.4° to 2.0°C). The percent of the total ischemia that undergoes the various degrees of temperature change is depicted by the *shaded areas* on the area curves and the thermograms. (Reproduced with permission from T. Stegmann et al.[16])

air emboli. The tolerance for carbon dioxide is approximately 30 times that of air for a single event and 50 times that of air for the sum of multiple episodes of emboli.[18-20] One of the problems of using carbon dioxide is the difficulty in achieving a high concentration in the operative field.

After coronary embolization, foam and small air bubbles appear in the coronary sinus. Thus, the management of coronary air emboli has been directed toward improving the transit of air through the coronary circulation. Increasing the flow rate while on cardiopulmonary bypass to raise coronary perfusion pressure is an effective method for reversing the effect of coronary air emboli. A systemic vasoconstrictor is useful, but is not as effective as a drug with inotropic and chronotropic effects as well.[19] Aortic clamping and compression of the aorta and left ventricle are also effective methods of improving the transit of air through the coronary circulation.[21] Retrograde perfusion of the coronary circulation through the coronary sinus has been advocated as an effective method of preventing entry of air into the coronary circulation and as a method of clearing air from the coronary arterial circulation.

The presence of air in the ventricular chamber was once believed to decrease stroke volume because of its compressible characteristics. This effect was shown to be of no importance when an air-filled balloon

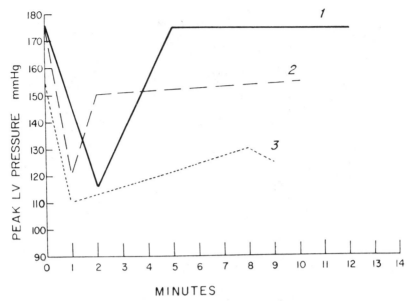

Figure 9.4. This figure shows the time course of the peak left ventricular pressure following successive injections of 2-cc boluses of air into the aortic root. The pressure returns to normal 5 minutes following the first injection. The second and third injections are followed by successive depression of systolic pressure with sustained depression (Reproduced with permission from C. Justice et al.[19])

in the ventricle was found to have minimal effect on stroke volume.[21]

Pulmonary Air Emboli

Air in the pulmonary circulation is tolerated much better than air in the systemic circulation. Air frequently enters intravenous lines and their connections or is inadvertently introduced, as evidenced by the frequent detection of air in the innominate vein or pulmonary artery by cardiac surgeons.

Pulmonary artery air emboli may be a complication of any procedure in which the pulmonary artery is opened or vented. Any procedure requiring opening the right ventricle or right atrium may also result in air in the pulmonary artery. Large amounts of air may be tolerated by the pulmonary circulation. The LD$_{50}$ for intravenous injection of air is 3 cc/kg in the dog.[22]

The pulmonary circulation has been considered relatively resistant to the passage of gas emboli to the venous side of the pulmonary vascular bed.[23] Thus, pulmonary air emboli rarely result in any systemic effects.

Presumably most of the gas is removed by the pulmonary alveoli.

Pulmonary arterial hypertension due to increased vascular resistance is an immediate consequence of pulmonary air emboli.[3, 4] The rise in pulmonary vascular resistance may be particularly pronounced in the presence of pulmonary vascular disease.[24] The rise in resistance may be transient, lasting 15 to 30 minutes, but pulmonary hemorrhage and edema may last for hours to days.[3, 4, 25]

Respiratory motion has been shown to increase the amount of air in the pulmonary circulation when the pulmonary artery is open during cardiopulmonary bypass. Clamping the pulmonary artery to prevent the entry of air has been recommended, but this precludes venting the left atrium and ventricle through the pulmonary artery.[24]

OXYGENATORS AS A SOURCE OF AIR EMBOLI

Improved design of oxygenators and the use of arterial filters has diminished the number of microemboli generated by the heart-lung machine. There is always the possibility of massive air embolus from the heart-lung machine. As the priming volume of oxygenators decreases, the risk of pumping air from the oxygenator increases. Thus, the small volume oxygenator has the advantage of lessening the need for blood priming, but it requires increased diligence by the perfusionist (Fig. 9.5).

Arterial line air embolism is second only to disseminated intravascular coagulation as a complication of pump oxygenator use.[26] Among the causes of air embolism in Stoney's survey were ruptured arterial line or connector; air pumped through vent by reversal of pump or tubing; leaking, pressurized, or burst oxygenator, and rupture of pulsatile assist device and reversal of arterial and venous lines (Fig. 9.6). Use of a low level alarm system is essential with a rigid shell bubble oxygenator. A collapsible bag oxygenator is less likely to be a source of air when pumped dry.

Other accidental causes of air emboli from the pump oxygenator include pressurization of the cardiotomy reservoir and detachment of oxygenator lines during cardiopulmonary bypass (Fig. 9.7). Clotting of the oxygenator due to inadequate heparinization may also lead to air emboli. A kink in the arterial line proximal to the pump head may allow air to enter at artery line connections between the kink and the pump head.[27] A common cause of pumping the oxygenator dry is unrecognized turning of the arterial pump head. Fatigue of the perfusionist is a major factor in the occurrence of pump oxygenator accidents. Unexplained "runaway" pump head presumably due to electrical surges or faulty electronic controls may cause rapid emptying of the oxygenator.[28]

Alarms

Alarms may be activated by a photocell that transmits light across a portion of the oxygenator that is without blood. Sensors that weigh the oxygenator will sense low levels and may be set up to adjust pump rates to preserve safe oxygenator levels. Valves that remain open when filled with fluid, but which close when filled with air, are also useful. The advantage of the valve system is that it is inexpensive and not dependent on an electrical circuit. Infrared

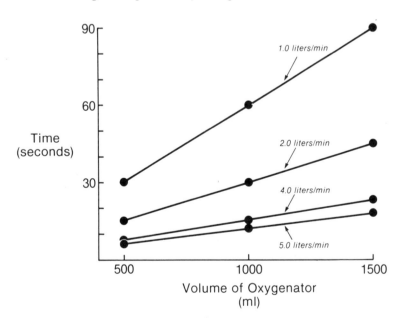

Figure 9.5. The time required to empty an oxygenator as a function of the flow rate and volume of the oxygenator is shown in this figure. The risk of pumping the oxygenator dry is less at low flow rates.

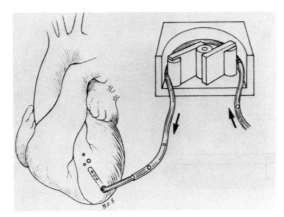

Figure 9.6. Reversal of the pump head may be a cause of air embolization into the heart. (Reproduced with permission from N. L. Mills and J. L. Ochsner.[27])

and capacitance sensors may also detect air in the arterial line.[29]

There is less risk of air emboli to the cerebral circulation from the pump oxygenator if the femoral artery is cannulated than if the ascending aorta is cannulated.[30]

OPERATIVE CONSIDERATIONS IN PREVENTING AIR EMBOLI

Prior to Cardiopulmonary Bypass

The presence of septal defects, especially if there is right to left shunting, increases the possibility of systemic air emboli from air in systemic veins prior to cardiopulmonary bypass. Low right atrial pressure, low intrathoracic pressure, and respiratory motion or diaphragmatic contractions may cause air to enter the right atrium at the time of cannulation which may embolize through a septal defect.

Cardiac Rhythm

The axiom "never open a beating heart" has been used for many years when ventricular fibrillation without aortic clamping is employed. The fibrillatory current should be applied continuously because of the tendency of the heart to defibrillate spontaneously. The use of cardioplegia arrest with aortic clamping has lessened the risk of air embolism following cardiotomy. The rapid return of sinus rhythm and ventricular

ejection following cardioplegia arrest requires that air removal procedures be performed prior to removing the aortic clamp, and that any vents for air evacuation be in place and functioning before aortic clamp removal.

Aortic Valve Procedures

The problems of air evacuation may be great following aortic valve procedures. Evacuating blood from the left ventricle by left ventricular, left atrial, or even the pulmonary artery vents may leave virtually the entire left heart, including pulmonary veins, atrium, ventricle, and aorta filled with air. One of the advantages of cannulating the coronary arteries for repeated doses of cardioplegia is that this avoids the entry of air from the aortic root into the coronary circulation. The author allows the left side of the heart fill with blood as the last sutures are tied on the aortic valve. As the aortotomy is closed, the aortic root is allowed to fill. Since the aortotomy is a high point in the left heart, it will be one of the last parts to fill. The lungs are slowly and completely inflated as the aortotomy is closed to push air from pulmonary veins into the aorta. Suction is stopped on the pulmonary artery, left ventricular, or left atrial vents as the heart is being filled. After closure of the aortotomy, the patient's head is lowered. An aspirating needle vent is placed in the ascending aorta, or the cardioplegia needle

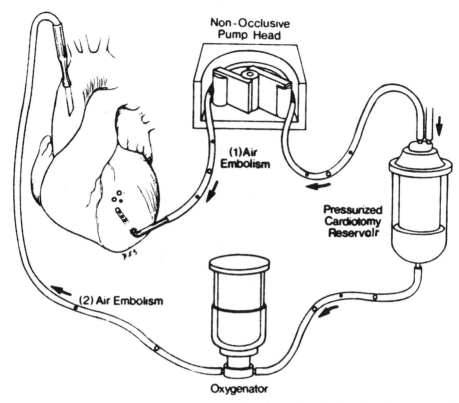

Figure 9.7.   Pressurization of a reservoir may lead to air embolization via a nonocclusive pump head or via an arterial cannula. (Reproduced with permission from N. L. Mills and J. L. Ochsner.[27])

is used. The aortic clamp is slowly removed. Air is aspirated from the right superior pulmonary vein and the apex of the left ventricle. A partially occluding aortic clamp is placed between the aortic needle vent and the arterial cannula. With the needle vent pulling blood from the ascending aorta, the ventricle is allowed to eject as the left heart is filled with blood. The lungs are ventilated, the patient is rotated from side to side by tilting the operating table, and the heart is massaged to mobilize any air trapped in the left heart. As cardiopulmonary bypass is discontinued, the partially occluding clamp is removed, but the aspirating needle vent is left in the ascending aorta and the patient's head remains down until several minutes after cardipulmonary bypass is terminated. If air bubbles are observed in the aortic needle vent, the period of Trendelen-

burg position and aortic venting is prolonged.

Mitral Valve

Mitral valve replacement with the aorta clamped allows entry of air into all parts of the left heart. After replacement or repair of the mitral valve, a device to produce incompetence of the valve should be placed so that air may be evacuated before the ventricle can eject into the aorta against a competent valve. A single red rubber catheter is sufficient for a ball or disc prosthetic valve, and we have used a small soft T tube for porcine heterograft valves. Multiple hole vent catheters and caged or spiral tubes may be used to keep a repaired valve incompetent[31] (Fig. 9.8). If there is any possibility that the valve may not be created temporarily insufficient by such a device,

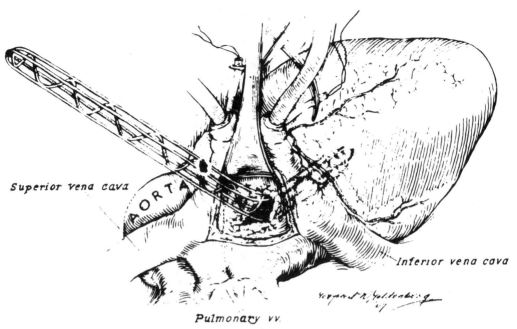

Superior vena cava

AORTA

Inferior vena cava

Pulmonary vv.

Figure 9.8. The figure shows a caged device placed across the mitral valve to create mitral valve incompetence while air is being removed from the left ventricle. (Reproduced with permission from A. Kantrowitz and J. D. Haller.[31])

then the atriotomy should be closed and the heart filled with blood before the aortic clamp is removed.

As closure of the atriotomy is begun, the atrium and ventricle should be allowed to fill with blood from the pulmonary veins. If the aorta is clamped, the aortic vent should not be placed on suction until the atriotomy is closed. Otherwise, the atrium and ventricle may be emptied of blood into the aorta. The vent in the left ventricle, atrium, or pulmonary artery should be removed or suction stopped to allow the left heart to fill. As the atriotomy suture is tied, the lungs should be inflated to evacuate air from the pulmonary veins as the atriotomy is visibly filled. The aortic clamp may then be safely removed with the head lowered and an aspirating vent in the ascending aorta.

If the aortic clamp is removed before closing the atriotomy to decrease ischemic time, the left heart should be allowed to fill with blood, and the mitral valve must be kept incompetent to prevent ejection into the aorta. If mitral valve incompetence cannot be achieved, the ventricle may be fibrillated

to prevent ejection of air. If the heart is beating and the mitral valve is made incompetent, the atriotomy is closed so that sutures are placed to be pulled tight to complete the closure as the device producing mitral valve incompetence is removed. As the catheter is removed and the mitral valve becomes competent, the sutures to close the atrium must be covered by a level of blood or saline and should be pulled up quickly to prevent air entry into the atrium.

A series of maneuvers including inversion of the atrial appendage, ventilation of the lungs, and aspiration from the aorta and/or apex of left ventricle with the head lowered should be carried out as in aortic valve procedures.

Congenital Heart Procedures

Air may enter the left heart with most congenital heart procedures. Procedures similar to those described for mitral valve surgery may be used to fill the left heart and evacuate air at the high point of closure of the left heart as an intraventricular or atrial repair is closed. In order to shorten ischemic time it may be advisable to remove the aortic clamp before the systemic atrium and ventricle are completely closed (Fig. 9.9). This is particularly true after Mustard or Senning procedures combined with VSD closure and/or pulmonic valvotomy for transposition of the great vessels. When these procedures are performed, the closure of the pulmonary venous atrium should be performed so that the level of blood covers the systemic atrioventricular valve as soon as possible if the heart is beating. The other alternative is to fibrillate the ventricles. In small infants aspiration from a vent catheter in the ascending aorta may be difficult because of the small diameter of the aorta. A small stab incision in the high point of the aorta, allowing this site to bleed into the pericardium may be a means of evacuating air ejected into the aorta in infants.

Pulmonary Artery Air

After repair of right-sided lesions or septal defects, the pulmonary circulation should be allowed to fill with blood as the cardiac incisions are closed. If a pulmonary artery vent is used, it may be placed on low suction to evacuate air as the heart is filled with blood. Excessive suction on a pulmonary artery vent catheter or cardiotomy suction in the right side of the heart may increase the amount of air in the right heart and increase the difficulties in getting the right heart to fill with blood. Excessive pulmonary artery suction may be a cause of systemic air emboli[27] (Fig. 9.10).

Operative Management to Prevent Embolization of Intracardiac Air

The maneuvers undertaken by the surgeon to prevent air emboli include the detection of intracardiac air, prevention of entry of air into the heart or cerebral circulation, prevention of ejection of air, mobilization of air from cardiac structures, filling of the heart with fluid or soluble gas, and removal of air from the heart.[26, 27, 32–36]

Detection of Intracardiac Air

The surgeon is certain of the presence of intracardiac air after operations in which

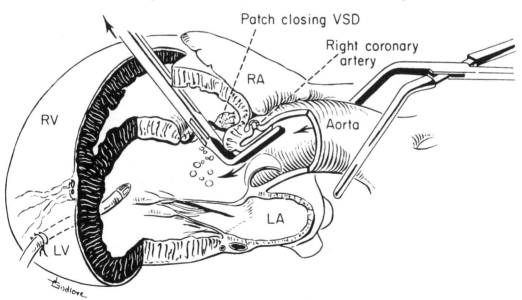

Figure 9.9. The figure shows a technique for creating aortic valve incompetence before removing the aortic clamp. The transient production of aortic insufficiency has the advantage of removing air from the aortic root and allowing the left ventricle to fill with blood. The aortic pressure should be lowered by reducing pump flow to prevent foaming of blood as this procedure is performed. (Reproduced with permission from D. C. McGoon.[32] Copyright © 1968 by Year Book Medical Publishers, Inc., Chicago.)

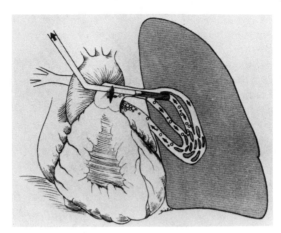

Figure 9.10. Excessive suction on a pulmonary artery vent of cardiotomy suction may cause air to enter the left heart from the lung or coronary arteriotomies. (Reproduced with permission from N. L. Mills and J. L. Ochsner.[27])

the left atrium or ventricle have been opened. The probability of air gaining entry to the left side exists any time the left heart is vented. The author has detected air in the aorta that entered through a coronary arteriotomy when the left ventricle, aorta, atrium, or pulmonary artery is vented.

Ultrasonic transducers have been used to detect micro- and macro-air emboli in blood.[37–41] These techniques have been useful in gaining understanding of the pathogenesis of microembolization during cardiopulmonary bypass. They have shown that air emboli may be mobilized for minutes to hours after cardiopulmonary bypass. The ultrasonic detection of microemboli in the arterial line or carotid artery is not helpful in terms of prevention, however, because the emboli detected are already in the arterial circulation.

Recent studies have shown that echocardiography may be useful in detecting intracardiac air before it has been mobilized to become an embolism.[42] Duff et al.[42] showed that in dogs M mode echocardiography could detect air in the left ventricular cavity (Fig. 9.11). The intracardiac air produced a stippled, granular pattern or a loss of the discrete linear echos or decreased far field echoes. The sensitivity and specificity was 100% when 1.0 cc of air was present. When 0.2 cc of air was injected into the left ventricle, the sensitivity and specificity fell to 86 and 58%, respectively. Borik et al.[43] found that as little as 0.04 cc of air could be detected in the dog heart. The elevation of the left ventricular apex and localization of air in the apex appeared to increase the sensitivity (Fig. 9.12).

Prevention of Air Entry into the Heart

Prevention of air entering the heart is best accomplished by not opening cardiac chambers while the heart is beating. While on cardiopulmonary bypass with low atrial pressures the ventricle can easily fill with air during diastole because insufficient blood is available to fill the capacitance of the ventricle. The mitral valve is more likely to "suck" air if the aortic pressure is less than 30 mm Hg.[35]

One of the advantages of the "no vent" technique for coronary artery surgery is the avoidance of air entry into the heart. Use of low suction, a one-way valve, or no suction on vent catheters may minimize the amount of air entering the heart.[44]

The axiom, "Never open a beating heart" has been used by surgeons for years. Induced ventricular fibrillation prior to cardiotomy was employed commonly in the past prior to the use of aortic clamping and cold cardioplegia. With induced asystole the risk

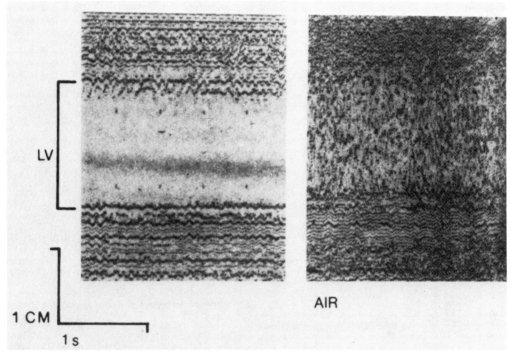

Figure 9.11. The panel on the *left* shows the intraoperative echocardiogram with the heart filled with blood. On the *right* are the changes which are detected with the heart filled with air. (Reproduced with permission from H. J. Duff et al.[42])

of air entry or cerebral embolization at the time of cardiotomy is eliminated.

Prevention of Air Entry into the Cerebral Circulation

The aorta or head vessels should be clamped anytime the circulation is arrested with deep hypothermia.[36] The surgeon should be certain that all cannulation sites that have access to the cerebral circulation are air-tight. Clamping the aorta as a part of cold cardioplegia techniques has the advantage of preventing the access of intracardiac air to the cerebral circulation.

Lowering the head when the heart begins to eject and as cardiopulmonary bypass is discontinued takes advantage of the buoyancy of air. The buoyant air does not tend to enter the cerebral circulation if the head is kept low.[45] This is particularly effective if used with an aortic vent placed in the high point of the aorta. Digital compression of the carotid arteries may also prevent emboli

from entering the cerebral circulation (Fig. 9.13).

MOBILIZATION OF AIR FROM CARDIAC STRUCTURES

In preparation for discontinuing cardiopulmonary bypass, the surgeon attempts to mobilize all air in the heart to the site where the most effective air evacuation is occurring. If the left ventricle or aorta are the site of air evacuation, elevation of the ventricle and massage of the ventricle helps to mobilize air from the left atrium into the left ventricle.[34, 46] The left atrial appendage is inverted to push air out. The heart or the chest may be shaken to dislodge bubbles or foam that may be adherent to the endocardium.[34] Air is evacuated from the pulmonary veins by ventilating the lungs and rotating the patient from side to side. The anatomic studies of Fishman and colleagues[47] have shown how the anterior pulmonary veins may be sites of trapping of air

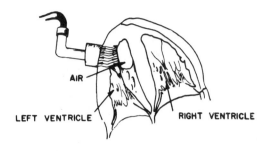

AIR

LEFT VENTRICLE   RIGHT VENTRICLE

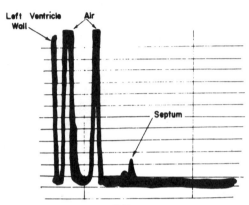

Left Ventricle   Air
Wall

Septum

Figure 9.12. The figure shows the localization of left ventricular air at the apex of the ventricle prior to detection by Doppler techniques. (Reproduced with permission from S. Borik et al.[43])

bubbles (Figs. 9.14 and 9.15). The apex of the left ventricle may be a high point trapping air (Fig. 9.16).

If the left atrium is the principal site of air evacuation then a device to produce mitral incompetence and allow air evacuation from the left ventricle into the left atrium and prevent ejection into the aorta is useful.[35, 48]

FILLING THE HEART WITH BLOOD OR SOLUBLE GAS

Prior to closing the left side of the heart, there is usually enough blood in the pulmonary veins to fill the chambers if the suction on the vent catheter is stopped. Additional filling may be accomplished by inflating the lungs to push more blood into the left heart. Saline may be poured into the atrium, ventricle, or aorta to fill the chamber completely. The aortic valve may be made

incompetent as the aortic clamp is removed to fill the left ventricle as the closure of congenital ventricular septal defect is completed.[32] The aortic pressure should be lowered by lowering the flow from the pump oxygenator to avoid the foaming of blood in the left ventricle. Foam may be difficult to remove.

Carbon Dioxide

Because of its great solubility carbon dioxide has been used to fill the aorta and left heart chamber to prevent air embolization. Carbon dioxide emboli appear to disappear from the blood as if dissolved and are not observed to pass through the capillary bed as are air emboli. Experimentally, large volumes of carbon dioxide may be injected into the pulmonary veins without producing death.[49] Carbon dioxide may also be used to purge filters of the extracorporeal circuits[50] (Fig. 9.17). Carbon dioxide flooding the operative field may be returned to the oxygenator through the cardiotomy suction and produce a hypercapnic acidosis.[51] This may be prevented by using autotransfusion apparatus for suction, such as the Cell-saver. Continuous purging of the cardiotomy reservoir with oxygen or air may eliminate the carbon dioxide, but this carries the danger of pressurizing the reservoir and causing air emboli through a vent or nonocclusive pump head.

The limitation of the technique of flooding the field with carbon dioxide is in achieving a high concentration of gas within the heart. Experimental studies have shown that the optimum technique includes a flow rate of 5 liters/min delivered through two nozzles at least 0.5 cm in diameter. The carbon dioxide need be used only immediately before closure of the heart and not continuously while the heart is open. The cardiotomy suction should be kept outside the cardiac incision while the carbon dioxide is being insufflated. The nozzles should be directed slightly downward in the pericardial cavity. The concentration of carbon dioxide should be measured to assure a high concentration.[52] Other studies have shown that carbon dioxide insufflated through the

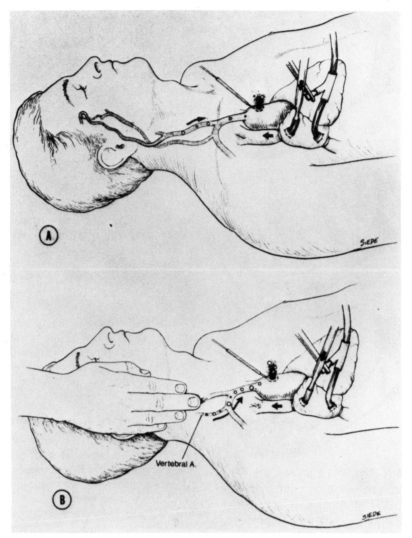

Figure 9.13. (*A*) During the period when air may be ejected from the heart into the aorta. (*B*) Digital occlusion of the carotid arteries may prevent cerebral embolus. (Reproduced with permission from N. L. Mills and J. L. Ochsner.[27])

interstices of a knitted Dacron graft may have advantages over an end hole nozzle. Excessive flow rates may produce turbulence and a fall in concentration.[53]

Removal of Air from the Heart

Aspiration of air and blood from portions of the left heart before and after the termination of cardiopulmonary bypass is a significant part of air evacuation.[33, 54] Before terminating cardiopulmonary bypass, the pump flow may be decreased and the right heart allowed to fill. As the right ventricle begins to fill, the lungs are slowly ventilated, the heart manipulated, and suction applied to high portions of the left heart, including ascending aorta, left ventricular apex, left atrium, and pulmonary veins (Fig. 9.18). The technique preferred by the author is to apply continuous suction to the ascending aortic needle vent and to aspirate left ven-

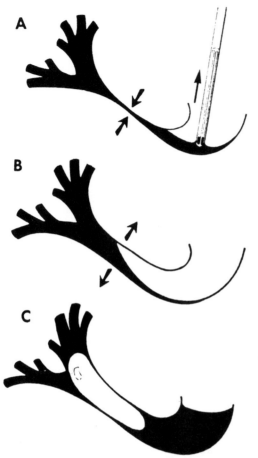

Figure 9.14. This figure shows the effect of pulmonary ventilation on pulmonary venous volume. Increased lung volume and increased intrathoracic pressure results in diminished pulmonary venous volume (*A* and *B*). At end expiration, an air bubble remains in the pulmonary veins (*C*). (Reproduced with permission from N. H. Fishmann et al.[47])

tricular apex, left atrium and pulmonary veins with an 18-gauge needle.

The original technique of aortic venting was to let the vent bleed into the pericardium and harvest the blood with the coronary suction.[55, 56] Modifications of this technique have included needles that evacuated the highest point of the aorta and controlled the direction of bleeding into the pericardium.[57, 58]

Using the aortic needle vent as the main site for air evacuation places the right coronary artery at greatest risk of air embolization. The occurrence of air embolization may be monitored by the surgeon by seeing or hearing the air bubble in the suction applied to the aortic vent or seeing a bubble in a right ventricular branch of the right coronary artery. Air ejected in the central stream of the aorta may pass the aortic vent without being evacuated.[34] The aortic vent will be better able to evacuate the air if left ventricular stroke volume is small in relation to the volume of the ascending aorta. Therefore, discontinuing cardiopulmonary bypass slowly rather than abruptly may be useful when this technique is used. The cerebral circulation may be protected by partially clamping the aorta above the aortic vent catheter, forming a pocket to catch the air[59] (Fig. 9.19).

Studies of the efficiency of various forms of aortic venting have shown that the most effective evacuation of air from the ascending aorta is accomplished by applying continuous suction to a fenestrated catheter in the aorta[60, 61] (Fig. 9.20).

Surface-Active Agents

The tendency for air bubbles to remain adherent to endocardial surfaces has been observed by several investigators. Although studies of surface-active agents have shown them effective in lowering the surface tension of blood, they have never been widely used clinically. Among the agents effective in nontoxic concentrations include saline, streptokinase, streptodornase, stroma-free hemoglobulin, dimethicone, ethyl alcohol, polyvinyl alcohol, acetylcystrine, and paraldehyde. Paraldehyde was found to be most effective.

TREATMENT OF AIR EMBOLI

The treatment of air emboli is dependent mainly on whether the coronary or cerebral circulation is the principal area involved.

Coronary Air Emboli

Coronary air emboli usually have a benign course if the circulation is supported

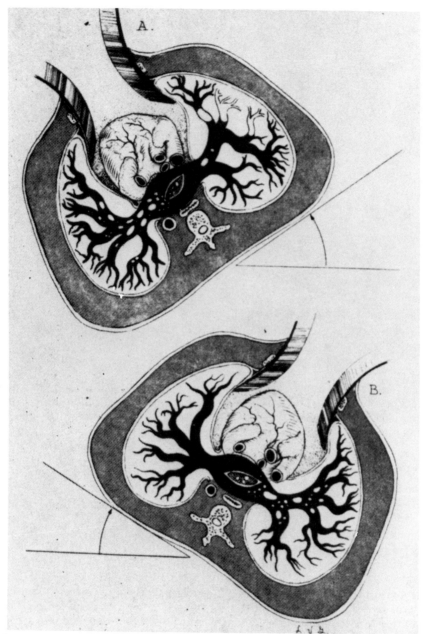

Figure 9.15. The air is evacuated from pulmonary veins by rotating the operating table and inflating the lungs. The removal of air from anterior veins is facilitated by the rotation of the chest. (Reproduced with permission from N. H. Fishmann, et al.[47])

by cardiopulmonary bypass until air is cleared from the coronary circulation.[62] Cardiopulmonary bypass should be instituted and the coronary perfusion pressure elevated by increasing flow, pharmacologic constriction of the systemic vessels, or partially clamping the aorta distal to the arterial line in the ascending aorta. Increasing the

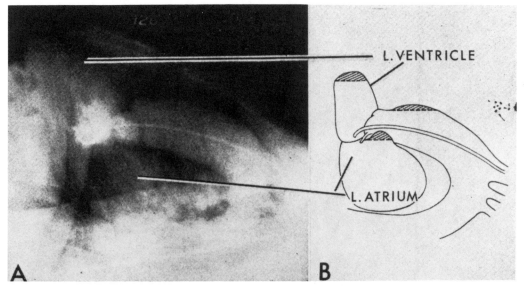

Figure 9.16. The radiograph (A) and drawing (B) show the left ventricle, left atrium, and aorta in a patient with mitral valve insufficiency. The highest point in this patient in the supine position is the apex of the left ventricle. (Reproduced with permission from R. E. Taber et al.[54])

inotropic state of the myocardium with epinephrine, isoproterenol, or calcium chloride infusion may increase the rate of transfer or air through the coronary circulation. Antiarrhythmic drugs, pacemakers, and cardioversion may be necessary to manage ventricular arrhythmias or atrioventricular block.

Cerebral Embolization

When massive air embolization into the ascending aorta occurs the surgeon is often the first to notice this with air coming from suture lines and cannulation sites in the ascending aorta. The surgeon should immediately make a stab incision into the ascending aorta, lower the head of the patient, and instruct the anesthesiologist to occlude the carotid arteries. If the heart-lung machine is the source of the air, it should be stopped. If the heart is the source of air, the heart-lung machine should be slowed to a very low flow to prevent the pushing of air into the cerebral circulation. The pericardium should be filled with saline and the heart and great vessels rigorously massaged

to evacuate air. Air must be evacuated from the heart-lung machine and arterial line if it has been the source of the emboli. The patient and the pump oxygenator should be ventilated with 100% oxygen to increase the resorption of nitrogen from the air emboli.

As cardiopulmonary bypass is reestablished, consideration should be given to using the heart-lung machine to achieve deep hypothermia or for retrograde perfusion of the cerebral circulation.

Hypothermia has the advantage of decreasing the size of gas bubbles.[63] Hypothermia also increases the solubility of gases and decreases the tissue requirement for oxygen.[64] With massive emboli, deep systemic hypothermia may be accomplished with the heart-lung machine for a period of recovery immediately after the massive air embolus. Moderate systemic hypothermia may be useful for several days following cerebral air emboli.

Retrograde cerebral perfusion may be performed by removing the arterial perfusion cannula from the ascending aorta and using the cannulation site for evacuation of

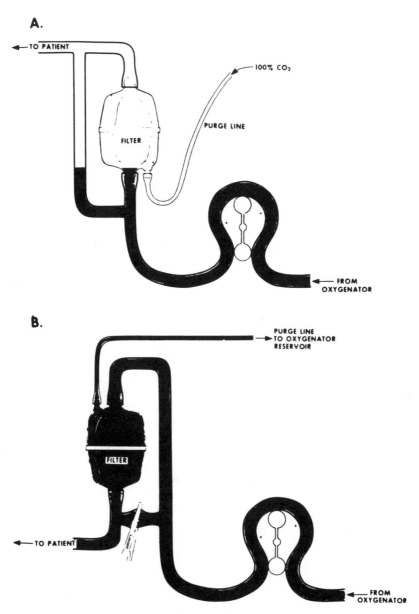

Figure 9.17. (*A*) The filter is inverted and 100% CO_2 is passed through the purge line to displace the air. Priming fluid is then pumped through the filter. (*B*) After the filter is filled, the device is turned to the upright position and the purge line is connected to the arterial reservoir of the oxygenator. (Reproduced with permission from H. A. Wellons and S. P. Nolan.[50])

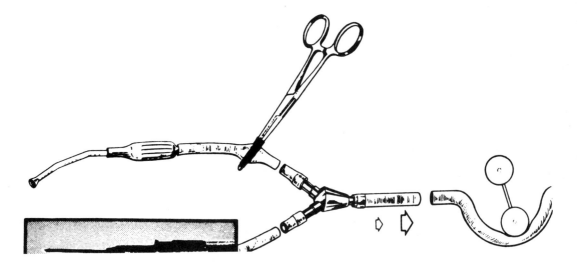

Figure 9.18. The figure shows a cardiotomy suction connected to an aspirating needle. (Reproduced with permission from R. E. Taber.[46])

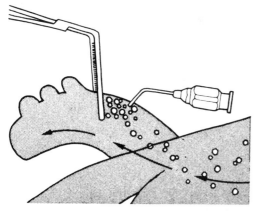

Figure 9.19. A partial clamp is placed distal to the site of air aspiration from the ascending aorta to create a pocket to trap air and to prevent air from passing to the cerebral circulation. (Reproduced with permission from G. M. Lemole and G. C. Pindder.[59])

blood and air from the aorta. The arterial cannula is attached to the divided superior vena caval cannula which is secured by a caval tourniquet. Flow rates of 1.0 to 2.0 liters/min at 20°C are used for 2 minutes into the superior vena cava (Fig. 9.21). Tem-porary compression of the carotid arteries may allow purging of the vertebral system. If air has filled the distal arterial tree the retrograde perfusion of the inferior vena cava may be used with the head vessels clamped to prevent entry of air into the cerebral circulation.[27]

Dexamethasone is given immediately and continued postoperatively. The patient is warmed slowly, and cardiopulmonary bypass is discontinued. No nitrous oxide is used to prevent the expansion of gaseous emboli. Sodium pentobarbital is given to protect the brain.

Pentobarbital may depress myocardial function, and inotropic drugs may be used to counteract this effect. Intracranial pressure monitoring may be used to determine effective cerebral perfusion pressure. Nitroprusside and other vasodilators which vasodilate the cerebral vessels and increase intracranial pressure should be avoided. Blood pressure control is best accomplished with Arfonad and propranolol.

Hyperbaric oxygenation has been recommended in the postoperative treatment of air embolism.[65, 66] Hyperbaric oxygenation increases oxygen delivery and increases the solubility of gas emboli. Experimental stud-

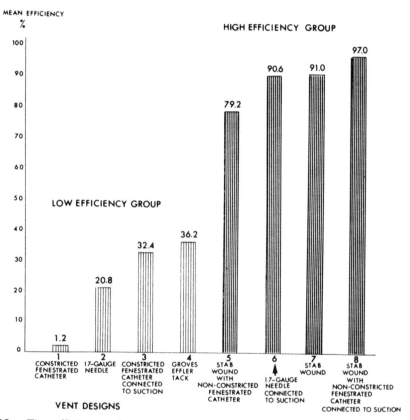

Figure 9.20. The efficiency of removal of air from the ascending aorta is shown. Components of the most efficient techniques included stab wound, nonconstricted fenestrated catheter, and suction. (Reproduced with permission from W. I. Brenner et al.[60])

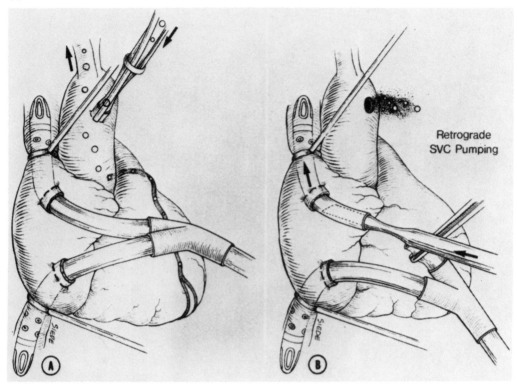

Figure 9.21. *A* shows massive air embolus into the ascending aorta via the aortic cannula. *B* shows the technique of perfusion retrograde into the superior vena caval cannulae with simultaneous venting through the ascending aorta. (Reproduced with permission from N. L. Mills and J. L. Ochsner.[27])

ies have shown improved cerebral function in rabbits treated with hyperbaric oxygen following gas embolus. Hyperbaric treatment has been shown to have rather dramatic effect when used clinically.[65]

SUMMARY

The greatest risks of air embolization during cardiac surgery are due to the effects on the heart and brain. The principles of preventing and treating air emboli are reviewed. The techniques important to the surgeon and perfusionist include avoiding emboli from the heart-lung machine, preventing entry of air into the heart, mobilization of air from within the heart, evacuation of air from the heart, and protection of the cerebral circulation.

References

1. Gomes OM, Pereira SN, Castagna RC, Bittencourt D, Amaral RVG, Zerbini EJ: The importance of the different sites of air injection in the tolerance of arterial air embolism. J Thorac Cardiovasc Surg 65:563, 1973.
2. Benjamin RB, Turbak CE, Lewis FJ: The effects of air embolism in the systemic circulation and its prevention during open cardiac surgery. J Thorac Cardiovasc Surg 34:548, 1957.
3. Nicks R: Air embolism in cardiac surgery: Incidence and prophylaxis. Aust NZ J Surg 38:328, 1969.
4. Nicks R: Arterial air embolism. Thorax 22:320, 1967.
5. Landew M, Bowles LT, Gelman S, Lowenfels AB, Tepper R, Lord JW Jr: Effects of intra-arterial microbubbles. Am J Phys 199:485, 1960.
6. Chase WH: Anatomical and experimental observations on air embolism. Surg Gynecol Obstet 59:569, 1934.
7. Warren BA, Philp RB, Inwood MJ: The ultrastructural morphology of air embolism: Platelet adhesion to the interface and endothelial damage. Br J Exp Pathol 54:163, 1973.
8. Fries CC, Levowitz B, Adler S, Cook AW, Karlson KE, Dennis C: Experimental cerebral gas embolism. Ann Surg 145:461, 1957.
9. Meldrum BS, Papy J-J, Vigouroux RA: Intracarotid air embolism in the baboon: Effects on cerebral

blood flow and the electroencephalogram. Brain Res 25:301, 1971.

10. Kennedy JH, Hwang NHC, Von Miller SG, Hartman A: Factors influencing distribution of cerebral gas embolism. Cryobiology 11:483, 1974.

11. Worman LW, Seidel B: Treatment of cerebral air embolism in the dog. Am J Surg 111:820, 1966.

12. Menkin M, Schwartzman RJ: Cerebral air embolism. Arch Neurol 34:168, 1977.

13. Spencer FC, Rossi NP, Yu S-C, Koepke JA: The significance of air embolism during cardiopulmonary bypass. J Thorac Cardiovasc Surg 49:615, 1965.

14. Glenn WWL, Sewell WH Jr: Experimental cardiac surgery. IV. The prevention of air embolism in open heart surgery; repair of interauricular septal defects. Surgery 34:195, 1953.

15. Rukstinat G: Experimental air embolism of the coronary arteries. JAMA 96:26, 1931.

16. Stegmann T, Daniel W, Bellmann L, Trenkler G, Oelert H, Borst HG: Experimental coronary air embolism. Assessment of time course of myocardial ischemia and the protective effect of cardiopulmonary bypass. Thorac Cardiovasc Surg 28:141, 1980.

17. Fornaro M, Hess O, Benoist F, Turina M: Myocardial damage in coronary air embolism. Thoraxchirurgie 26:190–193, 1978.

18. Eguchi S, Bosher LH Jr: Myocardial dysfunction resulting from coronary air embolism. Surgery 51:103, 1962.

19. Justice C, Leach J, Edwards WS: The harmful effects and treatment of coronary air embolism during open-heart surgery. Ann Thorac Surg 14:47, 1972.

20. Goldfarb D, Bahnson HT: Early and late effects on the heart of small amounts of air in the coronary circulation. J Thorac Cardiovasc Surg 46:368, 1963.

21. Geoghegan T, Lam CR: The mechanism of death from intracardiac air and its reversibility. Ann Surg 138:351, 1953.

22. Holt EP, Webb WR, Cook WA, Unal MO: Air embolism. Hemodynamics and therapy. Ann Thorac Surg 2:551, 1966.

23. Emerson LV, Hempleman HV, Lentle RG: The passage of gaseous emboli through the pulmonary circulation. Respir Physiol 3:213, 1967.

24. Anderson RM, Fritz JM, O'Hare JE: Pulmonary air emboli during cardiac surgery. J Thorac Cardiovasc Surg 49:440, 1965.

25. Chandler WF, Dimcheff DG, Taren JA: Acute pulmonary edema following venous air embolism during a neurosurgical procedure. J Neurosurg 40:400, 1974.

26. Stoney WS, Alford WC Jr, Burrus GR, Glassford DM Jr, Thomas CS Jr: Air embolism and other accidents using pump oxygenators. Ann Thorac Surg 29:336, 1980.

27. Mills NL, Ochsner JL: Massive air embolism during cardiopulmonary bypass. J Thorac Cardiovasc Surg 80:708, 1980.

28. Kurusz M, Shaffer CW, Christman EW, Tyers GFO: Runaway pump head: New cause of gas embolism during cardiopulmonary bypass. J Thorac Cardiovasc Surg 77:792, 1979.

29. Beullens T, van Ypersele de Strihou C: Air embolism during haemodialysis. Lancet 1:209, 1972.

30. Gomes OM, Bittencourt D, Pereira SN, et al: Perfusao femural como ator de protecao contra embolia aerea arterial em cirurgia cardiaca. Arq Bras Cardiol 26:131, 1973.

31. Kantrowitz A, Haller JD: Cage device for preventing air embolism during open mitral valve surgery. Am J Surg 188:476, 1969.

32. McGoon DC: Title. Curr Prob Surg 68:3, 1968.

33. Lawrence GH, McKay HA, Sherensky RT: Effective measures in the prevention of intraoperative aeroembolus. J Thorac Cardiovasc Surg 62:731, 1971.

34. Padula RT, Eisenstat TE, Bronstein MH, Camishion RC: Intracardiac air following cardiotomy. Location, causative factors, and a method for removal. J Thorac Cardiovasc Surg 62:736, 1971.

35. Lam CR, Gahagan T, Isaac B, Manzor A: Air-induced Complications of Open Heart Operations. An Experimental Study. VII Congress of the International Cardiovascular Society, Sept. 15–18, 1965, pp. 173–178.

36. Tsuji HK, Redington JV, Mendez A, Kay JH: The prevention of air embolism during intracardiac surgery. J Thorac Cardiovasc Surg 59:484, 1970.

37. Gallagher EG, Pearson DT: Ultrasonic identification of sources of gaseous microemboli during open heart surgery. Thorax 28:295, 1973.

38. Austen WG, Howry DH: Ultrasound as a method to detect bubbles or particulate matter in the arterial line during cardiopulmonary bypass. J Surg Res 5:283, 1965.

39. Patterson RH, Kessler J: Microemboli during cardiopulmonary bypass detected by ultrasound. Surg Gynecol Obstet 129:505, 1969.

40. Manley DMJP: Ultrasonic detection of gas bubbles in blood. Ultrasonics 7:102, 1969.

41. Lichti EL, Simmons EM Jr, Almond CA: Detection of microemboli during cardiopulmonary bypass. Surg Gynecol Obstet 134:977, 1972.

42. Duff HJ, Buda AJ, Kramer R, Strauss HD, David TE, Berman ND: Detection of entrapped intracardiac air with intraoperative echocardiography. Am J Cardiol 46:255, 1980.

43. Borik S, Davey TB, Kaufman B, Smeloff EA, Miller GE Jr: A new method for intraoperative detection of intracardiac air prior to discontinuance of bypass. Ann Thorac Surg 16:344, 1973.

44. Jones RD, Cross FS: A vent valve to minimize air embolism during open-heart surgery. J Thorac Cardiovasc Surg 48:310, 1964.

45. Bagdonas AA, Stuckey JH, Dennis C, Piera J, Amer NS, Domingo RT, Cappelletti RR: The role of position in the development of cerebral air embolism following air injection at the base of the aorta. Surg Forum 10:653, 1960.

46. Taber RD: Intracardiac air aspiration. Ann Thorac Surg 14:79, 1972.

47. Fishman NH, Carlsson E, Roe BB: The importance of the pulmonary veins in systemic air embolism following open-heart surgery. Surgery 66:655, 1969.

48. Starr A: The mechanism and prevention of air embolism during correction of congenital cleft mi-

tral valve. J Thorac Cardiovasc Surg 39:808, 1960.

49. Moore RM, Braelton CW Jr: Injections of air and of carbon dioxide into a pulmonary vein. Ann Surg 112:212, 1940.

50. Wellons HA, Nolan SP: Prevention of air embolism due to trapped air in filters used in extracorporeal circuits. J Thorac Cardiovasc Surg 65:476, 1973.

51. Burbank A, Ferguson TB, Burford TH: Carbon dioxide flooding of the chest in open-heart surgery. A potential hazard. J Thorac Cardiovasc Surg 50:691, 1965.

52. Ng WS, Rosen M: Carbon dioxide in the prevention of air embolism during open-heart surgery. Thorax 23:194, 1968.

53. Selman MW, McAlpine WA, Albregt H, Ratan R: An effective method of replacing air in the chest with CO_2 during open-heart surgery. J Thorac Cardiovasc Surg 53:618, 1967.

54. Taber RE, Maraan BM, Tomatis L: Prevention of air embolism during open-heart surgery: A study of the role of trapped air in the left ventricle. Surgery 68:685, 1970.

55. Janke WH, Esfahani AA: Air embolism following open heart surgery. Mich Med 69:761, 1970.

56. Groves LK, Effler DB: A needle-vent safeguard against systemic air embolus in open-heart surgery. J Thorac Cardiovasc Surg 47:349, 1964.

57. Geldof WCP, Aytug Z, Brom AG: Die entluftung der aorta nach extrakorporalem kreislauf. Thoraxchirurgie 20:218, 1972.

58. Mulch J, Asai N, Iida M, Hehrlein FW: Eine modifizerte form der aortenentluftung zur verhutung von luftembolien in der offenen herzchirurgie. Thoraxchirurgie 21:55, 1973.

59. Lemole GM, Pindder GC: A method of preventing air embolus in open-heart surgery. J Thorac Cardiovasc Surg 71:557, 1976.

60. Brenner WI, Wallsh E, Spencer FC: Aortic vent efficiency. A quantitative evaluation. J Thorac Cardiovasc Surg 61:258, 1971.

61. Brenner WI, Wallsh E, Spencer FC: Efficiency of aortic vents in the prevention of air embolism. Surg Forum 21:139, 1970.

62. Nichols HT, Morse DP, Hirose T: Coronary and other air embolization occurring during open cardiac surgery. Surgery 43:236, 1958.

63. Friedman IH, Gelman S, Lowenfels AB, Landew M, Lord JW Jr: The effects of intra-arterial microbubbles on normothermic and hypothermic dogs. J Surg Res 2:19, 1962.

64. Steward D, Williams WG, Freedom R: Hypothermia in conjunction with hyperbaric oxygenation in the treatment of massive air embolism during cardiopulmonary bypass. Ann Thorac Surg 24:591, 1977.

65. Takita H, Olszewski W, Schimert G, Lanphier EH: Hyperbaric treatment of cerebral air embolism as a result of open-heart surgery. Report of a case. J Thorac Cardiovasc Surg 55:682, 1968.

66. Meijne NG, Schoemaker G, Bulterijs: The treatment of cerebral gas embolism in a high pressure chamber. An experimental study. J Cardiovasc Surg (Torino) 4:757, 1963.

CHAPTER 10

MICROEMBOLI AND THE USE OF FILTERS DURING CARDIOPULMONARY BYPASS

L. HENRY EDMUNDS, JR., M.D.
WILLIAM WILLIAMS, C.C.P.

Microemboli are gaseous or solid particles that obstruct circulation to the microvasculature. By microvasculature we mean arterioles, precapillaries, capillaries, and venules which range from 8 to 40 μm in diameter. The body contains a huge number of microvessels; for instance, the cross-sectional area of the capillary bed is estimated to be 800 times that of the aorta. As the arterial tree subdivides, myriads of branches are formed so that the number of branches 40 μm or less in diameter is incalculable. For microemboli to cause detectable organ damage, thousands, perhaps millions of arterioles, precapillaries, and capillaries must be obstructed. Extracorporeal perfusion systems can produce the vast numbers of microemboli needed to produce organ damage from occlusion of the microcirculation; however, more damage can be caused by fewer emboli if the emboli are larger than 35 to 40 μm. These larger emboli obstruct small arteries and larger arterioles and thus stop circulation to organ and tissue segments before these vessels arborize into the microvasculature; axiomatically, the larger the embolus, the larger the segment of an organ or tissue rendered ischemic. Emboli greater than 35 to 40 μm in diameter have been causally related to some of the morbidity associated with cardiopulmonary bypass. However, no morbidity has been conclu-sively demonstrated from emboli smaller than 35 to 40 μm.

Current technology does not consistently exclude microemboli less than 35 to 40 μm in diameter from most extracorporeal perfusion systems. Although it is logical to assume that any embolus is detrimental, the term microemboli when used in the context of extracorporeal perfusion refers to gaseous or particulate emboli 35 to perhaps 400 μm in diameter. These particles may be present in large numbers within extracorporeal perfusion systems, are too small to see with the naked eye, do not exclusively obstruct the microvasculature as defined by physiologists, but are capable of obstructing larger arterioles and even small arteries to cause ischemic necrosis of hundreds and thousands of cells per embolus. These "microemboli" are the subject of this chapter.

SOURCES OF EMBOLI

Emboli that develop within extracorporeal perfusion systems can be divided into three broad categories: gaseous, blood-derived, and foreign material.

Gaseous Emboli

Massive air embolism occurs in 1.1 to 2.2 patients per 1,000 perfused.[1, 2] Approximately one-half of these instances result in

Table 10.1
Causes of Air Embolism*

1. Inattention to oxygenator blood level
2. Unexpected resumption of heartbeat
3. Reversal of vent or perfusion lines in pump head
4. Pressurized cardiotomy reservoir
5. Opening a beating heart
6. Clotted oxygenator
7. Runaway pump head
8. Kink in arterial line proximal to pump head
9. Break in integrity of lines or oxygenator
10. Detachment of oxygenator during perfusion
11. Faulty technique during circulatory arrest
12. Unnoticed rotation of arterial pump head

* Reprinted with permission from N. L. Mills and J. L. Ochsner.[2]

permanent neurologic damage or death. Causes of massive air embolism are listed in Table 10.1.[2] Large amounts of air can enter the circulation either through the bypass system or via a cardiotomy, and Mills and Ochsner[2] have described steps to prevent this. Filters cannot prevent massive air emboli.[3] If massive air embolism occurs cerebral damage may be reduced by hyperbaric compression and hypothermia[4, 5] in addition to standard pharmacologic methods to reduce brain swelling. Massive air embolism is a definite risk of extracorporeal perfusion, but like air travel the risk can be reduced by training, equipment selection, maintenance, and careful attention to details.

Microgaseous emboli (400 μm or less) are inherent in bubble oxygenator systems wherein gas bubbles are directly introduced into flowing venous blood.[6] Bubble oxygenators are designed to remove the microbubbles and foam produced by the oxygenating process by a combination of filtration, settling, and chemical modification of the surface tension of the gas in blood (antifoam compounds). In spite of these measures, thousands of microbubbles, as counted by ultrasonic techniques,[6–10] are present within the arterial line during clinical perfusions with bubble oxygenators. Since carbon dioxide is rapidly soluble in blood and since oxygen, though more slowly soluble, is also a metabolite, microemboli of these gases are less likely to cause ischemic damage than nitrogen which is poorly soluble in blood

and is not a metabolite. Microbubbles formed by field aspiration of air and blood in the cardiotomy suction system contain mostly nitrogen, dissolve slowly, and are likely to obstruct the microvasculature to produce ischemic damage.

The number of gaseous microemboli produced within the extracorporeal perfusion system is influenced by several factors. Bubble oxygenators produce more arterial line gaseous emboli when reservoir levels are low[11–13] or when gas to blood flow ratios are high. Although oxygen flows must be sufficient to fully saturate blood, modern bubble oxygenators achieve adequate oxygenation at 1:1 gas to blood flow ratios. Blows to the oxygenator release microbubbles.[10, 12] Negative pressure within the perfusion system causes cavitation and microbubbles within the blood.[12, 14] Centrifugal pumps produce fewer gaseous emboli than do roller pumps,[15] and membrane oxygenators produce far less gaseous emboli than bubble oxygenators.[6] Microbubbles develop in membrane oxygenators from small tears and pinholes in the membrane, detachment of small surface bubbles that remain after priming, and from areas of positive transmembrane gas/blood pressure ratios. It is estimated that approximately half of microemboli produced by membrane oxygenators are gaseous.

Oxygen, carbon dioxide, and nitrogen are more soluble in cold blood than in warm blood. Rapid rewarming of cold blood results in the release of microbubbles as dissolved gases come out of solution. Temperature gradients of more than 14°C result in the release of dissolved gases. During cooling, cold arterial blood leaving the heat exchanger enters the still warm patient. This blood with its dissolved gases is rapidly warmed to the patient's temperature, and microbubbles may be released within the patient's circulatory system. During rewarming when cold blood from the patient is rapidly warmed in the heat exchanger, bubbles may be released in the perfusion system. Production of these bubbles has led to the caution of avoiding temperature differences of more than 14°C between patient and arterial blood. However, when warmed arterial blood reaches the still cold patient, microbubbles are likely to dissolve and cause no harm. These considerations emphasize that the threat of gaseous microembolism due to temperature changes during perfusion are more likely to occur during *cooling* rather than rewarming. The general impression is the reverse.

Emboli from Blood Elements

Emboli also develop from the formed and unformed elements of circulated blood. Fibrin can form within extracorporeally circulated blood if the coagulation cascade is not adequately inhibited.[16] When blood contacts a foreign surface Factor XII is activated to Factor XIIa, and the coagulation cascade is initiated. Heparin in adequate doses inhibits serine esterases and blocks the coagulation at four or five different points.[17] Most importantly heparin potentiates the action of antithrombin III and thus inhibits conversion of fibrinogen to fibrin by thrombin produced by the coagulation cascade. Conventionally 3 $\mu g/kg$ of beef-lung heparin is used to prevent coagulation within extracorporeal perfusion systems, but this amount does not always completely inhibit fibrin formation during bypass.[18] Rates of heparin metabolism and sensitivity to the drug vary between patients.[19, 20] To ensure adequate heparinization, activated clotting times should be measured. Activated clotting times greater than 400 seconds are considered adequate to prevent fibrin formation within extracorporeal circuits.[21]

Fibrin tends to form in areas of stagnant flow, on rough surfaces, and in areas of turbulence and cavitation. Current bypass circuits contain numerous areas of non-streamlined blood flow and intraluminal projections which can develop fibrin deposits if anticoagulation is inadequate.[18] Fibrin deposits are prone to develop at connections, within oxygenators,[22] and in arterial line filters.[23, 24] Bubble and blood gas oxygenators form more fibrin emboli than do membrane oxygenators.[25]

Plasma proteins are denatured during contact with extracorporeal synthetic surfaces and during passage through membrane and bubble oxygenators.[27] Denaturation of plasma proteins alters immunologic

proteins[28] and complement[29] and affects adhesion of platelets to synthetic surfaces.[26, 30] There are no conclusive data that denatured proteins form aggregates and microemboli.

Cardiopulmonary bypass causes generation of macro- and microscopic fat emboli. Fat globules are routinely observed in pericardial blood which is aspirated and returned to the perfusion system.[31] This fat is undoubtedly released by trauma to fat cells in the epicardium and wound.[32, 33] Fat emboli as measured by increases in total lipids, free fatty acids, triglycerides, and serum lipase develop after median sternotomy or thoracotomy even without cardiopulmonary bypass.[32] Clark has found that two-thirds of fat emboli that develop within extracorporeal perfusion systems enter via the cardiotomy suction system.[33]

Fat emboli also develop from blood passed through extracorporeal perfusion systems, particularly those that contain bubble oxygenators.[27, 31, 33] Membrane oxygenators may produce fewer fat emboli than bubble oxygenators,[33] but this conclusion is challenged.[34] Zapol et al.[35] found that membrane oxygenators cause less denaturation of canine proteins and lipoproteins than bubble oxygenators. Fat emboli which develop from blood result from denaturation of plasma lipoproteins and lipids that cause fat to come out of solution. These emboli are aggregates of chylomicrons[27] or free fat and contain principally triglycerides and cholesterol.[33] Size may vary from 4 to 200 μm.[31] Fat emboli are easily stained in tissue with oil red O or osmium tetroxide stains. Hemodilution reduces generation of immiscible fat during bubble oxygenation,[33] but there are no means to completely prevent generation of fat emboli during cardiopulmonary bypass.

Contact between blood and synthetic surfaces activates platelets and causes the formation of platelet aggregates.[36, 37] Most platelet aggregates probably disaggregate in the microcirculation[38]; however, some platelet aggregate emboli have been observed in the central nervous system of patients who have died after open heart surgery. Experimentally, aggregated leukocytes have been found in the lungs of dogs following cardiopulmonary bypass.[38, 40] Leukocyte aggregates may release lysosomal enzymes which in turn cause extravasation of plasma into surrounding tissues. Pharmacologic inhibitors of platelets such as PGE_1 or PGI_2 can largely prevent the formation of platelet aggregates during cardiopulmonary bypass, but because of vasodilatory properties cannot be used routinely.[41] At present there are no means to prevent leukocyte aggregation during bypass; however, aside from the lung, organ damage due to leukocyte aggregation has not been demonstrated.

Cardiopulmonary bypass reduces the ability of red cells to change shape during passage through the microcirculation.[42] Although hypothermia and hypotension may cause stagnant flow and red cell sludging in the capillary circulation, altered red cells have not been shown to permanently obstruct capillaries during cardiopulmonary bypass.

Emboli from Foreign Material

Foreign materials may be introduced into extracorporeal perfusion systems from a variety of sources. Donor blood contains platelet and leukocyte aggregates,[37] bits of fibrin, red cell debris, and lipid precipitates.[43] During the first 24 hours of storage of citrated blood (4°C), most particles are platelet aggregates.[37] Particles increase with the duration of storage.[37] Within 1 week, each unit contains nearly 2 million particles 40 μm or greater in diameter.[44, 45] Particles can be removed by filtration or washing. Dacron wool or microfilters (20 μm pore size) are preferable to standard 170-μm screen filters.[37, 46] Crystalloid solutions also contain inorganic debris which should be removed by filtration before introduction into extracorporeal perfusion circuits.[47, 48]

Foreign particles may also be present on blood contact surfaces of commercial perfusion system components. Reed et al.[47] has demonstrated large numbers of foreign particles within various commercially available oxygenators that are sterile and ready for use. Antifoam compounds used to enhance dissolution of bubbles in early bubble oxygenators can form emboli.[49] Particles within unprimed perfusion systems can be removed by washing and filtration prior to priming.[47]

Roller pumps can cause small bits of the compressed pump tubing to break off and form emboli.[50] This process, called spallation, can produce large numbers of emboli up to 300 μm in diameter.[51] Spallation is more likely to occur with silicone rubber tubing than with polyvinyl or polyurethane.[50]

The largest source of microemboli during open heart surgery is the cardiotomy sucker system. Field-aspirated blood may contain fibrin, fat, cellular debris, calcium, muscle, talc, suture material, and any particulate material that reaches the surgical field. In addition, aspiration of large amounts of air creates thousands of microbubbles which largely contain nitrogen. Many studies have shown that field-aspirated blood is the largest single source of microemboli during operations involving cardiopulmonary bypass.[9, 33, 34]

DETECTION OF MICROEMBOLI

Several methods have been used to detect microemboli less than 400 μm in diameter in extracorporeal perfusion systems. These methods are summarized as follows: detection of changes in organ function; release of injured tissue markers; histologic examination; ultrasound; filters, particle counting, and blood analysis. Each method has advantages and disadvantages; none are suitable for reliably detecting all emboli during the period of bypass.

The brain is more likely to reflect functional changes due to multiple scattered microemboli than other organs. Functional measurements of kidney, liver, and heart are not sufficiently sensitive to detect microembolic phenomena. Although the eye is very sensitive to microemboli,[52] this organ receives only a miniscule percentage of the cardiac output and, therefore, the occurrence of microemboli is subject to serious sampling errors. Measurements of cerebral function, using various psychomotor tests before and after bypass, have shown small changes postoperatively.[7, 53–55] These studies usually show measurable changes in cerebral function during the first few days after óperation, but few changes weeks or months later.[54] Acute changes may be related to microemboli, but it is difficult to rule out other causes of cerebral dysfunction, such as cerebral edema, drugs, sleep deprivation, and psychologic considerations. Measurement of cerebral function before and after bypass is a sensitive but nonspecific method for detecting microemboli.

Recently, measurement of creatinine phosphokinase enzymes with brain-specific isoenzyme fractions in the cerebrospinal fluid of dogs has been used to detect brain injury associated with cardiopulmonary bypass.[56, 57] Experimentally, the increase in CPK enzymes correlates with the number of microemboli present in the arterial blood during bypass.

Microemboli from extracorporeal perfusion systems were first discovered from histologic examination of kidney, brain, and other organs[31, 34, 49, 58] which have relatively high blood flows per unit mass. Since the brain receives approximately 14% of the cardiac output, histologic studies of this organ are as likely to show emboli as studies of other high flow organs. These studies, of course, require tissue which is rarely obtained by biopsy. Special stains are available to identify the composition of the emboli found within blood vessels. This method provides only qualitative information with respect to the number and size of emboli, cannot detect gaseous emboli, but does indicate composition and provides proof of tissue injury.

In experimental animals the infusion of lamp-black into carotid arteries or arterial perfusion lines just prior to euthanasia has been used to detect areas of cerebral ischemia.[59] Occasionally microemboli may be detected by opthalmic examination of the retinal disc.[52]

Ultrasonic methods are very sensitive indicators of those microemboli that have an acoustical interface in blood.[6, 23, 60] These detectors count both gaseous and solid emboli and provide semiquantitative data of both size and number of emboli. The Doppler method does not reliably count solids,[8] and pulsed-echo systems may count some particles more than once.[8, 10, 59] A continuous wave ultrasonic device is relatively insensitive to flow, hematocrit and temperature changes, and can monitor emboli continuously.[8] The method does not accurately size particles of different composition and

does not distinguish between different solids or between solids and gas.[33] Ultrasound is the only method to detect gaseous emboli and is very sensitive. The extreme sensitivity of the method limits its usefulness, since counts rise precipitously with minor interventions, such as addition of drugs or fluids to the venous reservoir.[10]

Aliquots of perfusate can be removed from different locations in the extracorporeal perfusion circuit and counted for solid particles in an electronic particle counter.[37] This method measures only solid particles but can be adjusted to indicate both size and numbers of particles. The total volume of solid particles can also be calculated. The counter does not discriminate between the composition of the particles. The perfusate must be diluted and red cells hemolyzed before counting.

Many investigators have used in-line filters, sometimes in series, to trap solid microemboli during extracorporeal perfusion. Sometimes filters are used to merely sample the extracorporeally circulated blood[24]; more often, filters are analyzed following perfusion by particle counting, weighing, scanning electron microscopy (Fig. 10.1), histochemical staining, and biochemical analysis of the retained material.[33, 36, 61] The material trapped on filters is the best method for detecting the composition and relative amounts of solid microemboli formed during cardiopulmonary bypass. This method, more than others, has led to the identification of the various sources of solid emboli found in extracorporeally circulated blood.

A variant of the filter method involves passage of aliquots of perfusate through a standard screen with 20-μm holes at a constant rate.[62] Upstream pressure is measured over a 10-second period to determine the screen filtration pressure, which is an index of the number of solid microemboli present in the aliquot.

ORGAN DAMAGE BY MICROEMBOLI

Proof that microemboli cause organ damage has largely focused on the brain, although early histologic studies revealed embolic material in kidneys, heart, liver, lung, and spleen.[31, 49, 61] In 1969, Hill et al.[34] pub-

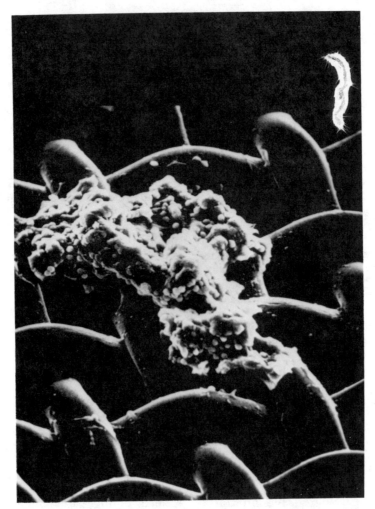

Figure 10.1. Scanning electron microscopy of platelet aggregates on a nylon mesh arterial filter.

lished a comprehensive study of 133 patients who died after open heart surgery. Histologic sections revealed fibrin, fat, fibrin-platelet aggregates, muscle fragments, and calcium emboli within the vasculature of brain sections. Eighty percent of patients who died after open heart surgery had fat emboli in the brain, but only 31% of these patients had nonfat emboli. The incidence of fat emboli was independent of all perfusion variables, whereas the incidence of nonfat emboli increased in patients perfused longer than 90 minutes.[34]

More recent studies have attempted to correlate changes in cerebral function with the occurrence of microemboli in the arterial perfusion line. Lee et al.[55] found that 23% of patients who had open heart surgery had postoperative neurologic deficits and 14% had psychiatric complications. Carlson et al.[7] found that 63% of patients perfused with a bubble oxygenator system and 36% perfused with a membrane oxygenator system had worse Bender-Gestalt visual motor test scores shortly after operation. Scores correlated roughly with ultrasonic counts of emboli in the arterial perfusion line (Table 10.2). Aberg and Kihlgren[54] also found temporarily decreased performance on psychomotor tests shortly after open heart surgery

Table 10.2
Bender-Gestalt Visual Motor Test:
Summary of Scores (47 Patients)*

	Percent of Worse Scores	
	Membrane Oxygenator	Bubble Oxygenator
No Filter	36	63
Filter	13	43

* Reprinted with permission from R. G. Carlson et al.[7]

and improved results when measures were taken to reduce the number of microemboli.

In dogs Taylor et al.[57] measured the brain-specific isoenzyme CPK-B in the cerebrospinal fluid. One hour of cardiopulmonary bypass causes a marked increase in this enzyme by the end of bypass. A 40-μm pore filter in the arterial line largely prevents the increase in the brain-specific isoenzyme.

From these and other studies,[53, 59, 64] accumulated data indicate that solid microemboli do block small arterial capillaries and do cause at least temporary cerebral damage as determined by brain-specific isoenzyme studies in dogs and psychomotor tests in patients. It is not known whether or not microemboli are related to the incidence of postoperative psychiatric disturbances, which in the past have occurred in up to 41% of patients.[65] Whether or not gaseous microemboli produce brain damage is not clear. In bubble oxygenator systems, microbubbles, which contain mostly oxygen, are infused in large numbers along with solid particles. Psychomotor test scores improve when the total number of infused emboli are reduced.[7, 53, 54] Since gaseous microbubbles are not selectively reduced, it is possible, but perhaps not probable, that the improvement is independent of the reduction in gaseous emboli and due only to a reduction in solid emboli.

PREVENTION OF MICROEMBOLI DURING EXTRACORPOREAL PERFUSION

Recognition of microemboli and the potential for organ damage has stimulated means to prevent their occurrence. The development of in-line filters is an important but not exclusive means for reducing microemboli during extracorporeal perfusion. Other measures relate to the choice of perfusion components and operation of the system.

Proper priming procedures can reduce the number of foreign particles entering the system. Crystalloids, colloids, and blood should be filtered (20 to 40 μm pore filters) to remove foreign particles.[43, 44, 47, 48] Additionally, the perfusate should be recirculated through the entire circuit and through a temporary filter to remove particles attached to the blood contact walls of the system.[47] Since small air bubbles can remain attached to dry, solid surfaces, the system ideally should be flushed with 100% CO_2 to reduce the amount of nitrogen within attached microbubbles before priming solutions are added.[66] This step is routine for membrane oxygenator systems, but also has merit for the smaller but still large solid surface areas of bubble oxygenator systems.

Membrane oxygenators produce far fewer microemboli than do bubble oxygenators.[7, 9, 36, 67] Although temperature changes, areas of cavitation, turbulence, and small tears and pinholes allow some gaseous emboli to form, properly primed and properly operated membrane oxygenators produce few gaseous microemboli.[7] There is also evidence that membrane oxygenators also produce less fat emboli,[33] but this possibility is not definite.[34] Early experimental studies indicate that membrane oxygenators cause less denaturation of proteins and lipoproteins[35] and also produce fewer nonfat particulate emboli.[9, 25, 36, 67]

During bypass, large temperature differences (>14°C) between arterial blood and patient should be avoided during both cooling and rewarming. Gas flow to blood flow ratios in bubble oxygenators should adequately saturate blood, but approach 1:1. The oxygenator should not be jostled or hit during operation, and several hundred milliliters of perfusate should be maintained in the reservoir.[10, 11] Only oxygen and carbon dioxide should be used in the gas line. With membrane oxygenators blood pressure should always exceed gas pressure within the device. The perfusionist must always be alert for membrane tears and holes during priming and operation and must be careful not to have poor connections or open stop-cocks through which air can enter the system.

Spallation from roller pump boots can be avoided by use of centrifugal pumps.[15, 51] Fibrin formation can be minimized by designs which favor streamlined flow paths and minimize areas of stagnation and turbulent flow. Most importantly, heparin anticoagulation must be adequate to prevent fibrin formation. Measurement of activated clotting times after the initial dose of heparin before starting bypass and at 30-minute intervals during bypass reduces the possibility of inadequate anticoagulation. Additional heparin is recommended when activated clotting times are less than 400 seconds. Drugs such as prostacyclin, that inhibit platelet activation and aggregate formation, have not been used routinely because of vasodilator properties which can reduce systemic blood pressure during perfusion below 50 mm Hg (mean).[68]

FILTERS IN THE CARDIOTOMY SUCTION SYSTEM

The cardiotomy suction system is the largest single source of solid particulate microemboli.[8, 9] Solis et al.,[9] using particle-counting techniques, found the concentration of microemboli in blood aspirated by the cardiotomy suction return system to be over 20 times the concentration in the arterial line (Fig. 10.2). After documenting the number and composition of microemboli found in brain sections of patients who died after open heart surgery, Hill and his colleagues[34, 64] introduced the Swank Dacron wool filter in the cardiotomy suction return line. They observed a significant decrease in postoperative mortality and also a decrease (from 30 to 4%) in the percentage of nonsurviving patients with nonfat emboli present in brain sections.[34, 64] The percentage of patients with fat emboli in brain sections did not change.[34]

Cardiotomy suction return filters are made of Dacron wool, polyurethane foam, or synthetic mesh and are incorporated within plastic reservoirs to form integral units. Dacron wool produces a three-dimensional (depth) filter with a large solid surface

area that effectively removes solid and gaseous particles down to 20 μm. Polyurethane foam can be made in varying pore sizes and combined to produce stratified depth filters, with pore sizes of 175, 75, and 27 μm.[34] Both Dacron wool and polyurethane foam filters cause the perfusate to traverse an irregular pathway through the thickness of the filter. Mesh filters are usually made of nylon and are woven to produce two-dimensional screens with uniform pores between 20 and 40 μm. Screens are usually pleated to increase the surface area of the filter.

Comparative studies of various commercial cardiotomy filtration systems indicate that all units are equally effective in removing solid particles greater than 40 μm, but vary in ability to remove smaller particles.[69, 70] In one study Dacron wool filters removed 89% of particulate emboli aspirated from the field, whereas nylon mesh (40-μm pores) and stratified polyurethane foam filters removed about 60% of these emboli.[9] Clarke et al.[33] found that Dacron wool filters also could remove fat emboli; however, in spite of filtration, fat emboli still develop downstream[71] as lipids and lipoproteins are denatured.

Removal of gaseous emboli is enhanced by increasing settling time of blood within the cardiotomy reservoir, reducing the amount of air aspirated, and adding a second filter downstream to the cardiotomy suction reservoir.[70, 72] In spite of these measures, a few gaseous emboli still enter the main perfusion circuit.[70]

Current commercial cardiotomy suction reservoir filters are designed to remove gaseous and solid particles greater than 20 μm in diameter. All contain some defoaming compound, and all utilize three-dimensional (depth) filters alone or in combination with a two-dimensional screen or mesh filter. Systems vary in reservoir volume, hold-up time, pressure gradients across the filter(s), and tendency to channel perfusate through the filter. Although no systematic comparative study has been performed, current commercial cardiotomy suction filtration systems adequately and effectively remove the majority of gaseous and solid microemboli greater than 40 μm in diameter.

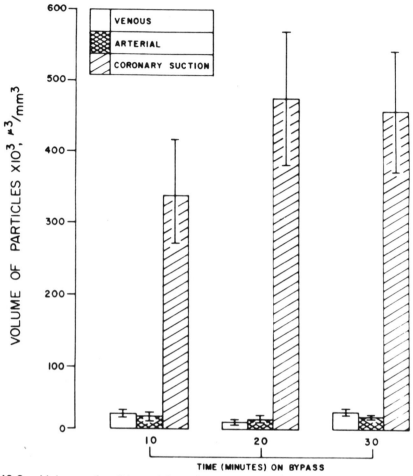

Figure 10.2. Volume of solid particles 13 to 80 μm in diameter in venous, arterial, and cardiotomy return line blood measured during first 30 minutes on cardiopulmonary bypass with membrane oxygenation (N = 19) (mean ± 1 SE). (Reproduced with permission from R. T. Solis et al.[9] and the American Heart Association, Inc.)

Passage of field-aspirated blood through filters capable of removing solid particles larger than 40 μm is now mandatory. The histologic studies of Hill et al.[34] and the results of psychomotor testing[7, 53, 54] indicate less morbidity (and perhaps mortality) if field-aspirated blood is filtered. Analysis of cardiotomy reservoir filters,[33] ultrasonic measurements,[7, 10] and particle counts[9, 36] confirm the efficacy of microfiltration of field-aspirated blood. Since field-aspirated blood is a priori severely traumatized, further damage to platelets, red cells, and leukocytes by the reservoir filter is inconsequential, unless very high negative pressures are used.[73] Clogging of these filters is not a problem. Although the need for even finer filters (20-μm pore size) has not been demonstrated, no disadvantage of these finer filters in the cardiotomy suction system has developed. For most open heart operations, recovery and autotransfusion of field blood is necessary to decrease requirements of homologous, stored blood. Microfiltration of heparinized, field-aspirated blood makes this possible.

ARTERIAL LINE FILTERS

In early extracorporeal perfusion systems, stainless steel arterial line filter-bubble traps were standard. These filters had pore sizes of 400 μm and thus did not prevent infusion of microemboli into the patient. Later, bubble oxygenator manufacturers introduced 170-μm pore filters within the oxygenator. Micropore filters were first introduced into arterial lines in the late 1960s.[64, 74] Initially, Dacron wool arterial filters developed high transfilter pressure differences and often needed to be changed during bypass.[74]

With the discovery of the organ damage and morbidity caused by microemboli produced during cardiopulmonary bypass,[7, 22, 25, 45, 49, 53–55, 58, 59, 75] improved microfilters were developed. Suitable arterial line filters were manufactured using a nylon or polyester mesh, polyurethane foam, or Dacron wool.[9, 10] The Dacron wool filter is highly efficient[9, 10] and is most effective in removing emboli less than 32 μm[37]; however, occasional instances of clogging during perfusion occur.[10] Efficiencies of arterial polyurethane foam and screen filters are similar.[10, 37] Currently most arterial line filters are screen filters with pore sizes of 20 to 40 μm and surface areas between 650 and 800 cm^2. Priming volume is approximately 200 ml and flow rates up to 6 liters/min are tolerated at pressure differences of 25 mm Hg or less.[10] The flow path is designed to encourage trapping of microbubbles at the top of the unit.

Both bubble and membrane oxygenator systems produce microemboli, but the concentration is far less than that found in cardiotomy suction return systems.[7, 9] All components of the system, including venous reservoirs, heat exchangers, and filters may produce solid emboli composed of fat, platelet aggregates, leukocytes, and amorphous material.[9, 33, 36] Bubble oxygenators produce large numbers of oxygen-carbon dioxide emboli and substantial numbers of particulate emboli.[7, 10, 23, 54] Membrane oxygenators produce a few gaseous emboli[7] and fewer particulate emboli.[9, 36, 76] (Fig. 10.3). Several studies indicate that bubble oxygenator systems produce far more solid and gaseous microemboli than do membrane oxygenator systems.[7, 9, 25, 33, 35, 36]

Arterial line filters are designed to remove emboli produced in the bypass system, those that escape blood priming solution

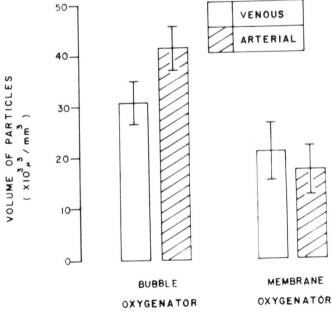

Figure 10.3. Volume of particles 13 to 80 μm in diameter in venous and arterial blood during first 10 minutes on cardiopulmonary bypass with bubble (N = 35) and membrane (N = 19) oxygenation (mean ± 1 SE). (Reproduced with permission from R. T. Solis et al.[9] and the American Heart Association, Inc.)

and cardiotomy suction return filters, and those produced by spallation of the pump boot. For bubble oxygenator systems, an arterial line filter significantly reduces the ber of microemboli perfused into the patient.[7, 9, 10, 23, 53, 54, 77] Although the filter removes both solid and gaseous emboli, the principal benefit is removal of gaseous microemboli which are produced in large numbers.[7, 10, 53, 54] Following bypass, analysis of filters for solid particles reveals primarily leukocyte and platelet aggregates,[16, 36, 71, 76, 78] rare fibrin,[79] occasional fat,[33] and some amorphous material.[36, 71] Variable amounts of solid emboli are trapped by the filter, and sometimes the amount may be small and consist principally of leukocytes.[78]

Arterial line filters also reduce the number of emboli perfused into the patient with membrane oxygenator systems.[7, 36, 53, 76] Ultrasonic counts downstream to membrane oxygenators are similar to counts downstream to arterial line filters of bubble oxygenator systems.[7, 53] Although an arterial line filter with a membrane oxygenator can further reduce the number of microemboli entering the patient, the benefit from this further reduction has not been measured.

Arterial line filters which require 200 ml to prime may be the source of microemboli and may contribute to the injury of formed blood elements.[79] Initial Dacron wool filters caused significant thrombocytopenia and hemolysis,[64] but improved models do not cause detectable changes in formed blood elements.[10] However, analyses of nylon mesh filters usually show large numbers of leukocyte aggregates which may have formed through the activation of complement[29] by the nylon mesh.[16] Since it is now possible to reduce the numbers of solid microemboli within extracorporeal perfusion systems by filtration of priming fluids and cardiotomy suction return blood, by rinsing the system before priming and by using a centrifugal pump, the benefits of arterial line filters must be carefully assessed.

Arterial line filters are recommended for bubble oxygenator systems to reduce the large numbers of gaseous emboli that would otherwise enter the patient. Although the

morbidity of these oxygen and carbon dioxide microemboli is not really known, arterial filtration results in improved early postoperative psychomotor test scrires[7, 53, 54] and reduction of a brain-specific isoenzyme in the cerebrospinal fluid of experimental animals.[57] As yet, the need to filter microemboli below 40 μm in diameter is not established. Logically, smaller pore filters should be better if the number of platelet and leukocyte aggregates is not increased, if red cells are not damaged, and if large pressure differences and clogging do not occur during perfusion.[79]

The need for arterial line filters in membrane oxygenator systems is less clear. Membrane oxygenators produce far fewer gaseous and solid emboli.[7, 23, 36, 76] Psychomotor tests have not shown benefits when an arterial line filter is added to a membrane oxygenator system.[7, 53] If established measures are taken to reduce the number of solid emboli within the circuit, and if a centrifugal pump is used, an arterial line filter does not materially change the number of solid microemboli entering the patient.

Based upon available information, the use of filters during short-term cardiopulmonary bypass can be summarized succinctly. Arterial filters are recommended for bubble oxygenator systems, but are optional for membrane oxygenator systems. However, cardiotomy suction return filters are mandatory. Optionally, a single arterial filter can be used in lieu of a cardiotomy suction return filter,[10] but this system is less effective than direct filtration of cardiotomy return blood.

References

1. Stoney WS, Alford WC Jr, Burrus GR, Glassford DM Jr, Thomas CS Jr: Air embolism and other accidents using pump oxygenators. Ann Thorac Surg 29:336, 1980.
2. Mills NL, Ochsner JL: Massive air embolism during cardiopulmonary bypass. J Thorac Cardiovasc Surg 80:708, 1980.
3. Kurusz M, Shaffer CW, Christman EW, Tyers GFO: Runaway pump head: New cause of gas embolism during cardiopulmonary bypass. J Thorac Cardiovasc Surg 77:792, 1979.
4. Kindwall EP: Massive surgical air embolism treated with brief recompression to six atmospheres fol-

lowing by hyperbaric oxygen. Aerospace Med 44:663, 1973.

5. Steward D, Williams WG, Freedom R: Hypothermia in conjunction with hyperbaric oxygenation in the treatment of massive air embolism during cardiopulmonary bypass. Ann Thorac Surg 24:591, 1977.

6. Kessler J, Patterson RH Jr: The production of microemboli by various blood oxygenators. Ann Thorac Surg 9:221, 1970.

7. Carlson RG, Lande AJ, Landis B, Rogoz B, Baxter J, Patterson RH Jr, Stenzel K, Lillehei CW: The Lande-Edwards membrane oxygenator during heart surgery. Oxygen transfer, microemboli counts and Bender-Gestalt visual motor test scores. J Thorac Cardiovasc Surg 66:894, 1973.

8. Clark RE, Deitz DR, Miller JG: Continuous detection of microemboli during cardiopulmonary bypass in animals and man. Circulation 54(Suppl. III):74, 1976.

9. Solis RT, Kennedy PS, Beall AC Jr, Noon GP, DeBakey ME: Cardiopulmonary bypass, microembolization and platelet aggregation. Circulation 52:103, 1975.

10. Loop FD, Szabo J, Rowlinson RD, Urbanek K: Events related to microembolism during extracorporeal perfusion in man: Effectiveness of in-line filtration recorded by ultrasound. Ann Thorac Surg 21:412, 1976.

11. Streczyn MV: Gas emboli arterial line filtration efficiencies of the Pall and JJ filters under stress conditions. AmSECT Proceedings 5:6, 1977.

12. Kamaryt JA, Jobgen EA, Naffah PH: Aeroemboli in the extracorporeal circuit. AmSECT, 14th International Conference, Atlanta, Georgia, 1980.

13. Miller SS, Mandl JP: Comparison of the effectiveness of various extracorporeal filters at reducing gaseous emboli. AmSECT Proceedings 5:55, 1977.

14. Bass RM, Longmore DB: Cerebral damage during open heart surgery. Nature 222:30, 1969.

15. Mandl JP: Comparison of emboli production between a constrained force vortex pump and a roller pump. AmSECT Proceedings, 1977, pp. 27–31.

16. Kurusz M, Schneider B, Conti VR, Williams EH: Scanning electron microscopy of arterial line filters following clinical cardiopulmonary bypass. Presented at the First World Congress on Open-Heart Technology, Brighton, England, July 13–17, 1981.

17. Rosenberg RD: Heparin action. Circulation 49:603, 1974.

18. Davies GC, Sobel M, Salzman EW: Elevated plasma fibrinopeptide A and thromboxane A_2 levels during cardiopulmonary bypass. Circulation 61:808, 1980.

19. Bull BS, Korpman RA, Huse WM, Briggs BD: Heparin therapy during extracorporeal circulation: Problems inherent in existing heparin protocols. J Thorac Cardiovasc Surg 69:674, 1975.

20. Young JA, Kisker CT, Doty DB: Adequate anticoagulation during cardiopulmonary bypass determined by activated clotting time and the appearance of fibrin monomer. Ann Thorac Surg 26:231, 1978.

21. Bull BS, Huse WM, Brauer FS, Korpman RA: Hep-

arin therapy during extracorporeal circulation: The use of a drug response curve to individualize heparin and protamine dosage. J Thorac Cardiovasc Surg 69:685, 1975.

22. Allardyce DB, Yoshida SH, Ashmore PG: The importance of microembolism in the pathogenesis of organ dysfunction caused by prolonged use of the pump oxygenator. J Thorac Cardiovasc Surg 52:706, 1966.

23. Abts LR, Beyer RT, Galletti PM, Richardson PD, Kairon D, Massimino R, Karlson KE: Computerized discrimination of microemboli and extracorporeal circuits. Am J Surg 135:535, 1978.

24. Dutton RC, Edmunds LH Jr: Measurement of emboli in extracorporeal perfusion systems. J Thorac Cardiovasc Surg 65:523, 1973.

25. Ashmore PG, Cvitek V, Ambrose P: The incidence and effects of particulate aggregation and microembolism in pump oxygenator systems. J Thorac Cardiovasc Surg 55:691, 1968.

26. Lee WH Jr, Hairston P: Structural effects on blood proteins at the gas-blood interface. Fed Proc 30:1615, 1971.

27. Lee WH, Krumhaar D, Fonkalsrud E, Schjeide OA, Maloney JV Jr: Denaturation of plasma proteins as a cause of morbidity and death after intracardiac operation. Surgery 50:29, 1961.

28. Clark RE, Beauchamp RA, Magrath RA, Brooks JD, Ferguson TB, Weldon CS: Comparison of bubble and membrane oxygenators in short and long perfusions. J Thorac Cardiovasc Surg 78:655, 1979.

29. Chenoweth DE, Cooper SW, Hugli TE, Stewart RW, Blackstone EH, Kirklin JW: Complement activation during cardiopulmonary bypass. N Engl J Med 304:497, 1981.

30. Vroman L, Adams AL, Klings M, Fischer G: Fibrinogen, globumin, albumin and plasma at interfaces. Adv Chemistry 145:255, 1975.

31. Wright ES, Sarkozy E, Dobell ARC, Murphy DR: Fat globulinemia in extracorporeal circulation. Surgery 63:500, 1963.

32. Arrants JE, Gadsden RH, Huggins MB, Lee WH Jr: Effects of extracorporeal circulation upon blood lipids. Ann Thorac Surg 15:230, 1973.

33. Clark RE, Margraf HW, Beauchamp RA: Fat and solid filtration in clinical perfusions. Surgery 77:216, 1975.

34. Hill JD, Aguilar MJ, Baranco A, deLanerolle P, Gerbode F: Neuropathological manifestations of cardiac surgery. Ann Thorac Surg 7:409, 1969.

35. Zapol WM, Levy RI, Kolobow T, Sprogg R, Bowman RL: In vitro denaturation of plasma alpha lipoproteins by bubble oxygenator in the dog. Curr Top Surg Res 1:449, 1969.

36. Dutton RC, Edmunds LH Jr, Hutchinson JC, Roe BB: Platelet aggregate emboli produced in patients during cardiopulmonary bypass with membrane and bubble oxygenators and blood filters. J Thorac Cardiovasc Surg 67:258, 1974.

37. Solis RT, Noon GP, Beall AC Jr, DeBakey ME: Particulate microembolism during cardiac operation. Ann Thorac Surg 17:332, 1974.

38. Hicks RE, Dutton RC, Reis CA, Price DC, Edmunds LH Jr: Production and fate of platelet aggregate

emboli during veno-venous perfusion. Surg Forum 24:250, 1973.

39. Connell RS, Page US, Bartley TD, Bigelow JC, Webb MC: The effect on pulmonary ultrastructure of dacron wool filtration during cardiopulmonary bypass. Ann Thorac Surg 15:217, 1973.

40. Ratliff NB, Young WG Jr, Hackel BB, Mikat E, Wilson JW: Pulmonary injury secondary to extracorporeal circulation. J Thorac Cardiovasc Surg 65:425, 1973.

41. Edmunds LH Jr, Addonizio VP Jr: Platelet physiology during cardiopulmonary bypass. In *Pathophysiology and Techniques of Cardiopulmonary Bypass*, edited by JR Utley, Vol. 1. Baltimore, Williams & Wilkins, 1981, pp. 106–119.

42. Starling JR, Murray GF, Adams K, Painter JC, Johnson G Jr: Erythrocyte filterability and lysosomal enzymes in patients requiring cardiopulmonary bypass. Surgery 77:562, 1975.

43. Swank RL: Alteration of blood on storage: Measurement of adhesiveness of "aging" platelets and leukocytes and their removal by filtration. N Engl J Med 265:728, 1961.

44. Donham RT: Rationale and indications for microfiltration of blood and emergency medicine. Med Instrum 11:344, 1977.

45. Connell RS, Swank RL: Pulmonary microembolism after blood transfusion—an electron microscope study. Ann Surg 177:40, 1973.

46. Moseley RV, Doty DB: Changes in the filtration characteristics of stored blood. Ann Surg 171:329, 1970.

47. Reed CC, Romagnoli A, Taylor DE, Clark DK: Particulate matter in bubble oxygenators. J Thorac Cardiovasc Surg 68:971, 1974.

48. Garvan JM, Gunner BW: The harmful effects of particles in intravenous fluids. Med J Aust 2:1, 1964.

49. Evans EA, Wellington JS: Emboli associated with cardiopulmonary bypass. J Thorac Cardiovasc Surg 48:323, 1964.

50. Kurusz M, Christman EW, Williams EH, Tyers GFO: Roller pump induced tubing wear: Another argument in favor of arterial filtration. J Extracorporeal Tech 12:49, 1980.

51. Hubbard LC, Kletschka HD, Olsen DA, Rafferty EH, Clausen EW, Robinson AR: Spalachian using roller pumps and its clinical implications. AmSECT Proceedings 3:27, 1975.

52. Gutman FA, Zegarra H: Occular complications in cardiac surgery. Surg Clin North Am 51:1095, 1971.

53. Landis B, Baxter J, Patterson RH Jr, Tauber CE: Bender-Gestalt evaluation of brain dysfunction following open-heart surgery. J Pers Assess 38:556, 1974.

54. Aberg T, Kihlgren M: Cerebral protection during open-heart surgery. Thorax 32:525, 1977.

55. Lee WH Jr, Miller W, Rowe J, Hairston P, Brady MP: Effects of extracorporeal circulation on personality and cerebration. Ann Thorac Surg 7:562, 1969.

56. Aberg T: Discussion of reference 2.

57. Taylor KM, Devlin BJ, Mittra SM, Gillan JE, Brannan JJ, McKenna JM: Assessment of cerebral damage during open-heart surgery: A new experimental model. Scand J Thorac Cardiovasc Surg 14:197, 1980.

58. Brierley JB: Brain damage complicating open heart surgery (a neuropathologic study): Proc R Soc Med 60:858, 1967.

59. Patterson RH Jr, Wasser JS, Porro RS: The effect of various filters on microembolic cerebrovascular blockade following cardiopulmonary bypass. Ann Thorac Surg 17:464, 1974.

60. Austen WG, Howry DH: Ultrasound as a method to detect bubbles on particulate matter in the arterial line during cardiopulmonary bypass. J Surg Res 5:283, 1965.

61. Katsumoto K, Watanabe S, Tanaka S: Evaluation of micropore filter in the extracorporeal circulation. Jpn Circ J 37:785, 1973.

62. Swank RL: The screen filtration pressure method in platelet research: Significance in interpretation. Ser Haematol 1:146, 1968.

63. Miller JA, Fonkalsrud EW, Latta HL, Maloney JV: Fat embolism associated with extracorporeal circulation in blood transfusion. Surgery 51:448, 1962.

64. Osburn JJ, Swank RL, Hill JD, Aguilar MJ, Gerbode F: Clinical use of a dacron wool filter during perfusion for open heart surgery. J Thorac Cardiovasc Surg 60:575, 1970.

65. Javid H, Tufo H, Najafi H, Dye WS, Hunter JA, Julian OC: Neurologic abnormalities following open heart surgery. J Thorac Cardiovasc Surg 58:502, 1969.

66. Wellons HA Jr, Nolan SP: Prevention of air embolization due to trapped air in filters used in extracorporeal circuits. J Thorac Cardiovasc Surg 65:476, 1973.

67. Page US, Bigelow JC, Carter CR, Swank RL: Emboli (debris) produced by bubble oxygenators. Ann Thorac Surg 18:164, 1974.

68. Ellison N, Addonizio VP Jr, Niewiarowski S, MacVaugh H III, Harken AH, Colman RW, Edmunds LH Jr: Platelet protection during cardiopulmonary bypass with albumin prime and prostaglandin E_1 infusion. Anesthesiology 53:S168, 1980.

69. Solis RT, Horak J: Evaluation of a new cardiotom blood filter. Ann Thorac Surg 28:487, 1979.

70. Pearson DT, Watson BG, Waterhouse PS: An ultrasonic analysis of the comparative efficiency of various cardiotomy reservoirs and micropore blood filters. Thorax 33:352, 1978.

71. Katsumoto K, Watanabe S, Tanaka S: Evaluation of micropore filter in the extracorporeal circulation. Jpn Circ J 37:785, 1973.

72. Maserko JJ, Sinkewich MG: Comparison of cardiotomy reservoirs with microaggregate filters. Proc Am Acad Cardiovasc Perfusion 1:9, 1980.

73. deJong JCF, ten Duis HJ, Smit Sibinga C Th, Wildevuur RH: Hematologic aspects of cardiotomy suction in cardiac operations. J Thorac Cardiovasc Surg 79:227, 1980.

74. Egeblad K, Osborn JJ, Burns W, Hill JD, Gerbode F: Blood filtration during cardiopulmonary bypass. J Thorac Cardiovasc Surg 63:384, 1972.

75. Brennan RW, Patterson RH Jr, Kessler J: Cerebral blood flow and metabolism during cardiopulmonary bypass. Evidence of microemboli encephalopathy. Neurology 21:665, 1971.

76. Guidoin RG, Kenedi RM, Trudell L, Galletti P, Blais P: Thrombus formation and microaggregate removal during extracorporeal membrane oxygenation. J Biomed Mater Res 13:317, 1979.

77. Hill JD, Osborn JS, Swank RL, Aguilar MJ, de-Lanerolle P, Gerbode F: Experience using a new dacron wool filter during extracorporeal circulation. Arch Surg 101:649, 1970.

78. Culliford AT, Gitel SN, Starr N, Thomas ST, Baumann FE, Wesler S, Spencer FC: Lack of correlation between activated clotting time and plasma heparin during cardiopulmonary bypass. Ann Surg 193:105, 1981.

79. Heimbecker R, Robert A, McKenzie FN: The extracorporeal pump filter—saint or sinner. Ann Thorac Surg 21:55, 1976.

CHAPTER 11

VENTING DURING CARDIOPULMONARY BYPASS

JOE R. UTLEY, M.D.
D. BARTON STEPHENS, C.C.P.

The advantages and disadvantages of ventricular venting have become a matter of controversy, particularly for coronary artery operations. Although the prevention of embolism by removing air was one of the reasons for venting the left ventricle in the past, more recently the risk of air embolism from venting has been a reason for not venting during coronary artery surgery.[1, 2]

EFFECTS OF VENTING OR DISTENTION

Ventricular venting may improve the ability of the surgeon to expose intracardiac structures during congenital heart or valve procedures. A properly functioning ventricular vent produces a dry operative field, improving exposure of the mitral valve, ventricular septal defect, and other intracardiac structures. Furthermore, retraction of the ventricle for exposure of posterior branches of the circumflex coronary artery or its main trunk in the atrioventricular groove may be facilitated by direct ventricular venting.[3] The decompressed ventricle requires less force and pressure for retraction, and myocardial injury may be diminished by venting.

Myocardial Effects

Elevations in intraventricular pressure in the fibrillating or ischemic myocardium increases oxygen consumption, increases sar-

comere length, and reduces coronary blood flow, particularly in the subendocardium. Distention of the left ventricle increases myocardial lactate production, elevates myocardial hydrogen ion concentration, and increases the efflux of potassium from the myocardium.[3] When the sarcomere is stretched beyond 2.2 to 2.4 μm, the ability to develop force decreases as the myofilaments become partially disengaged. At a length of 3.65 μm, the actin and myosin filaments are completely disengaged, and developed tension drops to zero.

Certainly, ventricular venting must be considered when the heart is fibrillating with or without aortic clamping. Hottenrott and Buckberg[43] showed that venting of the spontaneously or electrically fibrillated ventricle diminished left ventricular oxygen consumption. Distention produced increased subendocardial flow in the spontaneously fibrillating ventricle and decreased subendocardial flow in the electrically fibrillating ventricle. The endocardial to epicardial flow ratios were diminished by distention in both spontaneously and electrically fibrillating hearts, however (Fig. 11.1). Total ventricular flow was increased with both types of fibrillation with distention. Ventricular distention diminished coronary A-V O_2 differences and produced a transmural heterogeneity of flow with greater flow to the epicardium. Hottenrott also found increases in coronary sinus hydrogen

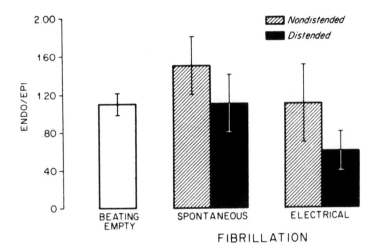

Figure 11.1. The ratio of endocardial to epicardial blood flow in the beating and fibrillating heart is shown. Ventricular distention diminished the relative subendocardial flow in both spontaneous and electrical fibrillation. (Reproduced with permission from C. Hottenrott and G. Buckberg.[43])

ion, lactate, and potassium concentration with distention (Fig. 11.2). He found that the biochemical and coronary flow changes with distention were followed by depression of left ventricular function curves following reperfusion.[4]

High intraventricular pressure produces high interstitial pressure in the subendocardial layers of the left ventricle. This high tissue pressure impedes coronary flow by increasing coronary venous pressure and compressing the coronary vascular bed.[5] This distention during delivery of cardioplegia may impede delivery of cardioplegia to the subendocardial areas.

The "payback" of the metabolic and oxygen diet incurred by a period of ischemia is facilitated by left ventricular venting.[4] The clinical study of Olinger and Boncheck[6] showed better ventricular function curves in patients who had ventricular venting than in those who did not. These studies were not performed with cardioplegia. The groups vented and not vented were operated upon in different hospitals with different surgeons, different anesthetic techniques, and different equipment was used for the studies.[7] The study does not seem conclusive regarding the benefits of venting.

Pulmonary Effects

High pulmonary venous pressure during cardiopulmonary bypass may contribute to pulmonary edema and lung dysfunction particular in patients with preoperative left ventricular failure or chronic pulmonary disease. Thus, either preexisting pulmonary disease or left ventricular dysfunction may be a selective indication for ventricular venting. Experimental studies have shown that no vent techniques produced higher left atrial pressures but no increase in lung water.[8]

Ventricular venting may diminish the rate of warning of the myocardium and may be used to cool the subendocardium by infusing cold saline through a cuff on the vent tube.[9] Venting may be selectively used for complex procedures requiring valve replacement with severe coronary disease which might limit the ability to deliver cardioplegia and cool the myocardium.

Evaluating Valve Function

Direct ventricular venting may be used to evaluate aortic and mitral valve function. In patients with severe mitral valve dysfunction and aortic valve insufficiency of ques-

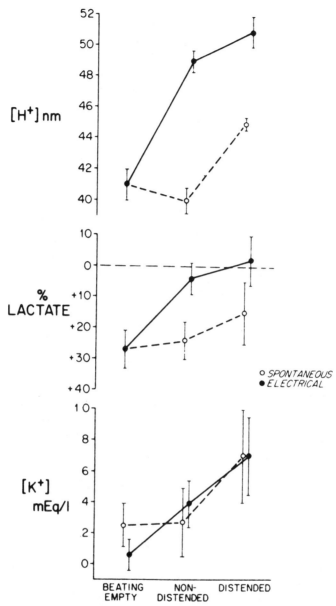

Figure 11.2. Distention of the spontaneously and electrically fibrillating ventricle increases the hydrogen ion, lactate, and potassium concentration of coronary venous blood. (Reproduced with permission from C. Hottenrott and G. Buckberg.[43])

tionable or indeterminant severity the flow from a vent in the left ventricular apex with the heart fibrillating and the aorta not clamped may be useful in determining the need for an aortic valve procedure. In patients with aortic insufficiency with congen-

ital ventricular septal defect, we have used this technique to evaluate aortic valve competence. Closure of the ventricular septal defect alone will occasionally correct the aortic insufficiency, whereas in other patients an aortic valvuloplasty is necessary to correct the aortic insufficiency. Thus, measurements of left ventricular vent flow permit one to determine the relative importance of VSD closure and aortic valvuloplasty in correcting the aortic insufficiency. Aortic pressure must be kept constant to make these observations valid, of course.

Infusion of blood into the left ventricle may be helpful in evaluating mitral valve function following mitral valve repair or replacement.[10] Nair and Yates[11] described a technique of infusion blood into the left ventricle to evaluate mitral valve function following reconstructive procedures. They recommended monitoring aortic and left ventricular pressures to avoid overdistention of the ventricle. Pomar and associates[12] used either a left ventricular catheter or an aortic catheter placed across the aortic valve to fill the ventricle and evaluate mitral valve function. These authors modified the cardiopulmonary bypass apparatus to allow infusion of blood through the vent catheter. King described a technique for creating flow into the left ventricle by advancing a catheter with multiple perforations from the left ventricular apex across the aortic valve. This technique was used to evaluate mitral valve leaks following mitral commissurotomy, repair of cleft mitral leaflet, and mitral valve replacement.

COMPLICATIONS OF VENTING

Left Ventricular Apex

Many complications have been reported following ventricular venting which have contributed to diminishing use of venting. Venting of the apex of the left ventricle has been associated with a significant incidence of myocardial injury, including new Q waves on postoperative electrocardiograms, contraction abnormalities, and elevation of myocardial enzymes.

Aintablian et al.[13, 14] found new Q waves after coronary bypass grafting in 22% of patients vented via the left ventricular apex, and in only 5% vented via the atrium. Postoperative ventriculogram did not always show contraction abnormalities in the region of the new Q wave, however.

Shaw et al.[15] found abnormalities of contraction of the left ventricular apex in 56%

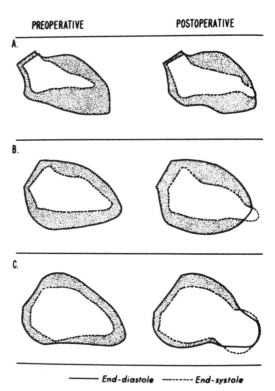

PREOPERATIVE　　　　　POSTOPERATIVE

——— End-diastole ---------- End-systole

Figure 11.3. The drawings show the end-systolic and end-diastolic contour of the left ventricle before and after venting through the apex of the left ventricle. The abnormalities range from minor contraction abnormalities to large ventricular aneurysms. (Reproduced with permission from R. A. Shaw et al.[15] and the American Heart Association, Inc.)

of patients with apical venting undergoing coronary artery bypass grafting and in none of the patients who did not have venting of the left ventricular apex (Fig. 11.3). Only 8% of patients having transventricular mitral commissurotomy with a Tubbs dilator showed contraction abnormalities. These data suggest that either the presence of coronary disease, associated cardiopulmonary bypass, or the length of time the device is in the left ventricular apex may be contributing factors in the development of contraction abnormalities. Apical left ventricular aneurysms were found in 32% of children having venting of the left ventricular apex for repair of congenital heart disease.[16] Al-

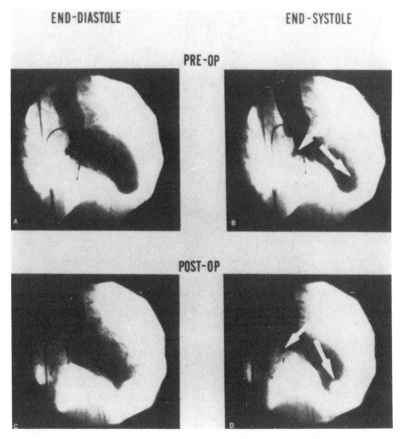

Figure 11.4.   The postoperative ventriculogram shows a mural thrombus at the site of left ventricular venting. (Reproduced with permission from A. Aintablian et al.[17])

though these contraction abnormalities are not often the cause of heart failure, mural thrombi have been observed at the site of apical left ventricular vent[17] (Fig. 11.4). Cerebral emboli may originate from the ventricular vent site.[18] False aneurysms of the left ventricle producing masses on chest x-ray have developed following left ventricular venting. These may require surgical excision and closure[19, 20] (Fig. 11.5). Factors which may contribute to postoperative contraction abnormalities include: elevated intracardiac pressures, hypertension, residual aortic stenosis or left ventricular outflow obstructions, size of cardiotomy, infection, and the use of inotropic drugs postoperatively.[21] Thus, injury of left ventricular myocardium is a risk of venting the left ventricular apex.

Air Emboli

Ventricular vents may introduce air into the left side which can become systemic air emboli. Zwart et al.[22] note 16% of patients had air introduced into the left ventricle by venting. The vent may be useful in removing air from the left ventricle. The introduction of air into the ventricle is particularly troublesome during coronary artery surgery. Left ventricular air will usually inevitably occur during congenital heart procedures or valve replacement procedure.

Bleeding

Other objections to venting include the time required to place and remove the vent, thus prolonging cardiopulmonary bypass,

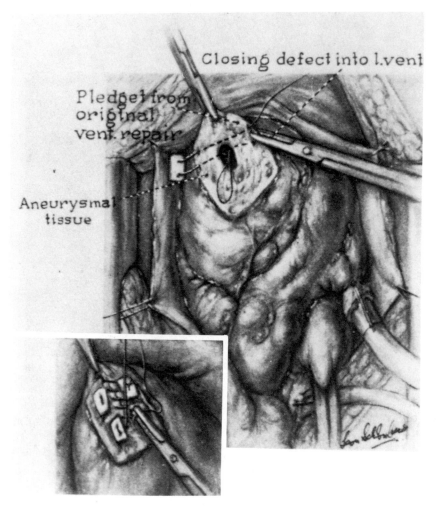

Figure 11.5. The figure shows a false aneurysm at the site of previous left ventricular venting. (Reproduced with permission from H. B. Robinson and J. S. Donahoo.[21])

and the occasional troublesome bleeding which may occur at a vent site. The left ventricular apex in the dilated and hypertrophied ventricle with increased wall tension may be a difficult site to control bleeding, especially following aortic valve replacement for chronic aortic insufficiency. Other infrequent complications of venting include perforation of the ventricle or atrium and obstruction of pulmonary veins at the site of vent insertion.

Arrhythmia

Arrhythmias from the presence of the vent or following removal of the transmy-

ocardial vent may occasionally be difficult problems. Vents within the left ventricle may contribute to postoperative left bundle branch blocks or hemiblocks on the electrocardiogram.

Summary of Relative Advantages

Figure 11.6 is an analysis of the relative advantages and disadvantages of various routes of ventricular venting. The greater advantage gained from direct venting of the left ventricle through the apex or atrium is associated with a greater incidence and severity of myocardial injury, introduction of

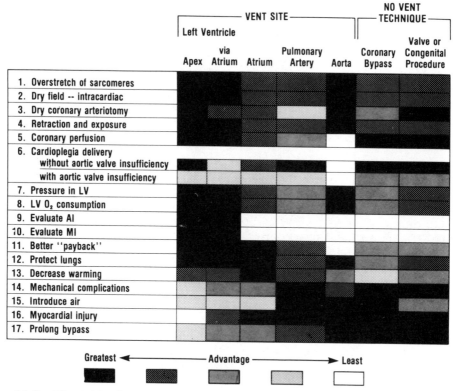

Figure 11.6. The table shows the authors' subjective assessment of the relative advantages or disadvantages of various forms of venting for types of cardiac surgical procedures in relation to the goals of venting and complications of venting.

air, and complications of closure of the cannulation site.

Valve Insufficiency

The presence of insufficiency of the aortic or mitral valve may affect the advantages gained from ventricular venting. During direct venting of the left ventricle, the vent may "steal" from the aortic root and diminish coronary flow or cardioplegia delivery. Thus, when infusing cardioplegia into the aortic root in the presence of aortic insufficiency one may choose to compress the ventricle occasionally to prevent distention rather than to aspirate blood directly from the left ventricle. Similarly, when both aortic insufficiency and mitral insufficiency are present cardioplegia injected into the aortic root may be aspirated from a left atrial or pulmonary artery vent catheter. On the other hand, decompression of the left ven-

tricle during postischemic recovery and payback may be particularly important in the presence of residual aortic insufficiency. Similarly, mild aortic insufficiency may make the use of intermittent clamping without ventricle venting result in high intraventricular pressure during reperfusion and pulmonary edema.

Venting of any site except the left ventricle is not useful when evaluating the severity of aortic or mitral valve insufficiency.

Cardioplegia

The main advantage of aortic venting is in combination with cardioplegia. The same needle used for cardioplegia may be used for aortic venting. The aortic vent is not helpful for venting during the period before or after aortic clamping or during cardioplegia infusion.

Pulmonary Artery Venting

The presence of complete mitral valve competence is the main failing of pulmonary artery venting. A completely competent mitral valve may allow ventricular distention with pulmonary artery venting.

NO VENT TECHNIQUE

A number of studies have been published showing the safety of "no vent" techniques for coronary and valve surgery.[2,22-28] The studies of Miller et al.[29,30] of the current practice of coronary artery surgery in 1975 and in 1980 showed that fewer surgeons were venting for coronary artery bypass procedures in 1980 than previously. He found that during this 5-year period, the percent of surgeons not venting for coronary artery surgery increased from 17.0 to 29.7% ($p < 0.001$). The percent who always vented decreased from 64.3 to 52.9%. The group who sometimes vented remained about the same, 18.9% in 1975 and 17.4% in 1980. The site of venting also changed during this period. A smaller percent of those venting used the left ventricular apex, and more used the right superior pulmonary vein or aortic root compared to 5 years previously. The right superior pulmonary vein was the most popular site of venting in both surveys, however. In 1975 it was noted that surgeons with larger caseloads were less likely to vent during coronary artery surgery.

Detecting Distention

Use of the "no vent" technique requires the surgeon to be alert to the development of distention to avoid complication of distention. The surgeon may determine the presence of distention by monitoring the left atrial or left ventricular pressure. Monitoring pulmonary artery pressure with a Swan-Ganz catheter may also detect distention. Visual observation and palpation of the ventricle may help one to determine early distention. Palpation of the pulmonary artery may be useful. The surgeon should carefully note the distention of any heart chamber during cardiopulmonary bypass.

Contraindications

Okies et al.[26] reported the safety of the no vent technique in coronary artery surgery using intermittent aortic clamping. He noted that the technique was contraindicated in the presence of aortic unsufficiency and that venting must sometimes be substituted to achieve a dry coronary arteriotomy.

Zwart's group[22] studied patients with and without ventricular venting during ventricular fibrillation and cardiopulmonary bypass. They found left ventricular, left atrial, and pulmonary artery pressures were higher without venting. They also found higher oxygen content in the pulmonary artery without ventricular venting, indicating retrograde flow through the pulmonary circulation. This is supportive of the efficacy of pulmonary artery venting.

Arom et al.[3] found that the incidence and severity of left ventricular distention was not great in dogs without ventricular venting unless caval slings were used. Thus, if the venous drainage from the heart into the venous lines is totally open without caval slings there is sufficient back flow to the caval cannulae, to decompress the left ventricle.

Nonventing Techniques of Ventricular Decompression

The distended left ventricle can be decompressed into the aorta by hand massage when the no vent technique is used.[23] When using the no vent technique for valve surgery, the surgeon must be particularly observant of the status of ventricular distention after the aortic clamp is removed and the ventricle is recovering from ischemia. Achieving a sinus rhythm and a regular ventricular contraction with sinus rhythm or a pacemaker diminishes the risk of distention because the heart can eject. If distention occurs, the surgeon may clamp the aorta and relieve the distention via the aorta. An aortic cardioplegia vent cannula is useful for this purpose. Distention during no vent techniques is more likely to occur with aortic valve insufficiency and higher perfusion pressures. Compressing the left ventricle and aorta prior to aortic clamping with no vent technique develops a capacitance in the chambers to allow filling with blood with high pressures or distention.

Air Emboli

Removal of air may be a problem with the no vent technique for valve replacement, although the risk of air embolus is low when air is carefully evacuated through the aortotomy or atriotomy.[23, 25]

Selective Use

The selective use of venting is becoming popular with many surgeons. Venting may be used selectively in coronary artery patients with aortic insufficiency, poor left ventricular function, and when cardioplegia is used. The use of aortic venting with cardioplegia is becoming a popular combination.[31, 32]

TECHNIQUES OF LEFT VENTRICULAR VENTING

Venting of the left ventricle may be accomplished by a variety of techniques which vary according to the type of suction or decompression, site of venting, and type of cannula or catheter.

Type of Suction or Evacuation

The most simple type of venting is merely an incision into the chamber, allowing the blood under pressure to exit from the incision. This is the technique often employed by making an atrial incision as cardioplegia is being infused. The left atrium is incised for mitral or aortic valve procedures and the right atrium is incised for congenital procedures in the presence of an atrial or ventricular septal defect.

Attaching the vent catheter or cannula to a side arm of the venous drainage system has the advantage of applying very low suction and thus diminishing the incidence and volume of air entry into the heart.[33] The method of siphon decompression into a separate reservoir independent of the cardiopulmonary bypass apparatus has been used effectively.[34] Intermittent or low suction pump drainage also has the advantage of minimizing the entry of air into the heart.[35, 36] Sump catheters with small side

arms that allow entry of air into the catheter but not into the heart may prevent the catheter holes from becoming obstructed against the side of the heart chamber without allowing air to enter the heart. Often air will enter around the catheter or cannula when negative pressure is applied to the vent system.

Venting with a cardiotomy suction apparatus is quite effective but usually allows entry of large volumes of air.

Site of Venting

Some of the complications and difficulties of various cannulation sites have been discussed previously.

LEFT VENTRICULAR APEX

Although venting by this route is effective in accomplishing the goals of venting, the incidence of complications, myocardial injury, and difficulties closing the vent site are such that fewer surgeons routinely use this route than in the past. Venting the apex with ventricular aneurysm repair has advantages with few complications (Fig. 11.7).

LEFT VENTRICULAR VENTING BY THE ATRIAL ROUTE

This was the most popular method of venting in coronary artery surgery in Mill-

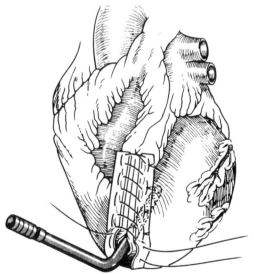

Figure 11.7. Venting through the repair of left ventricular aneurysm is a site of air removal with few complications.

er's survey of 1980. The catheter is introduced into the atria and advanced across the mitral valve into the left ventricle. Placing the right hand behind the ventricle may help deflect the catheter from the posterior left atrial wall and across the mitral valve. A rigid obturator in the catheter has been used but may increase the risk of atrial or ventricular perforation. Placement into the ventricle may be more difficult in previously operated patients because of adhesions. Delayed ventricular rupture following transatrial venting has been reported, especially in short patients.[37] The length of catheter should be carefully determined to avoid ventricular injury.

RIGHT SUPERIOR PULMONARY VEIN

This popular approach is usually performed by placing a purse string suture in the wall of the right superior pulmonary vein, often incorporating the adventitia of the adjacent atrial wall or interatrial groove.

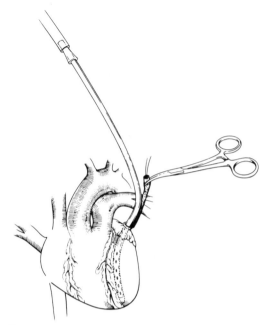

Figure 11.9. The left atrial appendage may be used as a site for placing a left atrial or left ventricular vent.

A stab incision in the purse string followed by a dilator creates a hole for insertion of the catheter.

The main disadvantage of this technique is the occasional difficulty encountered in closing the cannulation site. Pulmonary vein obstruction has been reported as a complication of this technique.

SUPERIOR APPROACH TO LEFT ATRIUM

This technique uses an approach to the atrium sometimes used for mitral valve exposure. This is a convenient and safe technique using a purse string similar to that used for the right superior pulmonary vein. If the patient has been previously operated upon, one must be careful to avoid the right pulmonary artery when the catheter is inserted.[38] The atrial incision is placed behind the atrial septal attachment between the aorta and superior vena cava (Fig. 11.8). Delayed left ventricular rupture has been described after transatrial venting of the left ventricle. This complication may be related to inserting the catheter too far into the ventricle and is perhaps more common in patients with short stature.

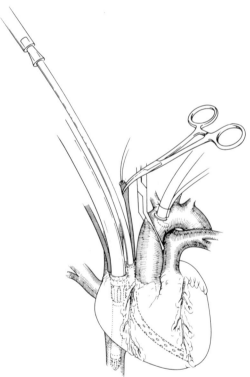

Figure 11.8. The superior approach to the left atrium between the superior vena cava and the aorta is a convenient way of venting the atrium or ventricle in some patients.

LEFT ATRIAL APPENDAGE

In some patients access to the left atrial appendage is easier than to the previously mentioned sites and either atrial or transatrial ventricular decompression may be performed through the left atrial appendage. This cannulation is usually most easily accomplished by amputating a small piece of the appendage for insertion of the catheter and closing it by ligation (Fig. 11.9).

TRANSATRIAL APPROACH

When wide exposure within the right atrium is being accomplished to perform a procedure requiring exposure of only the right side of the heart, a vent catheter may be introduced into the left atrium or the left ventricle across a patent foramen ovale or a stab in the fossa of the foramen ovale. Some of the procedures in which this technique may have some advantages include transatrial closure of ventricular septal defect and tricuspid valve replacement.

The site of venting of the atrium is a convenient site for placing a line for left atrial pressure monitoring postoperatively.

PULMONARY ARTERY VENTING

Pulmonary artery venting appears to be increasing in popularity, particularly with increased use of single venous drainage for cardiopulmonary bypass. The ease of insertion and closure is one of the great advantages of this technique. Its main drawback is the failure to decompress the left ventricle with a completely competent mitral valve. It also is not a useful site for air evacuation from the left side of the heart but may be very important in air evacuation from the pulmonary circulation following congenital heart procedures. Pulmonary artery air may be an important cause of transient pulmonary hypertension after repair of congenital heart defects.

The technique described by Heimbecker and McKenzie[39] is a form of pulmonary artery venting which creates incompetence of the pulmonary valve and drainage of the blood through the right ventricle.

AORTIC VENTING

The use of the aortic needle for venting after infusing cardioplegia is becoming in-

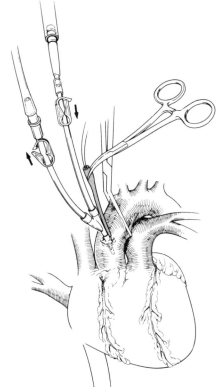

Figure 11.10. The needle placed in the ascending aorta for cardioplegia infusion is a convenient site for venting during aortic clamping. The vent is also useful for air evacuation.

creasingly popular[31, 32, 40, 41] (Fig. 11.10). This technique has certain disadvantages, including the ability to vent the ventricle when the aorta is clamped and the inability to vent the ventricle while cardioplegia is being infused. The venting may be by syphon into the pump oxygenator[31] or by attaching the needle to coronary suction.[32] Engelman and Rousou[40] employ a technique in which a multihole catheter is placed in the aorta for cardioplegia infusion. Some of the proximal holes are withdrawn from the aortic wall to allow decompression after cardioplegia is infused. When the vein grafts are attached to the aorta first the vein may be used as a means of venting the aorta after the aorta is clamped and cardioplegia is infused.[42]

RIGHT SIDED VENTING OF THE LEFT VENTRICLE

When an atrial and/or ventricular septal defect is present, an incision into the right atrium as cardioplegia is infused allowing the blood under pressure in the atria to escape is a useful and practical method of decompressing the heart and harvesting the cardioplegia solution from the right atrium. In patients with tetralogy of Fallot or ventricular septal defect, placing a cardiotomy suction through the ventricular septal defect into the left ventricle is a very effective means of achieving a dry operative field and decompressing the left ventricle.

References

1. Miller BJ, Gibbon JH Jr, Greco VF, Cohn CH, Allbritten FF Jr: The use of a vent for the left ventricle as a means of avoiding air embolism to the systemic circulation during open cardiotomy with the maintenance of the cardiorespiratory function of animals by a pump oxygenator. Surg Forum 4:29, 1953.
2. Charrett EJP, Salerno TA: Is left ventricular decompression necessary during coronary artery surgery? Can J Surg 22:121, 1979.
3. Arom KV, Vinas JF, Fewel JE, Bishop VS, Grover FL, Trinkel JK: Is a left ventricular vent necessary during cardiopulmonary bypass? Ann Thorac Surg 24:566, 1977.
4. Buckberg GD: The importance of venting the left ventricle. Ann Thorac Surg 20:488, 1975.
5. Utley JR, Michalsky GB, Mobin-Uddin K, Bryant LR: Subendocardial vascular distortion at small ventricular volumes. J Surg Res 17:114, 1974.
6. Olinger GN, Boncheck LI: Ventricular venting during coronary revascularization: Assessment of benefit by intraoperative ventricular function curves. Ann Thorac Surg 26:525, 1978.
7. Oldham HN Jr: Left ventricular venting during coronary bypass operation. Ann Thorac Surg 26:497, 1978.
8. Jara FM, Toledo-Pereyra LH: Lung water accumulation with and without left ventricular venting during cardiopulmonary bypass. Eur Surg Res 12:363, 1980.
9. Zumbro GL, Treasure RL: A simple and effective left ventricular vent tube. Ann Thorac Surg 21:458, 1975.
10. King H, Csicsko J, Leshnower A: Intraoperative assessment of the mitral valve following reconstructive procedures. Ann Thorac Surg 29:81, 1980.
11. Nair KK, Yates AK: Direct evaluation of mitral valve function during surgery following conservative procedures. J Thorac Cardiovasc Surg 73:684, 1977.
12. Pomar JL, Cucchiara G, Gallo I, Duran CMG: Intraoperative assessment of mitral valve function. Ann Thorac Surg 25:354, 1978.
13. Aintablian A, Hamby RI, Hoffman I, Weisz D, Voleti C, Wisoff BG: Significance of new Q waves after bypass grafting: Correlations between graft patency, ventriculogram, and surgical venting technique. Am Heart J 95:429, 1978.
14. Aintablian A, Hamby RI, Hoffman I, Weisz D, Voleti C, Wisoff BG: Significance of new Q waves after bypass grafting: Correlation between graft patency, ventriculogram, and surgical venting technique. Chest 70:418, 1976.
15. Shaw RA, Kong Y, Protchett ELC, Warren SG, Oldham HN, Wagner GS: Ventricular apical vents and postoperative focal contraction abnormalities in patients undergoing coronary artery bypass surgery. Circulation 55:434, 1977.
16. Weesner KM, Byrum C, Rosenthal A: Left ventricular aneurysms associated with intraoperative venting of the cardiac apex in children. Am Heart J 101:622, 1981.
17. Aintablian A, Hamby RI, Kramer RJ, Wisoff BG: Unusual complications of coronary bypass surgery. Am Heart J 96:17, 1978.
18. Murphy DA, Krause VW: Fatal cerebral embolus—a complication of left ventricular venting. Can J Surg 19:228, 1976.
19. Lee SJK, Ko PTH, Hendin D, Sterns LP: False left ventricular aneurysm as a complication of open heart surgery. Can Med Assoc J 115:45, 1976.
20. Fallah-nejad M, Abelson DM, Blakemore WS: Left ventricular pseudoaneurysm. Chest 61:90, 1972.
21. Robinson HB, Donahoo JS: Postoperative aneurysms of the heart. J Cardiovasc Surg 18:181, 1977.
22. Zwart HHJ, Brainard JZ, DeWall RA: Ventricular fibrillation without left ventricular venting. Ann Thorac Surg 20:418, 1975.
23. Salerno TA, Charrett EJP: Prospective analysis of valvular replacement without venting the left ventricle. J Thorac Cardiovasc Surg 78:131, 1979.
24. Salerno TA, Charrett EJP: Elimination of venting in coronary artery surgery. Ann Thorac Surg 27:340, 1979.
25. Najafi H, Javid H, Goldin MD, Serry C: Aortic valve replacement without left heart decompression. Ann Thorac Surg 21:131, 1976.
26. Okies JE, Phillips SJ, Crenshaw R, Starr A: "No-Vent" technique of coronary artery bypass. Ann Thorac Surg 19:191, 1975.
27. Molina JE: Rapid hypothermic cardioplegia and air venting with an aortic root cannula. Bull Texas Heart Inst 5:150, 1978.
28. Ullyot DJ: Current controversies in the conduct of the coronary bypass operation. Ann Thorac Surg 30:192, 1980.
29. Miller DW Jr, Hessel EA II, Winterscheid LC, Merendino KA, Dillard DH: Current practice of coronary artery bypass surgery. J Thorac Cardiovasc Surg 73:75, 1977.
30. Miller DW Jr, Ivey TD, Bailey WW, Johnson DD, Hessel EA: The practice of coronary artery bypass surgery in 1980. J Thorac Cardiovasc Surg 81:423, 1981.
31. Salomon NW, Copeland JG: Single catheter technique for cardioplegia and venting during coronary artery bypass grafting. Ann Thorac Surg 30:88, 1980.
32. Harlan BJ, Kyger ER III, Reul GJ Jr, Cooley DA: Needle suction of the aorta for left heart decompression during aortic cross-clamping. Ann Thorac Surg 23:259, 1977.
33. Cox WD, Sharp EH: Left ventricular venting with-

out suction in myocardial revascularization. J Thorac Cardiovasc Surg 64:472, 1972.

34. Lajos TZ, Lee AB, Schimert G: Decompression of the heart with siphon drainage. Ann Thorac Surg 25:454, 1978.

35. Ross IM, Theman TE: Intermittent venting of the left ventricle. Ann Thorac Surg 31:379, 1981.

36. Munnell ER, Grantham RN: Left ventricular decompression by sump drainage. Ann Thorac Surg 28:397, 1979.

37. Breyer RH, Lavender S, Cordell AR: Delayed left ventricular ruture secondary to transatrial left ventricular vent. Ann Thorac Surg 33:189, 1982.

38. Siderys H: The superior approach for operative decompression of the left side of the heart. Ann Thorac Surg 17:277, 1974.

39. Heimbecker RO, McKenzie FN: A new approach to left heart decompression. Ann Thorac Surg 21:456, 1976.

40. Engelman RM, Rousou JH: Left ventricular venting during cardioplegic arrest. Ann Thorac Surg 28:603, 1979.

41. Marco JD, Barner HB: Aortic venting. Comparison of vent effectiveness. J Thorac Cardiovasc Surg 73:287, 1977.

42. Bolgan FJ, Federico AJ, Guarino RL: An alternative method of left ventricular decompression during aortocoronary bypass. Ann Thorac Surg 23:476, 1977.

43. Hottenrott C, Buckberg G: Studies of the effects of ventricular fibrillation on the adequacy of regional myocardial flow. II. Effects of ventricular distention. J Thorac Cardiovasc Surg 68:626, 1974.

CHAPTER 12

PULSATILE FLOW DURING CARDIOPULMONARY BYPASS

WILLIAM Y. MOORES, M.D.

The existence of pulsations in the circulation has been recognized for many centuries. Pulsations were noted prior to the description of the circulation by Harvey and was alluded to by classic scholars.[1] Nonpulsatile flow during cardiopulmonary bypass has been most commonly practiced. This practice is due primarily to the ease of producing nonpulsatile flow compared to pulsatile flow during cardiopulmonary bypass. Early experience with these nonpulsatile roller pumps failed to reveal any major detrimental effects due to the lack of arterial pulsations, and generally good results were achieved.[2] The maintenance of renal function was a major concern, and several studies documented satisfactory renal function during nonpulsatile flow.[3–5]

Acceptable results were achievable with nonpulsatile flow; however, there was interest in the idea that perfusions could be improved if pulsatile flow was used. Some investigators noted that increasing peripheral resistance and lactic acidosis could be diminished with pulsatile cardiopulmonary bypass.[2] Most early studies concentrated on general circulatory effects, such as changes in vascular resistance, oxygen consumption, and lactate production. These clinical and experimental studies produced varied results but, in general, suggested a beneficial effect of cardiopulmonary bypass. The mechanism for these benefits was not conclusively established. However, there was a general feeling that the benefits were due to the increased energy in pulsatile flow at a given mean arterial pressure that resulted in improved lymph flow and more effective opening of capillary beds.[6, 7]

EFFECTS ON TISSUE PERFUSION

Adequate oxygen delivery is the *sine qua non* of acceptable circulatory support. Most authors showed that pulsatile flow increased oxygen consumption compared to linear flow.[8–10] The increased oxygen consumption during pulsatile flow was interpreted as being beneficial, especially because most studies showed decreased lactic production as well. A reduction in peripheral vascular resistance was also noted during pulsatile perfusion and was likewise interpreted as beneficial.[11, 12] The energy of pulsatile flow may be as much as 2.3 times the amount of energy in linear flow at the same mean arterial pressure. Many authors postulated that the decrease in peripheral resistance was due to more effective opening of the capillary bed from the increased energy available in pulsatile flow. Other investigators postulated that the decreased peripheral resistance was due to maintenance of more physiologic neurological reflex activity and/or catecholamine blood levels. Another detrimental effect of cardiopulmonary bypass was increased water accumulation, and pulsatile flow helped promote more effective lymphatic flow.[10,11,13]

Neurologic Effects

Direct observation of the cerebral circulation has been carried out in animal studies with both pulsatile and nonpulsatile flow with the finding of improved circulation with pulsatile flow.[14] Other studies have attempted to determine the adequacy of neurologic reflex activity and, again, have substantiated improved function when a pulse pressure is present.[15-18] Clinical investigations have been less conclusive but have shown earlier extubation of patients maintained on pulsatile flow during cardiopulmonary bypass.[19]

Myocardial Effects

Prior to the wide use of ischemic arrest with cold cardioplegia the myocardium was perfused from a nonpulsatile pump. This nonpulsatile perfusion might be provided for a beating nonworking heart, a beating partially working heart, or a fibrillating heart, depending on the operative situation. Preservation of myocardial function under these conditions was occasionally inadequate, and several investigations were initiated to determine whether the heart could be better preserved on cardiopulmonary bypass with pulsatile perfusion.

Beating Heart

In our laboratory, studies were done to determine whether pulsatile flow was important in preserving the function of the beating nonworking heart on cardiopulmonary bypass. Our initial study was carried out in a canine model in an attempt to determine the advantage of pulsatile flow in maintaining left ventricular function. This study showed a slight decrease in function that was not reversed by pulsatile flow.[20] The studies showed no difference in left ventricular dp/dt. The study showed no increase in peripheral resistance with linear flow. We did note a slightly increased lactate extraction when pulsatile flow was used, but this was not accompanied by any significant change in myocardial oxygen consumption. In an attempt to determine why a pulsatile flow failed to provide any advantage in a beating heart, further studies were performed using a swine model. Swine were chosen because the animal was obtainable in a more uniform size due to standards of agricultural breeding, and because the swine's coronary circulation appears to more closely approximate that of man, especially in terms of cardiovascular reserve and the lack of significant collateral flow. An initial study examining the beating swine myocardium supported by pulsatile and nonpulsatile flow, with and without a pressure load in the ventricle, was carried out. The surgical preparation for this study is presented in Figure 12.1. Phasic blood flow in the left coronary artery was monitored during these perfusion conditions, and it became apparent that pulsatile flow within the coronary circulation was well maintained, despite the presence or absence of a pulse pressure in the ascending aorta. Furthermore, this pulsation in the coronary arteries was maintained either with or without a pressure load in the left ventricle. Of interest was the fact that an augmentation of this flow pattern could not be substantiated with synchronized pulsatile flow. We quantitated the diastolic to systolic flow ratios in the left anterior descending coronary artery and noted that a flow ratio of approximately 3:1 was preserved in all conditions. All of the pulsatile modalities exemplified a diastolic to systolic flow ratio which was greater than the value of 2.6, which was the ratio we found in the coronary circulation without cardiopulmonary bypass. Typical examples of the wave forms during the studies are presented in Figure 12.2. The conclusion following this study[21] was that an artificially maintained pulse pressure appeared to have no major role in determining pulsatile flow within the coronary circulation. This impression was further substantiated by the failure to discern any difference in endocardial to epicardial flow ratios with the various perfusion modalities.

Ventricular Fibrillation

Standard linear perfusion of the myocardium during ventricular fibrillation had been shown to be detrimental by several investigators,[22] and it was postulated that these detrimental effects might be reversed by the institution of pulsatile perfusion. This

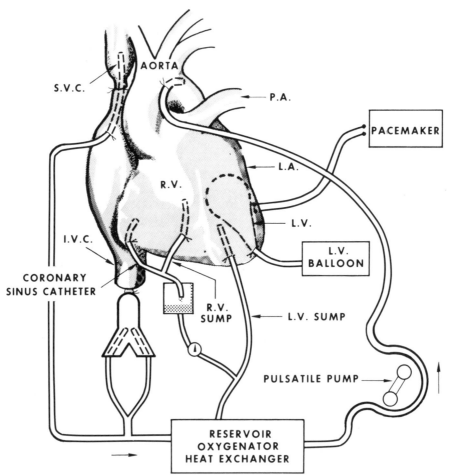

Figure 12.1. Diagram showing extracorporeal circuit for evaluation of pulsatile flow with a loaded and unloaded ventricle. *S.V.C.*, superior vena cava; *I.V.C.*, inferior vena cava; *R.V.*, right ventricle; *P.A.*, pulmonary artery; *L.A.*, left atrium; *L.V.*, left ventricle.

question was actively studied in our laboratory, again using a perfused swine model, with the finding that in these short-term perfusions no significant beneficial effect from pulsatile flow could be discerned.[23] In fact, it was impossible to negate this pulsatile coronary flow within the coronary circulation, even if the aortic root perfusion was 180° out of phase. This finding is illustrated in Figure 12.3, showing synchronized and unsynchronized pulsatile flow in the beating heart. With the heart supported during ventricular fibrillation, the flow within the coronary artery system is determined by the aortic root perfusion pressure. If this pressure is nonpulsatile, the coronary flow

is likewise nonpulsatile, but if pulsatile pressure is applied to the aortic root, this pressure is accompanied by pulsatile flow within the coronary bed. Pressure and flow wave forms depicting this phenomena are illustrated in Figure 12.4. This study again failed to substantiate any benefit to the myocardium in terms of endocardial flow when pulsatile perfusion was used in the fibrillation heart. During these short-term perfusions, fibrillation did cause a decrease in the endocardial to epicardial flow ratio, and this decreased ratio was not reversed with the institution of pulsatile flow. The question of the role of pulsatile perfusion in preserving left ventricle function following fibrillation

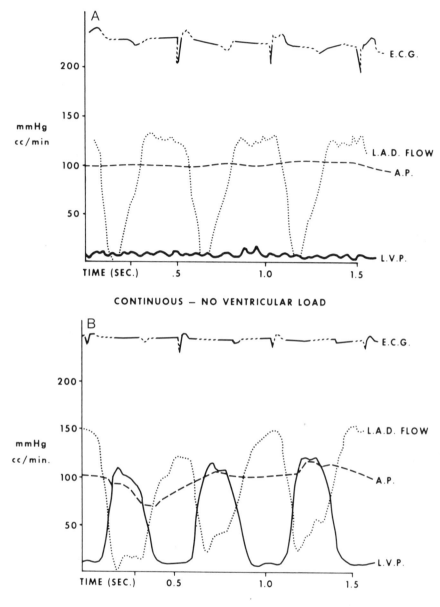

Figure 12.2. (A) Actual wave form tracings taken from an animal during continuous flow in an unloaded ventricle. Note continuation of pulsatile flow in the left anterior descending coronary artery even during continuous perfusion. (B) Wave form tracings from an animal during continuous flow in the beating heart with the ventricular pressure low. *L.A.D.*, left anterior coronary artery; *A.P.*, aortic pressure; *L.V.P.*, left ventricular pressure.

was addressed in an additional study using a right heart bypass preparation in swine.[24] This study, which examined a longer period of perfusion, revealed that hearts perfused with linear flow while in a state of fibrillation did manifest a decrease in stroke volume at a given end-diastolic pressure. This decrease did not occur if the fibrillating

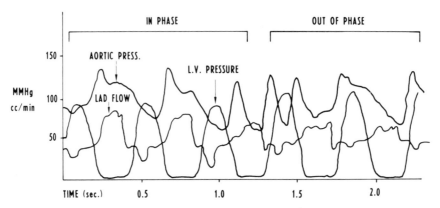

Figure 12.3. Wave form tracings taken from an actual animal showing pulsatile flow in the left anterior descending coronary artery with pulsatile perfusion which is initially in phase and subsequently out of phase. Note the continuation of pulsatile flow in the left anterior descending coronary artery; even the pump is out of phase. *LAD*, left anterior descending; *LV*, left ventricular.

hearts were supported with pulsatile flow. The stroke volume values for this study are seen in Table 12.1. Of interest was the finding that a decreased endocardial to epicardial flow ratio also accompanied the decreased stroke volume measurement following 1 hour of support of the fibrillating heart with continuous flow. These values are summarized in Table 12.2. The findings and conclusions from this study were confirmed and supported by an additional study by Dunn and his associates,[25] using a canine model with a balloon-loaded left ventricle. They also noted lower values in their left ventricular force measurements in fibrillating hearts supported with linear flow as opposed to pulsatile flow.

Abnormal Hearts

The role of pulsatile flow in providing a more adequate perfusion beyond a fixed coronary stenosis has been investigated with the finding of improved perfusion with pulsatile flow.[26]

The question of maintenance of adequate myocardial perfusion in hypertrophied hearts, with and without pulsatile flow, has been examined in some depth by Salerno and his associates.[27, 28] They found that during high flow rates pulsatile perfusion did not effect endocardial flow distribution.

Furthermore, at moderate to low flows, subendocardial ischemia with ventricular fibrillation occurred, and this ischemia was not reversed with pulsatile flow. Additional studies have failed to show any beneficial effect of pulsatile flow on myocardial oxygen consumption in the beating nonworking heart.[23, 29]

Clinical studies have appeared in the literature attempting to determine the importance of pulsatile perfusion during cardiopulmonary bypass. Results of these studies have been mixed, with some authors failing to find any significant difference in hemodynamics between perfusion modalities.[30-32] Maddoux and his associates,[33] in a study utilizing an intraaortic balloon pump to achieve pulsatile flow, did note an improved ejection fraction in patients supported with pulsatile flow during cardiopulmonary bypass in contrast to those supported with linear flow.

Other Organ Effects

Numerous studies, both clinical and experimental, have documented the beneficial effects of pulsatile cardiopulmonary bypass on several organ systems. Most of these studies have concentrated on kidney function and have substantiated an increased urine output with pulsatile flow as well as

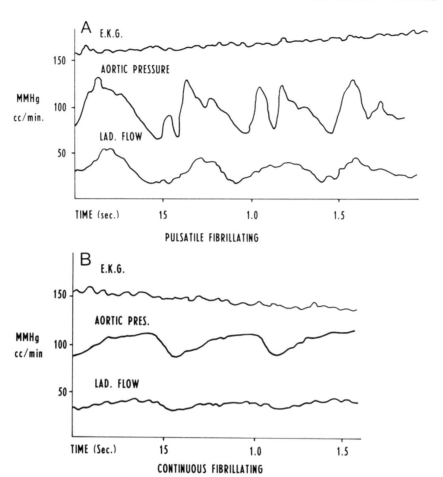

Figure 12.4. (A) Wave form tracing showing left anterior descending coronary artery flow present in the fibrillating heart when the aortic route is perfused with pulsatile pressure. Note the pulsatile flow occurring as aortic pressure is varied. (B) Wave form tracings taken from a typical animal during continuous perfusion of fibrillating heart. Note the absence of any significant pulsatile flow when there is no significant variation in aortic pressure. *LAD,* left anterior descending coronary artery.

Table 12.1
Stroke Volume (ml) at 8 mm Hg Left Ventricular End-Diastolic Pressure

	Beating		Fibrillating	
	Continuous	Pulsatile	Continuous	Pulsatile
Control	8.7 ± 1.6	9.7 ± 1.6	12.6 ± 1.4	9.4 ± 1.1
1 hr	9.8 ± 2.0	9.8 ± 2.5	9.2 ± 1.1*	9.0 ± 1.0
2 hr	7.2 ± 1.3	8.6 ± 2.2	9.1 ± 1.3*	9.3 ± 1.2

*$p < 0.025$ control *vs.* 1, 2 hours.

Table 12.2
Endocardial to Epicardial Flow Ratios

	Beating		Fibrillating	
	Continuous	Pulsatile	Continuous	Pulsatile
Control	1.35 ± 0.12	1.35 ± 0.12	1.22 ± 0.12	1.30 ± 0.07
1 hr	1.43 ± 0.17	1.39 ± 0.08	$1.03 \pm 0.08*$	1.32 ± 0.12
2 hr	1.31 ± 0.12	1.40 ± 0.04	1.29 ± 0.12	1.43 ± 0.07

* $p < 0.05$ control vs. 1 hour.

improved renal vein flow.[11, 34, 35] Some authors failed to substantiate these benefits if the mean arterial pressure was kept constant and at a sufficiently high value.[3-5,36] Some of this discrepancy may be due to the various methods of producing "pulsatile flow." The variation in energy values for various types of pulsatile flow production can vary considerably, as has been pointed out by Wright and his colleagues.[7] However, the finding of an increased urine output has been substantiated clinically in studies examining pulsatile flow with a compression device. These studies have attempted to find a significant hemodynamic advantage with pulsatile flow, but have generally concluded with the finding of increased urine output in patients supported with pulsatile flow during cardiopulmonary bypass.[37, 38]

The response of the lung to nonpulsatile flow was examined experimentally by Clark et al.,[39] who showed some detrimental effects from nonpulsatile flow. The oxygenation function of the lung was preserved, but alveolar thickening and an increase in pulmonary resistance was noted with linear flow. In an earlier study by Wesolowski et al.,[40] no difference in pulsatile or linear flow for the pulmonary circulation could be discerned. They substantiated the preservation of normal pulmonary function in spite of the perfusion modality used.

Isolated reports in the literature have examined the effects of pulsatile flow on other organ systems and have provided some evidence for improved organ function with pulsatile flow. We examined postperfusion amylase values in a clinical population following perfusion with pulsatile and nonpulsatile flow and found generally decreased values when pulsatile flow was employed.[41]

PULSATILE DEVICES

The earliest pulsatile pumps employed diaphragm systems that were driven by compressed air and employed one-way heart valves to facilitate forward flow. These devices were inherently more complicated and less reliable than standard roller pumps and consequently never found wide usage. Present pulsatile pumping systems almost always use a standard roller pump as the primary propulsive force. The pulsation in both flow and pressure are subsequently superimposed either by a tube compression system[37] or by a motor start and brake circuit that interrupts the normally continuous roller pump movement.[42] Both of these "modified" roller pump systems are provided with a synchronization system that allows the systolic pressure pulse to be delivered during the patient's diastole. The synchronization systems are identical with those presently used in intraaortic balloon pumping and, in fact, the compression devices can frequently be driven off a minimally modified intraaortic balloon pump. If these pulsatile perfusion systems are to be used during partial bypass when substantive flow through the patient's heart is occurring, then this synchronization is mandatory.

Other devices that are capable of producing pulsatile flow include systems that accentuate the normal pulsations in roller pumps by inserting either a very large caliber tube in the pump head or by inserting an asymmetric segment in the head.[43] The character of the pulse created by these simple devices may be quite adequate to provide the benefits of pulsatile flow during cardiopulmonary bypass when there is no flow through the heart, but the pulsatile feature of this system is of no value during partial bypass or during weaning of the patient from bypass.

Clinical Experience

Several authors have reported clinical experience with these simpler more effective pulsatile devices. Many of the authors in their enthusiasm for the devices have attempted to document major hemodynamic benefits with the devices but have generally not been able to reproduce the improvement in ventricular function that was noted by Maddoux and his associates[33] in their use of an intraaortic balloon to produce pulsatile flow. Bregman et al.[32] used his "PAD" pulsatile system in 300 patients and documented a significantly increased urine output and greater saphenous vein graft flow in those patients supported on pulsatile flow rather than on linear flow. He failed to document any substantive hemodynamic effect, and the increased urine and graft flows were not correlated with a significantly improved clinical course. Kaplitt and Tamari[38] used an almost identical device in 15 patients and also noted similar effects in terms of urine output and coronary bypass graft flow. The failure to produce a significant hemodynamic benefit with these devices was further emphasized by Frater et al.[30] in another clinical study.

Concern with central nervous system abnormalities prompted Williams and his associates[19] to use the Datascope PAD device in 15 patients and compare their response to a matched group of 15 patients undergoing linear perfusion. Their principal finding was that infants perfused with pulsatile flow had significantly shorter extubation times. More efficient perfusion of these infants was further supported by shorter warming times when a pulse pressure was provided. Higher urine flow were also noted during pulsatile perfusion, but again no hemodynamic effects were substantiated.

PULSED OR PULSELESS PERFUSION: DOES IT MAKE A DIFFERENCE?

The evidence currently available[44] argues for the value of pulsatile flow during car-

diopulmonary bypass. The issue becomes problematic because pulsatile flow using the modified roller pumps cannot be provided without some cost, either in terms of an additional dollar cost for a disposable compression device (*e.g.*, Datascope PAD system) or in terms of additional equipment costs and complexibility that many feel unnecessarily complicates generally acceptable clinical perfusions using nonpulsatile systems. Many of the earlier pump-related problems that prompted the investigations into the importance of preserving pulsatile flow have disappeared with improvements in oxygenators, priming solutions, and the general conduct of clinical perfusions. Almost all of these improvements have been in the absence of pulsatile perfusion. The decision to use or not to use pulsatile flow during cardiopulmonary bypass would seem to depend on how important the various organ flow benefits are for a particular patient in whom the added cost would be appropriate.

The major reason for lack of wider application of pulsatile flow in current practice would seem to revolve around the lack of any substantitive effect for the myocardium. With the widespread use of cardioplegic arrest the heart is effectively taken out of the perfusion circuit, and it becomes irrelevant what type of perfusion is being supplied. Fibrillation is now avoided in most circumstances and when the heart is returned to the perfusion circuit it is usually returned in a beating nonworking state. Our own work, as well as supporting data from other laboratories, has failed to substantiate any "myocardial preservation" effect with pulsatile flow. A review of the unique coronary flow characteristics in the beating heart, as well as our own investigations into the diastolic/systolic flow ratios during bypass with linear and pulsatile flow, seem to provide conclusive evidence of why a benefit should not be expected. It therefore appears that any benefit for the myocardium with pulsatile flow is limited to perfusion of the fibrillating heart. Artificially induced and maintained ventricular fibrillation is now rarely used, and the value of pulsatile flow for the heart fades into nonrelevance with its disappearance. It would seem logical that synchronized pulsatile partial bypass would still be appropriate for those patients that require additional cardiopulmonary bypass support following operation. Unfortunately, it is difficult to obtain data from any comparative study in either an appropriate patient population or animal model.

In conclusion, it can be stated that pulsatile perfusion does "make a difference." The question that remains is how important that difference is for the various clinical situations that are encountered during the conduct of cardiac surgery. If the "cost" of pulsatile perfusion in terms of "dollars" and complexity becomes lower and more appropriate, then one can probably anticipate a wider application of this mode of perfusion during cardiopulmonary bypass.

References

1. Harris CRS: *The Heart and Vascular System in Ancient Greek Medicine.* Oxford, Clarendon, 1973.
2. Trinkle JK, Helton NE, Wood TC, et al: Metabolic comparison of a new pulsatile pump and a roller pump for cardiopulmonary bypass. J Thorac Cardiovasc Surg 58:562, 1969.
3. Goodyer AVN, Glenn WL: Relation of arterial pulse pressure to renal function. Am J Physiol 167:689, 1951.
4. Selkut EE: Effects of pulse pressure and mean arterial pressure modification on renal hemodynamics and electrolyte and water excretion. Circulation 4:541, 1951.
5. Ritter ER: Pressure flow relationships in the kidney: Alleged effects of pulse pressure. Am J Physiol 68:480, 1952.
6. Shepard RC, Simpson DC, Sharp IF: Energy equivalent pressure. Arch Surg 93:730, 1966.
7. Wright G, Sanderson JM, Furness A: Pulsatile pumps for open-heart surgery. Lancet, January 28, 1978.
8. Shepard RB, Kirklin JW: Relation of pulsatile flow to oxygen consumption and other variables during cardiopulmonary bypass. J Thorac Cardiovasc Surg 58:694, 1969.
9. Ogata T, Ida Y, Nonoyama A, et al: A comparative study on the effectiveness of pulsatile and non-pulsatile blood flow in extracorporeal circulation. Arch Jpn Chir 29:59, 1960.
10. Dunn J, Kirsh MM, Harness J, et al: Hemodynamic, metabolic and hematologic effects of pulsatile cardiopulmonary bypass. J Thorac Cardiovasc Surg 68:138, 1974.
11. Nakayama I, Tamiya, Yamamoto K, et al: High amplitude pulsatile pump in extracorporeal circulation with particular reference to hemodynamics. Surgery 54:798, 1963.
12. Mendelbaum I, Burns WH: Pulsatile and non-pulsatile blood flow. JAMA 191:121, 1965.
13. Jacobs LA, Klopp EH, Seamone W, et al: Improved organ function during cardiac bypass with a roller pump to deliver pulsatile flow. J Thorac Cardiovasc Surg 58:703, 1969.
14. Matsumoto T, Wolferth CC Jr, Perlaman MH: Effects of pulsatile and non-pulsatile perfusion upon cerebral and conjunctival microcirculation in dogs. Am Surg 37:61, 1971.
15. Angell James JE: The effects of altering mean pressure pulse pressure and pulse and frequency of the impulse activity in baroreceptor fibres from the aortic arch and right subclavian artery in the rabbit. J Physiol (Lond) 214:65, 1971.
16. Angell James JE: Their responses of aortic arch and right subclavian baroreceptors of changes of non-pulsatile pressure and their modification by hypothermia. J Physiol (Lond) 214:201, 1971.
17. Angell James JE, de Burgh Daly M: Comparison of the reflex vasomotor responses to separate and combined stimulation of the carotid sinus and aortic arch baroreceptors by pulsatile and non-pulsatile pressures in the dog. J Physiol (Lond) 209:257, 1970.
18. Angell James JE, de Burgh Daly M: Effects of graded pulsatile pressure on the reflex vasomotor responses elicited by changes of mean pressure in the perfused sinus-aortic arch regions of the dog. J Physiol (Lond) 214:51, 1971.
19. Williams GD, Seifen AB, Lawson NW, Norton JB, Readinger RI, Dungan TW, Callaway JK: Pulsatile perfusion versus conventional high-flow nonpulsatile perfusion for rapid core cooling and rewarming of infants for circulatory arrest in cardiac operation. J Thorac Cardiovasc Surg 78:667, 1979.
20. Moores WY, Hannon JP, Tyberg JV, Crum JD, Rodkey WG, Willford DC: Synchronized pulsatile extracorporeal coronary perfusion: Its effects on preservation of left ventricular function in the beating non-working canine heart. Institute Report No. 57, Letterman Army Institute of Research, Presidio of San Francisco, 1979.
21. Moores WY, Hannon JP, Crum JD, Willford DC, Rodkey WG, Geasling JW: Coronary flow distribution during continuous and pulsatile extracorporeal perfusion in the pressure loaded and unloaded swine left ventricle. Fed Proc 35:599, 1977.
22. Hottenrott CE, Towers B, Kurkji HJ, et al: The hazard of ventricular fibrillation in hypertrophied ventricles during cardiopulmonary bypass. J Thorac Cardovasc Surg 66:742, 1973.
23. Moores WY, Hannon JP, Crum JD, Willford DC, Rodkey WG, Geasling JW: Coronary flow distribution and dynamics during continuous and pulstile extracorporeal circulation in the pig. Ann Thorac Surg 24:582, 1977.
24. Moores WY, Hannon JP, Crum JD, Willford DC: Continuous and pulsatile extracorporeal coronary perfusion in the beating and fibrillating swine myocardium: Effects on left ventricular function. Surg Forum 28:262, 1977.
25. Dunn J, Peterson A, Kirsh MM: Effects of pulsatile perfusion upon left ventricular function. J Surg Res 25:211, 1978.
26. Schaff HV, Ciardullo R, Flaherty JT, Brawley RK, Gott VL: Myocardial ischemia distal to critical cor-

onary stenosis during cardiopulmonary bypass: Fibrillating versus beating nonworking heart. Surg Forum 27:248, 1976.

27. Salerno TA, Shizal HM, Dobell ARC: Blood flow with roller vs. pulsatile pump during cardiopulmonary bypass in hypertrophied hearts. Surg Forum 25:141, 1974.

28. Salerno TA, Shizal HM, Dobell ARC: Pulsatile perfusion: Its effects on blood flow distribution in hypertrophied hearts. Ann Thorac Surg 27:559, 1979.

29. Kane JJ, Straub KD, Murphy ML, Peng CF, Bisset JK: Left ventricular wall thickness and epicardial ST segment mapping during acute ischemia and reperfusion. Clin Res 25:6a, 1977.

30. Frater RWM, Wakayama S, Oka Y, Becker R, Desai P: Pulsatile cardiopulmonary bypass: Failure to influence hemodynamics or hormones. Circulation 59,60(Suppl. II):34, 1979.

31. Trinkle JK, Helton NE, Bryant LR, Griffin WO: Pulsatile cardiopulmonary bypass: Clinical evaluation. Surgery 68:1074, 1970.

32. Bregman D, Bailin M, Bowman FO Jr, et al: A pulsatile assist device for use during cardiopulmonary bypass. Ann Thorac Surg 24:574, 1977.

33. Maddoux G, Pappas G, Jenkins M, et al: Effect of pulsatile and non-pulsatile flow during cardiopulmonary bypass on left ventricular ejection fraction early after aortocoronary bypass surgery. Am J Cardiol 37:1000, 1976.

34. Hooker DR: Study of isolated kidney: Influence of pulse pressure on renal function. Am J Physiol 27:24, 1910.

35. Hamel G: Die Bedeutung des Pulses fur den Blutstrom. Z Biol NSF:474, 1889.

36. Oelert H, Eufe R: Dog kidney function during total left heart bypass with pulsatile and non-pulsatile flow. J Cardiovasc Surg (Torino) 15:674, 1974.

37. Bregman D, Parodi EN, Haubert SM, et al: Counterpulsation with a new pulsatile assist device (PAD) in open heart surgery. Med Instrum 10:232, 1976.

38. Kaplitt MJ, Tamari Y: Clinical experience with the Tamari-Kaplitt pulsator: A new device to create pulsatile flow or counterpulsation during open heart surgery (abstr.). Am J Cardiol 39:620, 1977.

39. Clarke CP, Kahn DR, Dufek JH, et al: The effects of non-pulsatile blood flow on canine lungs. Ann Thorac Surg 6:450, 1968.

40. Wesolowski SA, Fisher JH, Welch CS: Perfusion of pulmonary circulation by non-pulsatile flow. Surgery 33:370, 1953.

41. Moores WY, Gago O, Morris JD, Peck CC: Serum and urinary amylase levels following pulsatile and continuous cardiopulmonary bypass. J Thorac Cardiovasc Surg 74:73, 1977.

42. Moores WY, Kahn DR, Kirsh MM, Gago O, Carr EA Jr, Abrams GD, Dufek J, Sloan H: Mechanical support of the circulation by a modified pulsatile roller pump. Ann Thorac Surg 12:262, 1971.

43. Ciardullo R, Schaff HV, Flaherty JT, et al: A new method of producing pulsatile flow during cardiopulmonary bypass using a standard roller pump. J Thorac Cardiovasc Surg 72:585, 1976.

44. Mavroudis M: To pulse or not to pulse. Ann Thorac Surg 25:259, 1978.

CHAPTER 13

CARDIOPLEGIC SOLUTION: WHAT COMBINATION OF ADDITIVES?

STEVEN R. WYTE, M.D.

In 1955 Melrose et al.[1] used chemical cardioplegia to induce cardiac arrest. Injecting potassium citrate (25 to 100 mg/ml) into the aortic root, arrest occurred within 5 minutes, but normal ventricular function postarrest could not be restored in some animals, even though microscopic examination of the cardioplegia-arrested tissue showed normal cellular architecture. The potassium citrate technique was abandoned when reports[2] appeared describing a high incidence of ventricular fibrillation without ventricular decompression, diffuse fatty degeneration, and myofibrillar necrosis following 30 minutes of ischemia.

Cardiac standstill was then introduced by anoxic aortic cross-clamping or by continuous electrical fibrillation.[3] Myocardial metabolic requirements were reduced by systemic[4] and topical hypothermia[5]; substrate and oxygen were supplied by intermittent coronary perfusion.[6]

Maloney and Nelson[7] reviewed the literature prior to 1975 and concluded that a 20-minute ischemic period at 32°C could be tolerated by the heart without the need for inotropic support (Fig. 13.1). Reducing myocardial temperature to between 16 and 20° extended the anoxic "safe period" to 30 minutes.

The use of hypothermia as an adjuvant to cardiac surgery reduces cardiac rate and myocardial oxygen consumption.[8] At 28°C,

stroke oxygen demand remains unchanged or increases with hypothermia-induced positive inotropy. Overall oxygen consumption decreases when heart rate falls. At lower temperatures coronary resistance increases and subendocardial flow decreases. Topical hypothermia selectively decreases myocardial temperature below systemic temperature, thereby increasing myocardial protection and decreasing the deleterious effects of hypothermia (Fig. 13.2). If a topically cooled heart is lifted out of the pericardial needle exposing the anterior surface to the operating room lights, a temperature gradient occurs between the endocardium and epicardium.[9] This gradient is exacerbated in patients with ventricular hypertrophy.

Continuous electrical fibrillation[3] produces a 50% rise in oxygen consumption, and a rapid fall in ATP, creatinine phosphate (CP), and glycogen stores. During coronary artery perfusion in a fibrillating heart, flow is diverted away from the subendocardial surface. Inadequate ventricular venting causes a rise in left ventricular end-diastolic pressure (LVEDP) and a further decrease in subendocardial flow.

Intermittent coronary perfusion provides inadequate myocardial oxygenation, metabolite substrate enhancement, or washout of catabolic products. Intermittent perfusion for 5 minutes followed by ischemia for 15 minutes decreases myocardial contractility, compliance, and increases myocardial edema. If the cyclical periods are prolonged beyond 90 minutes, there is a progressive fall in adenine nucleotides.

The need for longer periods of arrest and better myocardial preservation renewed interest in chemical cardioplegia.

Gay and Ebert[10] substituted potassium chloride for potassium citrate, reduced the potassium concentration to 25 mEq/liter, adjusted the pH to 7.5, and osmolality to 275 mOsmoles/liter. Following cardioplegic infusion and ischemic arrest microscopic ex-

amination revealed slight myocardial edema but otherwise normal architecture. Reidemeister et al.[11] and Kirsch et al.[12] also described effective cardioplegic solutions containing magnesium and procaine (Table 13.1).

Since the initial favorable reports, a proliferation of new techniques with different cardioplegic agents and substrates has produced confusion and raised questions concerning the most appropriate technique. The purpose of this report is to simplify and compare the various animal and human data available and to present a rational approach to the use of cardioplegia.

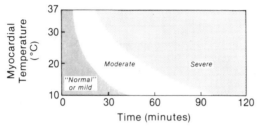

Figure 13.1. Composite of data from various authors comparing myocardial temperature to anoxic cross-clamp ties. (Reproduced with permission from J. V. Maloney and R. L. Nelson.[7])

Table 13.1
Chemical Principles for Inducing Cardiac Arrest*

1. Myocardial depletion of calcium.
2. Myocardial depletion of sodium.
3. Elevation of extracellular potassium.
4. Elevation of extracellular magnesium.
5. Infusion of local anesthetic agents.
6. Infusion of calcium and antagonistic agents.

* Reprinted with permission from D. J. Hearse et al.: *Protection of the Ischemic Myocardium: Cardioplegia.* New York, Raven Press, 1981.

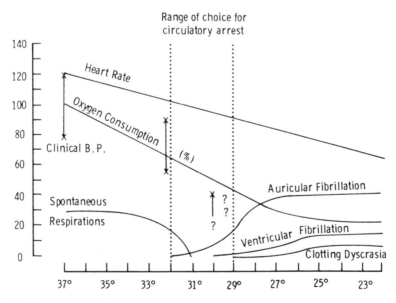

Figure 13.2. Effects of surface hypothermia on heart rate, respiration, blood pressure, and oxygen consumption. (Reproduced with permission from H. Swan.[8])

CARDIOPLEGIC COMPONENTS

Potassium

Potassium rapidly infused into the cross-clamped aorta depolarizes the myocardial cells, producing sustained diastole. Asystole decreased the amount of ATP consumption and reduced oxygen demand after cross-clamping. Hearse et al.[13] plotted a potassium dose-response curve in the isolated rat heart (Fig. 13.3). A concentration of 10 to 20 mEq/liter rapidly produced arrest, while a concentration exceeding 30 mEq/liter increased coronary vascular resistance due to a calcium-activated rise in left ventricular tension. Asanguineous cardioplegic solutions containing over 30 mEq of potassium per liter can cause severe intimal damage.[14] At 24°C arrest can be induced with 13 mEq/liter KCl. Although the dose-response curves suggest that optimal potassium cardioplegic concentration should be between 12 and 20 mEq/liter, Tucker et al.[15] and Ellis et al.,[16, 17] comparing hypothermic cardioplegic solutions containing 5 and 20 mEq/liter, found that ejection fractions, cardiac index, stroke work, oxygen consumption, and myocardial compliance measured after cardiopulmonary bypass were virtually identical. The group receiving 5 mEq of potassium per liter had a prolonged period to arrest (131 seconds) as compared to the high potassium group (54 seconds). The high potassium group had a higher incidence of AV dissociation arrhythmias. Ellis

suggests that 20 mEq of potassium per liter should be administered initially to produce asystole, and when repeated the infusion should contain 5 mEq/liter. Blood cardioplegia must contain 30 mEq/liter KCl to produce asystole at 20°C.[18] Prolonged ischemia reduces intracellular potassium and increases sodium ion intracellular flux. A fall in ATP concentration inactivates the sodium-potassium pump mechanism. Following an osmotic gradient, water enters the cell, causing cellular edema and reducing ventricular compliance. Potassium containing cardioplegia may reverse or partially negate this effect.

Magnesium

Elevating magnesium levels to a cardioplegic concentration (15 mEq/liter)[19] (Fig. 13.4) depresses both the inherent rhythmicity of pacemaker cells and myocardial contractility.[20] Pacemaker cells are unstable, due to a slow inward flux of sodium which eventually reduces action potential to the firing level. Magnesium blocks the inward flow of sodium into the cells and also interferes with systolic depolarization. Magnesium competes with calcium at activation sites at ATP, suppressing myocardial ATPase activity and decreasing myocardial contractility. Magnesium activates enzymes which transfer phosphate from ATP to ADP. It is an essential co-factor for many enzymes controlling cellular function and cellular energy transfer reactions. Magne-

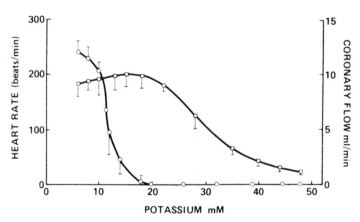

Figure 13.3. The effect of increasing potassium concentration on heart rate and coronary flow in the isolated rat heart. (Reproduced with permission from D. J. Hearse et al.[13] and the American Heart Association, Inc.)

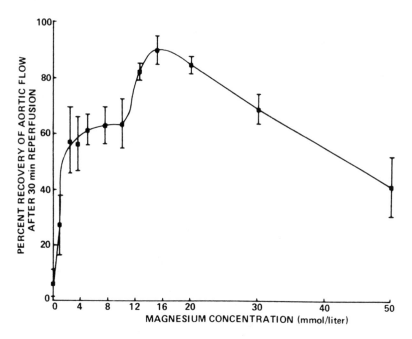

Figure 13.4. The effects of increasing magnesium concentration on percent recovery of aortic flow in the perfused isolated rat heart. (Reproduced with permission from D. J. Hearse et al.[19])

sium is involved with the production of cyclic AMP, a calcium channel activator.[21] Calcium and magnesium compete at receptor sites on the cell membrane to activate or slow neuromuscular transmission.[22] Magnesium inhibits the release of calcium by the sarcoplasmic reticulum. Calcium accumulates, thereby inhibiting calcium influx and stabilizing potassium channels.[23] Recent studies have suggested that many patients with left ventricular hypertrophy may suffer from hypomagnesemia. Pretreatment with oral magnesium salts and addition of magnesium sulfate to the pump prime may reduce the incidence of arrhythmias.[24] Kraft et al.[25] studied the effects of magnesium on the electrophysiologic effects of hyperkalemia. Magnesium attenuates the electrophysiologic response to an elevated potassium, protecting the myocardium during infusion of potassium cardioplegia and protecting the myocardial conducting system postbypass. If high noncoronary collateral flow is present, magnesium may be washed out of the coronary circulation and may inhibit neuromuscular transmission.

Calcium

Calcium is actively associated with excitation contraction in skeletal, smooth, and cardiac muscle.[26] Small quantities of extracellular calcium are necessary to activate cell membrane receptors which produce electrochemical activation of the cell. Following excitation, extracellular calcium enters the cell accompanied by sodium, and calcium is released from the lateral sacs of the sarcoplasmic reticulum (Fig. 13.5). Calcium binds to the tropin-tropomyosin complex, causing actinine and myocin to interact via crossbridge formation producing sarcomere shortening and tension develops. Following systole, diastole is initiated when the cytosolic calcium levels decrease through sequestration of calcium by the sarcoplasmic reticulum, active pumping of intracellular calcium into the extracellular compartment, and by calcium buffering. The uptake of calcium is ATP-dependent.[27] During ischemia myocardial mitochondrial function may be impaired, and the ATPase may lack substrate to drive calcium into the sarco-

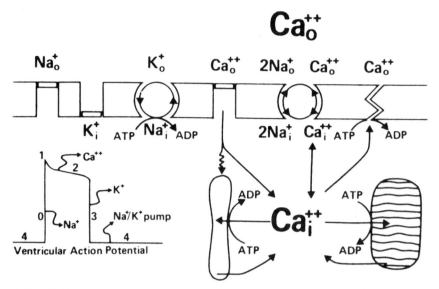

Figure 13.5. Cellular calcium regulation: Ion fluxes across the cell membrane and ventricular action potential. (Reproduced with permission from D. J. Hearse et al.: *Protection of the Ischemic Myocardium: Cardioplegia.* New York, Raven Press, 1981.)

plasmic reticulum. The extracellular excretion of calcium is related to the sodium-calcium exchange mechanism, so that the rate of relaxation is dependent upon the sodium gradient. Hearse et al.[28] perfused isolated rat hearts with high, intermediate, and low millimolar concentration of sodium with and without calcium. With a low concentration of extracellular sodium (30 mM/liter, 1.2 mM/liter of calcium), the compliance of the ventricle decreased rising left ventricular pressure. Ventricular contracture is also associated with continuous perfusion of calcium-free solution. A calcium "washout" from high affinity binding sites occurs in the basement membrane glycokalix. Reperfusion with calcium-containing solution causes cell membrane disruption, allowing calcium to enter the cell which stimulates massive contracture, swelling, and mitochondrial loss. A small quantity of calcium added to the perfusate will decrease the incidence of irreversible contracture. In order to reduce calcium to a critical "washout" level, a volume of 7,500 to 12,000 ml would be required in the 300-gm heart.[29] Acidosis protects the heart from the calcium paradox. Hypothermia delays the onset of the paradox. At 37°C, calcium contracture occurs 25 times more frequently than at 20°C. The interaction of the other ions and constituents of the cardioplegic solution also modifies the onset of the calcium paradox. If asanguineous cardioplegic solutions are used, noncoronary collateral flow may provide enough calcium to prevent the paradox. Likewise, sanguineous cardioplegic solutions also contain enough calcium to prevent the calcium damage.

Local Anesthetic Agents

Local anesthetic agents are critical components in many cardioplegic solutions. Local anesthetics act upon the cell membrane by blocking sodium, slow calcium channels, and the calcium channel of the sarcoplasmic reticulum. They induce rapid cardiac arrest by inhibiting extracellular calcium influx and blocking sarcoplasmic reticulum release of calcium. Local anesthetics "stabilize" cell membrane and reduce postarrest arrhythmias.[30] A procaine or xylocaine dose-response curve is bell-shaped.[31] A concentration of 0.05 mmoles/liter of procaine or xylocaine added to the standard St. Thomas cardioplegic solution increases ischemic protection by two-thirds. Higher concentrations of local anesthetic agents (1 to 2 mmoles/

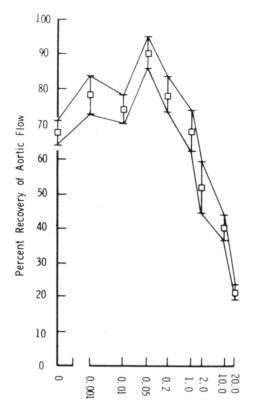

Figure 13.6. Protective effect of procaine added to St. Thomas's solution—isolated at heart. (Reproduced with permission from D. J. Hearse et al.[31])

liter) decrease protection (Fig. 13.6). Bixler et al.[32] compared potassium-induced arrest with procaine-induced arrest and found that postarrest ventricular function were identical, although the potassium solution produced less myocardial edema. Tyres et al.,[33] studying tetrodotoxin, a selective sodium blocker isolated from the pufferfish, found that intracoronary injection into the isolated rat heart produces rapid arrest with preservation of high energy phosphates.

Hypothermia

Cardiopulmonary bypass hypothermia has superceded body surface cooling in the adult. Either deep hypothermia (<20°C) or moderate hypothermia (28 to 30°C) is readily achieved. Topical myocardial hypothermia (4°C) further protects the myocardium during ischemic arrest.[34] Figure 13.7 graphically describes the advantages and disadvantages of hypothermia. The major disadvantages of hypothermia are evident at temperatures below 15°C. Hess et al.[35] studied the subcellular function of the hypothermic canine myocardium. Temperatures were reduced to between 10 and 16° following global ischemia, and ventricular samples were obtained at 30- and 60-minute intervals. Contractile protein function, myofibrillar ATPase activity, and glycogen stores were moderately depressed, but ventricular ejection was significantly compromised. In

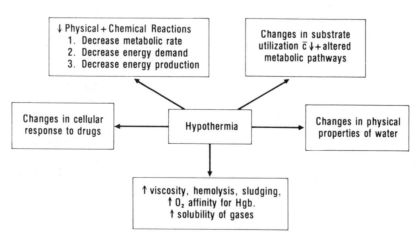

Figure 13.7. Effects of hypothermia.

contrast, there was only limited protection to processes involving excitation-contraction coupling. Lazar et al.[36] studied the effects of 45 minutes of normothermic ischemia in the dog on cardiopulmonary bypass. Group 1 continued to beat at normothermia; Group 2 had oxygen demand reduced by perfusing the heart to 18°C with blood for 10 minutes (the hypothermic beating heart); and Group 3 was arrested by potassium-containing blood cardioplegia at 37°C for 5 minutes. Groups 1 and 2 were weaned from cardiopulmonary bypass 30 minutes postischemia, but stroke work compliance and oxygen consumption were severely depressed. The group (3) receiving cardioplegia had the highest stroke work index, compliance, and ability to augment oxygen uptake. Lazar et al.[36] concluded that hypothermia postischemia depresses recovery and may delay metabolic processes responsible for reversal. Hess et al.[37] studied the effects of global ischemic arrest on normothermic, hypothermic, and hypothermic cardioplegia-treated canine hearts at 30- and 60-minute intervals. The normothermic group had significant depression of both sarcoplasmic reticular calcium uptake velocities and myofibrillar calcium ATPase activity. Hypothermic arrest protected sarcoplasmic reticulum but not myofibrillar function. The combination of hypothermia and cardioplegia demonstrated significant protection of both sarcoplasmic reticulum and myofibrillar function. Protection with the hypothermic cardioplegic solution lasted 30 minutes but at 60 minutes was lost in the absence of reperfusion. These findings were corroborated by the St. Thomas group in animals subjected to ischemia for 120 minutes at 20°C.[38] Grover et al.[39] suggested combining systemic hypothermic protection and cold cardioplegic protection. They concluded that moderate systemic hypothermia enhances myocardial protection by maintaining lower myocardial temperatures between 20-minute reinfusion periods. In conclusion, a combination of chemical cardioplegia plus myocardial hypothermia is additive, with each component preserving myocardial function at different sites of action.

Substrate Enhancement

An intriguing approach to the problem of myocardial preservation is from the "supply" side instead of the "preservation" side of the equation. Foker et al.[40] found that after 20 minutes of normothermic ischemia, ATP levels fell 60%, creatinine phosphate (CP) levels 12-fold, and the predicted rises in ADP, AMP, and adenosine are absent. Evidence of ADP, AMP catabolism were present. Coronary perfusion with adenosine increases coronary blood flow five times, but ATP production is unaffected. The infusion of EHNA, an inhibitor of adenosine deaminase, together with adenosine, results in recovery of ATP to 88% of preischemic levels. They conclude that ATP regeneration after ischemia is limited by the availability of ADP, AMP, and adenosine. Inhibition of adenosine catabolism and infusion of adenosine will enhance ATP production. Levitsky and Feinberg,[41] pursuing the same rationale, infused creatinine to elevate the creatinine phosphate pool during ischemia. Lazar et al.[42] infused L-glutamate with secondary blood cardioplegia and concluded that L-glutamate increased postischemic ATP production by stimulating oxidative metabolism through replenishing of the Kreb's cycle. Substrate enhancement with glutathione in cold blood cardioplegia did not improve or protect.[43]

Membrane Stabilization

The value of membrane stabilization with methylprednisolone is questionable. No advantage was noted when 500 mg were added to a liter of cardioplegic solution compared to a nonsteroid-containing solution.[44] Toledo-Pereyra[45] concluded that during normothermic ischemia, methylprednisolone given 2 hours prior to ischemia exerted a protective effect. The protective effects of steroids are controversial and require more data before drawing conclusions.

Cardioplegic Distribution

The major impediment to cardioplegic preservation is the inability to perfuse areas beyond severe obstructive lesions. Hilton et al.[46] studied ventricular wall motion and left ventricular function in dogs with occluded left anterior descending arteries prior to cardioplegia infusion and found significant impairment of the segment supplied by the LAD and decreased overall left ventricular function. A rational approach to the perfusion problem would be: (1) construct the proximal aortic vein anastomosis; (2) apply the aortic cross-clamp distal to the proximal vein anastomosis; (3) infuse cardioplegic solution until arrest; (4) anastomose the distal end to the most jeopardized area of myocardium; (5) perfuse cardioplegia after completion of each distal anastomosis; (6) if distal anastomoses are performed first, arrest the heart with cardioplegic solution, rapidly anastomose a distal graft into the most jeopardized area, and infuse cardioplegic solution through the proximal end with a syringe. Under the most ideal circumstances, poor ventricular contractility may prevent "weaning" from cardiopulmonary bypass. Lazer et al.,[47] using a secondary blood cardioplegic solution, demonstrated improved left ventricular function in dogs perfused with oxygenated blood cardioplegia at 37°C for 5 minutes prior to cessation of cardiopulmonary bypass. They concluded that hearts supplied with oxygen during arrest recovered more readily from the ischemic insult. In another study the authors added L-glutamate to the reperfusion cardioplegia and concluded that L-glutamate was beneficial.

Calcium Channel Blockers

Calcium channel blockers prevent the influx of calcium into the cell at different receptor sites on the calcium channel. Robb-Nicholson et al.[48] using isolated rat hearts compared the effects of potassium cardioplegia to Verapamil-induced cardioplegia (Fig. 13.8). Hearts treated with verapamil, 2 gm/cc, recovered 85% of LV function with normal ATP levels and CP levels reduced (40%). Potassium chloride-treated hearts recovered 95% function with equivalent high energy phosphate levels. Using a normothermic dog right heart bypass model, Lowe et al.[49] produced a flaccid heart with 60 minutes of ischemia. Those animals receiving a verapamil-containing cardi-

oplegic solution had a good return of LV function. Clark et al.[50] recently studied the effects of a nifedipine-containing cardioplegic solution (275 mg/liter) and found that LV function was improved, less CK-MB enzyme was released, and pyrophosphate scans showed less myocardial injury post cardiopulmonary bypass. Robb-Nicholson noted that the metabolic and physiologic effects of verapamil lasted 20 minutes longer compared to cardioplegia-containing potassium chloride. Verapamil is tightly bound to calcium channel receptor sites. If there is need to rapidly discontinue cardiopulmonary bypass then verapamil cardioplegia is disadvantageous. Verapamil produces ideal conditions for secondary blood cardioplegia perfusion in the non-beating heart.

Beta Blockers

Little material is available concerning beta blockers as components of cardioplegia. Lucas et al.[51] compared the additive myocardial protection afforded by propranolol. He found that propranolol added to potassium chloride and hypothermia improved myocardial protection compared to potassium chloride and hypothermia. The mechanism of action appears to be through inhibition of catecholamine effects. Beta blockers also "stabilize" the ventricular conduction system, reducing arrhythmias prior to cardiopulmonary bypass surgery. The use of beta blockers is widespread, and their major treatment potential may lie in the preoperative area.[53]

Secondary Additives to Cardioplegia

GLUCOSE

Hearst et al.[53] added glucose to the St. Thomas solution in the isolated rat heart, producing a dose-dependent reduction in cardioplegic protection. As an additive to cardioplegia in a normothermic pig bypass model, glucose had no significant effect on the stores of glycogen, CP, and ATP during cardiopulmonary bypass.[54] Lolley et al.[55] studied the effects of increasing preoperative glycogen level with a fat-loading diet and overnight glucose loading. Noting the

PERCENT RECOVERY

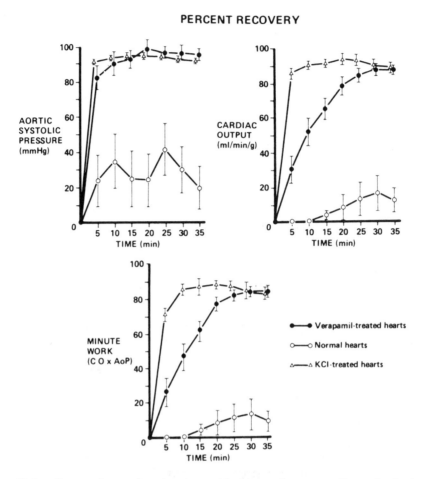

Figure 13.8. Comparison of potassium chloride and verapamil cardioplegia on aortic systolic pressure, cardiac output, and minute work. (Reproduced with permission from C. Robb-Nicholson et al.[48] and the American Heart Association, Inc.)

number of transmural myocardial infarctions, atrial or ventricular arrhythmias, and need for postbypass inotropic support, they concluded that patients with a high glycogen level prior to surgery and treated with potassium chloride cardioplegia did significantly better. The addition of glucose to the cardioplegic solution may stimulate glycolysis with the production of lactate and hydrogen ions. Its glycogen-sparing ability may be due to glucose utilization in lieu of glycogenolysis. Noncollateral coronary blood flow plus intermittent cardioplegia infusion at 16 to 20°C may negate the need for exogenous glucose utilization.

pH

Recent literature strongly suggests that optimal pH at 28°C should be 7.72.[56] Becker et al.[57] found that puppies kept at a pH of 7.4 during surface cooling had a decreased cardiac output associated with systemic lactic acidosis. At 22°C pH 7.4, and a PCO_2 40 torr, cerebral blood flow decreased 75%, left ventricular oxygen uptake decreased 80%, systemic vascular resistance increased, and left ventricular subendocardial blood flow decreased. Animals with pH adjusted to 7.75 by reducing PCO_2 (hypocapnea) had a two-fold increase in coronary blood flow and improved left ventricular subendocardial flow and oxygen utilization. They concluded that maintaining a pH of 7.4 decreases the myocardial protection afforded by hypothermic cardioplegia.

OSMOLALITY

Many cardioplegic solutions contain mannitol, sorbitol, plasma, albumin, dextran, and hydroxyethyl starch to create a normal or hyperosmolar cardioplegic solution. Two opposing views are presented in the literature. Hypoosmolar solutions can increase myocardial cell water, thereby decreasing compliance and redistributing coronary flow. Hyperosmolar solutions can cause cellular dehydration. It seems reasonable to formulate a normal osmolar solution or slightly hyperosmolar cardioplegic solution (370 to 400 mOsm).

Asanguineous vs. Sanguineous Solutions

The oxygen requirement of the chemically arrested heart at 15°C is 0.3 to 0.5 ml oxygen/min/100 gm. Is there a need to supply oxygen to the heart at this temperature? Can oxygen demands be met by oxygenating asanguineous solutions or can noncoronary collateral flow meet these minimal oxygen requirements? If an asanguineous solution is oxygenated to a Pa_{O_2} of 760 mm torr, 3.42 cc of oxygen are dissolved per 100 ml. In order to avoid an oxygen debt, 25 to 50 cc of flow would have to be delivered per minute per 100 gm myocardial tissue. Continuous perfusion can provide adequate flow. Noncoronary collateral flow estimated at 2 ml/min/100 gm with a hematocrit of 25% provides enough oxygen if there is no intermittent washout with cardioplegia. A cardioplegic solution containing 10 gm/100 ml of hemoglobin at 20°C equilibrated with a P_{O_2} of 400 mm will provide enough oxygen if flow is 50 to 80 cc/100 gm every 20 minutes. Hypothermia, an alkalotic pH, reduced 2 to 3 DPG, and banked blood increase oxygen affinity for hemoglobin and decrease solubility. Shapira et al.[58] compared blood cardioplegia with potassium crystalloid cardioplegia and found no significant advantage. Rose et al.[59] reviewed immediate and long-term effects (120 days)

of blood cardioplegia and crystalloid cardioplegia and found that immediate postbypass studies demonstrated no significant difference in contractility, but later studies showed improved contractility in the blood cardioplegic group. A higher concentration of potassium chloride 28 to 30 mEq/liter is required to produce asystole. Takamoto et al.[60] measured the effluent from the coronary sinus and noted that when blood cardioplegia with 25 mEq of potassium chloride per liter was infused, only 8 to 10 mEq/liter was recovered. When crystalloid solution was infused at 25 mEq/liter, the fluid recovered contained 20 to 25 mEq potassium chloride. A need for a higher potassium chloride concentrate in the blood cardioplegia may be due to potassium influx into the red blood cell. Excellent left ventricular function was seen in the multiple dose blood cardioplegia, but poor function was noted in the single dose blood cardioplegia group. Potassium chloride-containing crystalloid solution provided a more sustained and consistent result.[61] The failure of a single dose blood cardioplegia may be due to increased viscosity, rouleaux formation, or a combination in patients having multiple stenotic lesions.

OVERVIEW OF ISCHEMIC MYOCARDIAL PRESERVATION

In an excellent discussion of the cardioplegic controversy, Buckberg[62] concludes with the following quote: "The future does not lie in proving the value of cardioplegia, but understanding better the deleterious effects of ischemia and reperfusion injury so that current cardioplegic techniques can be modified to avoid these effects." In understanding these effects we must realize that cardioplegia is only a portion of the myocardial preservation problem (Fig. 13.9). Pretreating patients with pharmacologic agents may prevent intraoperative myocardial damage.[63] Beta-blocking agents such as propranolol may decrease oxygen consumption by decreasing heart rate and metabolically blocking catechol-induced ATP depletion. In addition, beta blocking these catecholamine effects may provide a more ad-

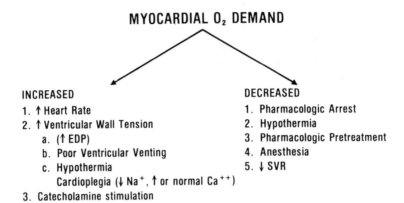

MYOCARDIAL O$_2$ DEMAND

INCREASED
1. ↑ Heart Rate
2. ↑ Ventricular Wall Tension
   a. (↑ EDP)
   b. Poor Ventricular Venting
   c. Hypothermia
      Cardioplegia (↓ Na$^+$, ↑ or normal Ca^{++})
3. Catecholamine stimulation

DECREASED
1. Pharmacologic Arrest
2. Hypothermia
3. Pharmacologic Pretreatment
4. Anesthesia
5. ↓ SVR

Figure 13.9. Factors which increase or decrease myocardial oxygen demand.

vantageous coronary flow distribution. Nitroglycerin infusion has been shown to dilate coronary vessels and thus reduce myocardial injury due to acute coronary occlusion. Nitroglycerin affects flow distribution by increasing coronary blood flow to periinfarction areas. Agents that increase myocardial blood flow, such as dipyridalomine (Persantine), may prevent regional blood flow maldistribution. Persantine also lowers microaggregate formation and decreases ATP depletion. Pretreatment with calcium channel blockers such as nifedipine may restrict the quantity of calcium in the cytosol and decrease flow through the calcium channels thereby decreasing left ventricular compliance. Increasing glycogen stores by fat loading prior to myocardial ischemia may be advantageous. Butchart et al.[64] stresses the importance of keeping glucose levels above 150 mg/100 ml prior to ischemic arrest in dogs, since control of this factor improved left ventricular function following ischemia. Glucose, insulin, and potassium[65] (GIK) have been utilized to prevent extension of myocardial infarction. Glucose facilitates anaerobic glycolysis, and potassium replenishes intracellular loss. In addition, GIK is a positive inotrope and may cause coronary vasodilation. Perhaps preoperative treatment with this combination would provide optimal substrate to better tolerate ischemia. Replenishment of oxygen and substrate prior to the cessation of bypass may reduce ischemia-induced left ventricular failure. Evidence is accumulating that continuous normothermic potassium-containing oxygenated blood cardioplegia with or without substrate enhancement is beneficial following hypothermic cardiac arrest.[66, 67] Anesthetic agents and techniques affect left ventricular function following cardiopulmonary bypass. Reduction of systemic vascular resistance and myocardial contractility prior to inducing anesthesia, at the time of laryngoscopy and intubation, and during sternal splitting will favorably effect the O$_2$ supply-demand equation.[68] Merin et al.[69] found that halothane causes a dose-dependent negative inotropic effect upon myocardial contractility accompanied by a decline in oxygen demand equal to or greater than the reduction in oxygen delivery. Gersen et al.[70] produced ischemia in dogs by left anterior descending artery occlusion. Using epicardial electrograms, he found that both halothane and nitroprusside reduced ST segment depression. The reduction in the halothane group was significantly greater than in the nitroprusside group. Unfortunately, coronary artery bypass surgery is palliative, and eventually patients succumb to arteriosclerotic heart disease. At autopsy grafts can be examined for patency. Moore and Hutchins[71] evaluated myocardial preservation or lack of preservation to the percent of graft patency, and amount of regional myocardial injury in 119 patients autopsied at Johns Hopkins Hospital. Patients receiving cold potassium cardioplegia had a higher graft patency rate and had less regional myocardial injury (Ta-

Table 13.2
Effect of KCl Cardioplegia on Percent of Occluded Coronary Grafts and Regional Myocardial Injury*

	No. of Patients	Anastomosed Arteries	No. (%) Occluded	No. (%) Regional Myocardial Injury
Normothermic anoxic arrest	20	44	15 (34)	24 (55)
Hypothermic anoxic arrest	21	41	7 (17)	26 (63)
Hypothermic ventricular, fibrillation	19	38	11 (29)	16 (24)
Combined and other	17	34	5 (14)	14 (41)
Cold potassium chloride cardioplegia	32	79	14 (17)	19 (24)†
Total	109	236	52	99

* Reprinted with permission from G. W. Moore and G. M. Hutchins.[71]
† Significantly less regional injury; $p < 0.001$.

ble 13.2). In conclusion, hypothermia cardioplegic infusion produces superior preservation of high energy phosphates and myofibrillar function. The components and concentration of the solutions are still being investigated in both isolated and whole animal preparations. Factors that may prove oxygen utilization, left ventricular function, and preserve high energy nucleotides in the preoperative, perioperative, and postoperative periods require further study.

References

1. Melrose DG, Dreyer B, Bentall HH, Baker JBE: Elective cardiac arrest. Lancet 269:21, 1955.
2. Helmsworth JA, Kaplan S, Clark LC, McAdams AJ, Matthews EC, Edwards FK: Myocardial injury associated with asystole induced with potassium citrate. Ann Surg 149:200, 1959.
3. Buckberg GD, Hottenrott CE: Ventricular fibrillation. Its effect on myocardial flow, distribution, and performance. Ann Thorac Surg 20:76, 1975.
4. Gollan F, Nelson IA: Anoxic tolerance of beating and resting heart during perfusion at various temperatures. Proc Soc Exp Biol Med 95:485, 1957.
5. Shumway NE, Lower RR, Stofer RC: Selective hypothermia of the heart in anoxic cardiac arrest. Surg Gynecol Obstet 109:750, 1959.
6. Ebert PA, Greenfield LJ, Austen WG, Morrow AG: Experimental comparison of methods for protecting the heart during aortic occlusion. Ann Surg 155:25, 1962.
7. Maloney JV, Nelson RL: Myocardial preservation during cardiopulmonary bypass. An overview. J Thorac Cardiovasc Surg 70:1040, 1975.
8. Swan H: Clinical hypothermia: A lady with a past and some promise for the future. Surgery 73:736, 1973.
9. Rosenfeldt JC, Watson DA: Development of an in vivo model of myocardial cooling: A study of the effects of cardiac size on cooling rate. Ann Thorac Surg 27:7, 1979.
10. Gay WA, Ebert PA: Functional, metabolic, and morphologic effects of potassium-induced cardioplegia. Surgery 74:284, 1973.
11. Reidemeister JC, Heberer G, Bretschneider HJ: Induced cardiac arrest by sodium and calcium depletion and application of procaine. Int Surg 47:535, 1967.
12. Kirsch V, Rodewald G, Kalmar P: Induced ischemic arrest in clinical experience with cardioplegia in open heart surgery. J Thorac Cardiovasc Surg 63:121, 1972.
13. Hearse DJ, Stewart DA, Braimbridge MV: Hypothermic arrest and potassium arrest, metabolic and myocardial protection during elective cardiac arrest. Circ Res 36:481, 1975.
14. Follette DM, Buckberg GD, Mulder DG, Fonkalsrud EW: Deleterious effects of crystalloid hyperkalemic cardioplegic solutions on arterial endothelial cells. Surg Forum 31:253, 1980.
15. Tucker WY, Ellis RJ, Mangano DT, Ryan CJM, Ebert PA: Questionable importance of high potassium concentrations in cardioplegic solutions. J Thorac Cardiovasc Surg 77:183, 1979.
16. Ellis RJ, Mavroudis C, Gardner C, Turley K, Ullyot D, Ebert PA: Relationship between atrioventricular arrhythmias and the concentration of K^+ ion in cardioplegic solution. J Thorac Cardiovasc Surg 80:517, 1980.
17. Ellis RJ, Mangano DT, Van Dyke DC, Ebert PA: Protection of myocardial function not enhanced by high concentrations of potassium during cardioplegic arrest. J Thorac Cardiovasc Surg 78:698, 1979.
18. Laks H, Barner HB, Kaiser G: Cold blood cardioplegia. J Thorac Cardiovasc Surg 77:319, 1979.
19. Hearse DJ, Stewart DA, Braimbridge MV: Myocardial protection during ischemic cardiac arrest: The importance of magnesium in cardioplegic infusates. J Thorac Cardiovasc Surg 75:877, 1978.
20. Skaredoff MN, Roaf E, Datta S: Hypermagnesaemia and anaesthetic management. Can Anaesth Soc J 29:35, 1982.
21. Lehr D, Chau R, Irene S: Possible role of magnesium loss in the pathogenesis of myocardial fiber necrosis. Recent Adv Stud Card Struct Metab 6:95, 1975.

22. Fedelesová M, Ziegelhöffer A, Luknárová O, Kostolanský S: Prevention by K$^+$, Mg^{2+}-aspartate of isoproterenol-induced metabolic changes in the myocardium. Recent Adv Stud Card Struct Metab 6, 1975.

23. Massry SG: Pharmacology of magnesium. Annu Rev Pharmacol Toxicol 17:67, 1977.

24. Krasner BS, Girdwood R, Smith H: The effect/of slow releasing and magnesium chloride on the QT internal of the electrocardiogram during open heart surgery. Can Anaesth Soc J 28:329, 1981.

25. Kraft LJ, Kathol RE, Woods WT, James TN: Attenuation by magnesium of the electrophysiologic effects of hyperkalemia on human and canine heart cells. Am J Cardiol 45:1189, 1980.

26. Fleckenstein A: Specific pharmacology of calcium in myocardium, cardiac pacemakers, and vascular smooth muscle. Annu Rev Pharmacol Toxicol 17:149, 1977.

27. St. Louis PJ, Sulakhe PV: Adenosine triphosphate dependent calcium binding and accumulation by guinea pig sarcolemma. Can J Biochem 84:946, 1976.

28. Hearse DJ, Humphrey SM, Boinsk ABTJ, Ruigrok TJC: The calcium paradox: Metabolic, electrophysiological, contractile and ultrastructural characteristics in four species. Eur J Cardiol 7:241, 1978.

29. Jynge P: Protection of the ischemic myocardium. Cold chemical cardioplegia, coronary infusates and the importance of cellular calcium control. J Thorac Cardiovasc Surg 28:310, 1980.

30. de Jong RH: *Local Anesthetics*, Ed. 2. Springfield, Ill., Charles C Thomas, 1977.

31. Hearse DJ, O'Brien K, Braimbridge MV: Protection of the myocardium during ischemic arrest: Dose-response curves for procaine and lignocaine solutions. J Thorac Cardiovasc Surg 81:873, 1981.

32 Bixler TJ, Gardner TJ, Flaherty JT, Goldman RA, Gott VL: Effects of procaine-induced cardioplegia on myocardial ischemia, myocardial edema, and postarrest ventricular function. A comparison with potassium-induced cardioplegia and hypothermia. J Thorac Cardiovasc Surg 75:886, 1978.

33. Tyers GFO, Todd GJ, Neely JR, Waldhausen JA: The mechanism of myocardial protection from ischemic arrest by intracoronary tetrodotoxin administration. J Thorac Cardiovasc Surg 69:190, 1975.

34. Hess ML, Krause SM, Greenfield LJ: Assessment of hypothermic, cardioplegic protection of the global ischemic canine myocardium. J Thorac Cardiovasc Surg 80:293, 1980.

35. Hess ML, Williams EL, Robbins AD, Poland J, Greenfield LJ: Subcellular function of the hypothermic myocardium. Surg Forum 31:301, 1980.

36. Lazar HL, Buckberg GD, Manganaro AM, Becker H: Myocardial energy replenishment and reversal of ischemic damage by substrate enhancement of secondary blood cardioplegia with amino acids during reperfusion. J Thorac Cardiovasc Surg 80:350, 1980.

37. Hess ML, Krause SM, Greenfield CJ: Assessment of hypothermic, cardioplegic protection of the global ischemic canine myocardium. J Thorac Cardiovasc Surg 80:293, 1980.

38. Braimbridge MV, Chayen J, Bitensky L, Hearse DJ, Jynge P, Čanković-Darracott S: Cold cardioplegia or continuous coronary perfusion? Report on preliminary clinical experience as assessed cytochemically. J Thorac Cardiovasc Surg 74:900, 1977.

39. Grover FL, Fewel JG, Ghidoni JJ, Trinkle JK: Does lower systemic temperature enhance cardioplegic protection? J Thorac Cardiovasc Surg 81:11, 1981.

40. Foker JE, Einzig S, Wang T, Anderson RW: Adenosine metabolism and myocardial preservation. Consequences of adenosine catabolism on myocardial high-energy compounds and tissue blood flow. J Thorac Cardiovasc Surg 80:506, 1980.

41. Levitsky S, Feinberg H: Protection of the myocardium with high-energy solutions. J Thorac Cardiovasc Surg 20:86, 1975.

42. Lazar HL, Buckberg GD, Manganaro AM, Becker H: Myocardial energy replenishment and reversal of ischemic damage by substrate enhancement of secondary blood cardioplegia with amino acids during reperfusion. J Thorac Cardiovasc Surg 80:350, 1980.

43. Standeven JW, Jellinek M, Menz LJ, Hahn JW, Barner HB: Cold-blood potassium cardioplegia. Evaluation of glutathione and postischemic cardioplegia. J Thorac Cardiovasc Surg 78:893, 1979.

44. Kirsh MM, Behrendt DM, Jochim KE: Effects of methylprednisolone in cardioplegic solution during coronary bypass grafting. J Thorac Cardiovasc Surg 77:896, 1979.

45. Toleo-Pereyra LH, Jara FM: Myocardial protection with methylprednisolone. Evaluation of viability of hearts subjected to warm ischemia before transplantation. J Thorac Cardiovasc Surg 77:619, 1979.

46. Hilton CJ, Teubl W, Acker M, Levinson HJ, Milland RW, Riddle R, McEnany MT: Inadequate cardioplegic protection with obstructed coronary arteries. Ann Thorac Surg 28:323, 1979.

47. Lazar HL, Buckberg GD, Manganaro AJ, Foglia RP, Becker H, Mulder DG, Maloney JV: Reversal of ischemic damage with secondary blood cardioplegia. J Thorac Cardiovasc Surg 78:688, 1979.

48. Robb-Nicholson C, Currie WD, Wechsler AS: Effects of verapamil on myocardial tolerance to ischemic arrest. Comparison to potassium arrest. Circulation 58(Suppl. 1):119, 1978.

49. Lowe JE, Kleinman LH, Riemer KA, Jennings RB, Wechsler AS: Effects of cardioplegia produced by calcium flux inhibition. Surg Forum 28:279, 1977.

50. Clark RE, Christlieb IY, Ferguson TB, Weldon CS, Marbarger JP, Biello DR, Roberts R, Ludbrook PA, Sobel BE: The first American clinical trial of nifedipine in cardioplegia. A report of the first 12 month experience. J Thorac Cardiovasc Surg 82:848, 1981.

51. Lucas SK, Magee PG, Flaherty JT, Gott BL, Gardner TJ: Additive myocardial protection during ischemic arrest with propranolol and potassium cardioplegia. Surg Forum 30:257, 1979.

52. Manning AS, Keogh JM, Shattock MJ, Coltart DJ, Hearse DJ: Long-term beta-blockade: Prolonged protective action on the ischaemic myocardium. Cardiovasc Res 15:462, 1981.

53. Hearse DJ, Stewart DA, Braimbridge MV: Myocar-

dial protection during ischemic cardiac arrest—possible deleterious effects of glucose and mannitol in coronary infusates. J Thorac Cardiovasc Surg 76:16, 1978.

54. Salerno TA, Chiong MA: Cardioplegic arrest in pigs. Effects of glucose-containing solutions. J Thorac Cardiovasc Surg 80:929, 1980.

55. Lolley DM, Ray JF, Myers WO, Sautter RD, Tewksbury DA: Importance of preoperative myocardial glycogen levels in human cardiac preservation. J Thorac Cardiovasc Surg 78:678, 1979.

56. White FN: A comparative physiological approach to hypothermia. J Thorac Cardiovasc Surg 82:821, 1981.

57. Becker H, Vinten-Johansen J, Buckberg GD, Robertson JM, Leaf JD, Lazar HL, Manganaro AJ: Myocardial damage caused by keeping pH 7.40 during systemic deep hypothermia. J Thorac Cardiovasc Surg 82:810, 1981.

58. Shapira N, Kirsh M, Jochim K, Behrendt DM: Comparison of the effect of blood cardioplegia to crystalloid cardioplegia on muocardial contractility in man. J Thorac Cardiovasc Surg 80:647, 1980.

59. Rose DM, Koch JP, Barnhart GR, Jones M: Early and late hemodynamic evaluation of crystalloid and blood cardioplegic solutions. Surg Forum 31:293, 1980.

60. Takamoto S, Levine FH, LaRaia PJ, Adzick NS, Fallon JT, Austen WG, Buckley MJ: Comparison of single-dose and multiple dose crystalloid and blood potassium cardioplegia during prolonged hypothermic aortic occlusion. J Thorac Cardiovasc Surg 79:19, 1980.

61. Cunningham JN, Adams PX, Knopp EA, Baumann FG, Snively SL, Gross RI, Nathan IM, Spencer FC: Preservation of ATP, ultrastructure, and ventricular function after aortic cross-clamping and reperfusion. J Thorac Cardiovasc Surg 78:708, 1979.

62. Buckberg GD: A proposed "solution" to the cardioplegic controversy. J Thorac Cardiovasc Surg 77:803, 1979.

63. Hickey PA: Prevention of intraoperative myocardial injury by pretreatment with pharmacological agents. Ann Thorac Surg 20:101, 1975.

64. Butchart EG, McEnany MT, Strich G, Sbokos C, Austen WG: The influence of prearrest factors on the preservation of left ventricular function during cardiopulmonary bypass. J Thorac Cardiovasc Surg 79:812, 1980.

65. Opie LH: Myocardial infarct size. Part 2. Comparison of anti-infarct effects of beta-blockade, glucose-insulin-potassium, nitrates, and hyaluronidase. Am Heart J 100:531, 1980.

66. Follette DM, Fey KH, Steed DL, Foglia RP, Buckbert GD: Reducing reperfusion injury with hypocalcemia, hyperkalemic, alkalotic blood during reoxygenation. Surg Forum 29:284, 1978.

67. Follette DM, Steed DL, Foglia RP, Fey KH, Buckberg GD: Reduction of postischemic myocardial damage by maintaining arrest during initial reperfusion. Surg Forum 28:281, 1977.

68. Kaplan J: *Cardiac Anesthesia.* Grune & Stratton, New York, 1979.

69. Merin RG, Kumazawa T, Luka NL: Myocardial function and metabolism in the conscious dog and during halothane anesthesia. Anesthesiology 44:402, 1976.

70. Gerson JI, Hickey RF, Bainton CR: Treatment of myocardial ischemia with halothane or nitroprusside-propranolol. Anesth Analg (Cleve) 61:10, 1982.

71. Moore GW, Hutchins GM: Coronary artery bypass grafts in 109 autopsied patients. Statistical analysis of graft and anastomosis patency and regional myocardial injury. JAMA 246:1785, 1981.

CHAPTER 14

POTASSIUM IN THE CARDIAC SURGICAL PATIENT

JOE R. UTLEY, M.D.

Managing potassium is an important aspect of the care of the cardiac surgical patient. Patients who have received chronic diuretic therapy may be potassium-depleted before the cardiac surgical procedure, whereas those with renal dysfunction may have hyperkalemia. The effect of cardiopulmonary bypass and surgical procedures on potassium concentration is complex and may contribute to hypokalemia or hyperkalemia. Drugs, acid-base alterations, diuresis, and endocrine effects may also contribute to the hypokalemia that often follows cardiac surgical procedures. The effect of potassium on the myocardium's rhythm and function may affect the patient's tolerance of cardiac drugs.

DIGITALIS AND POTASSIUM

Potassium is an important determinant of the patient's tolerance to digitalis. Maintaining the serum potassium at 7 to 8 mEq/liter in dogs increases the toxic dose of digitalis 240%.[1] Ventricular arrhythmias due to digitalis are less frequent and of shorter duration with elevated serum potassium. Administration of potassium controls all the disorders of rhythm and conduction produced by digitalis, but does not interfere with its inotropic effects. In experimental preparations, digitalis will reverse the depression of myocardial contractility produced by hyperkalemia. Although potassium administration may raise the toxic dose of digitalis by 240%, it raises the lethal dose by only 40%. Thus, the ratio of lethal to toxic dose is less with hyperkalemia. Potassium will suppress ventricular arrhythmias of any etiology. The therapeutic dose of potassium is the same regardless of the arrhythmia. The suppression of the arrhythmia may be transient and only during the phase of hyperkalemia.

Conversely, with potassium depletion, the toxic dose of digitalis is decreased to 40% of that before potassium depletion in experimental animals. Rapid diuresis may produce a rapid increase in sensitivity to digitalis. This was once thought to be due to "redigitalization" from the mobilization of digitalis from the interstitial space. The change in digitalis sensitivity produced by diuresis is proportional to the potassium content of the urine and can be prevented by potassium replacement. Digitalis intoxication may be produced by acute lowering of the serum potassium by infusion of sodium chloride, bicarbonate, glucose, or insulin.

The correlation of digitalis sensitivity to serum potassium is relatively poor. The sensitivity to digitalis is most directly related to the body content of potassium relative to other cell solids.[1]

Cardiopulmonary bypass may increase the tolerance of the digitalized animal to digitalis, whereas the nondigitalized animal has no change in digitalis tolerance. This suggests that cardiopulmonary bypass causes the loss of digitalis or inactivation of the drug, rather than change in myocardial responsiveness.[2] Digitalis concentration in atrial and skeletal muscle is typically decreased with cardiopulmonary bypass.[3]

Clinical studies of tolerance to acetyl strophanthidium have shown a diminished tolerance to digitalis in the early postoperative period that could not be related to potassium or acid-base changes.[4]

POTASSIUM AND ARRHYTHMIAS

Increased extracellular potassium decreases the transmembrane potassium gradient and lowers the resting membrane potential which slows conduction. Increased extracellular potassium also increases permeability to potassium. Decreased extracellular potassium increases the resting membrane potential of the ventricular fibers.

Increase of serum potassium from 5.5 to 7.5 mg/liter suppresses ventricular arrhythmias (Fig. 14.1). Atrioventricular conduction abnormalities are also common at these higher concentrations. Further increases in potassium result in prolonged P waves of lower amplitude. The P-R interval lengthens, and second and third degree heart block may appear. With greatly elevated serum potassium, the QRS widens. Death may be by cardiac standstill or ventricular fibrillation. Hypocalcemia aggravates the effect of hyperkalemia on atrioventricular and intraventricular conduction. Hyponatremia augments and hypernatremia counteracts the effect of hyperkalemia. Hypermagnesemia may also augment the effect of hyperkalemia.

Patients with hypokalemia have a high incidence of supraventricular and ventricular ectopic rhythms and beats. They may also have atrioventricular and intraventricular conduction disturbances. Hypopotassemia patients may also be more sensitive to vagal stimulation. Hypocalcemia counteracts the effect of hypokalemia, and hypercalcemia aggravates it.[5] Potassium supplementation may suppress atrial arrhythmias at lower concentrations than ventricular arrhythmias. Defibrillation of the atrium with rapid infusion of potassium may occur.

Rapid intravenous infusion of potassium may also defibrillate the ventricles. Cardiac pacemakers may demonstrate an elevated

7-7-65 SERUM K: 2.8 mEq/L

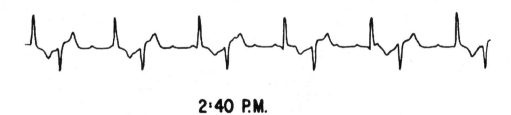

2:40 P.M.

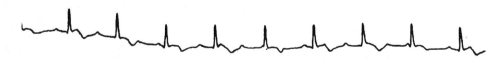

2:44 P.M. After 4 mEq potassium chloride I.V.

Figure 14.1. The figure shows the effect of intravenous potassium chloride on frequent ventricular premature contractions. (Reproduced with permission from C. A. Selmonosky and J. B. Flege Jr.[7])

stimulus threshold with either hypokalemia or hyperkalemia. Sudden elevation of potassium from low levels to normal levels may result in cardiac standstill.[5]

Arrhythmias after cardiac surgery are often related to hyperkalemia.[3,6] Ventricular arrhythmias which are unresponsive to lidocaine or Dilantin may respond to potassium.[6] Small doses of potassium have been effective in suppressing ventricular arrhythmias after cardiopulmonary bypass.[7]

PREOPERATIVE POTASSIUM DEPLETION

Potassium depletion is common in patients with chronic congestive failure and diuretic therapy. Significant depletion of total body potassium was found in four of ten patients undergoing valve replacement.[8] The duration of diuretic therapy is a significant determinant of total potassium depletion. Patients who had diuretic therapy more than 1 year have greater depletion of serum potassium.[9] The hypopotassemia after cardiopulmonary bypass was greater in patients who had received diuretics for more than 1 year. Patients on preoperative diuretics had a greater chance of arrhythmia postoperatively.[9] Attempts to increase total body potassium by preoperative supplementation have not been successful, although the patients studied were not shown to be depleted before supplementation.[10]

EFFECTS OF ANESTHETIC AGENTS ON POTASSIUM

Increases in serum potassium following the use of depolarizing muscle relaxants such as succinyl choline and suxamethonium have been described.[11–13] The increase in potassium may be diminished by previous treatment with a nondepolarizing relaxant, such as tubocurarine or gallamine. The rise in potassium is less with halothane or thiopentone anesthesia.[14] The hyperkalemic effects of depolarizing relaxants are exaggerated in the presence of renal failure.[13]

CARDIOPULMONARY BYPASS AND POTASSIUM

Hypokalemia is the most frequent change in potassium concentration observed during and after cardiopulmonary bypass[3,15,16] (Fig. 14.2). Hyperkalemia is also occasionally observed, particularly in the diabetic, uremic patient, or the patient receiving propranolol or potassium cardioplegia. Decrease in total body potassium during cardiopulmonary bypass was not proved by a study in dogs.[17] The fall in potassium may

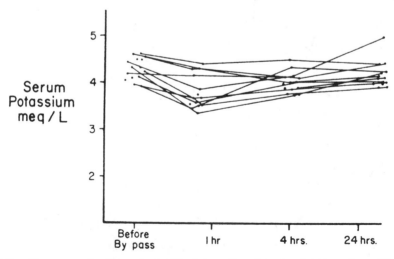

Figure 14.2. Serum potassium typically falls after the beginning of cardiopulmonary bypass and returns to prebypass levels in 24 hours. (Reproduced with permission from P. A. Ebert et al.[3] and the American Heart Association, Inc.)

be partially a function of the type of heart disease,[18] although the loss of potassium by diuresis is an important effect of cardiopulmonary bypass. The magnitude of urinary potassium loss is similar in cardiac surgical patients with and without cardiopulmonary bypass.[19]

PUMP PRIMING SOLUTION

The serum potassium is rapidly diluted by the pump-priming solution at the onset of cardiopulmonary bypass. This rapid change in serum potassium is rapidly compensated. Serum potassium then rises slowly to levels near those before the onset of cardiopulmonary bypass. Priming with whole blood rather than hemodilution with potassium-containing solutions may cause greater decreases in serum potassium.[20] Greater sodium concentration in the perfusate may lead to greater lowering of serum potassium.[6] Patients who were hypocalcemic during cardiopulmonary bypass had lower serum potassium than those who were normocalcemia.[21, 22] Within the range of hemodilution priming solutions currently used, the choice of priming solution probably has little effect on serum potassium concentration.

DIURESIS DURING CARDIOPULMONARY BYPASS

Potassium loss during cardiopulmonary bypass is linearly related to urine flow, indicating a relatively constant urine potassium concentration[23] (Fig. 14.3). The kaluresis may be diminished by the aldosteronal inhibitor, triamterene.[23] The increased potassium excretion continues into the postoperative period[24] (Fig.14.4). However, Vasko et al.[25] could not relate total volume to potassium depletion. The diuretics bumetamide and furosemide produce equal amounts of diuresis during cardiopulmo-

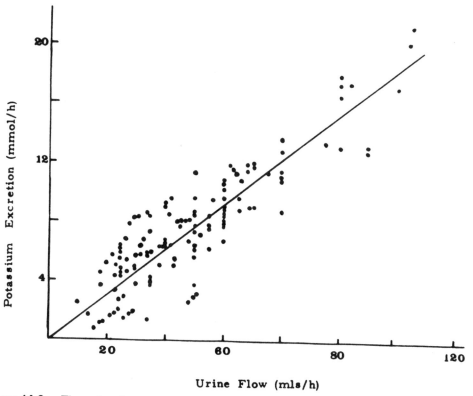

Figure 14.3. The rate of potassium excretion is related in a linear fashion to urine flow. (Reproduced with permission from J. Patrick and S. Siopragasam.[23])

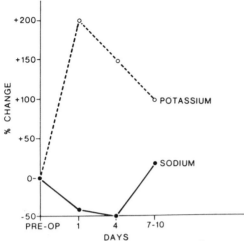

Figure 14.4. The percent change in excretion of potassium is increased in the postoperative period. Sodium excretion tends to be diminished compared to preoperative levels. (Reproduced with permission from L. H. Cohn et al.[24])

nary bypass, but bumetamide is associated with less potassium loss.[26]

HYPERVENTILATION

Respiratory alkalosis and hypocarbia may contribute to hypokalemia during cardiopulmonary bypass (Fig. 14.5). Potassium loss may be decreased by raising CO_2 tension in the gas mixture used in the pump oxygenator. The use of 3% carbon dioxide has been effective in preventing potassium loss due to hyperventilation.[27, 28] Postoperative hyperventilation may be associated with hypokalemia[29] (Fig. 14.6).

INTRACELLULAR SHIFTS OF POTASSIUM DURING CARDIOPULMONARY BYPASS

The studies of potassium balance during cardiopulmonary bypass have repeatedly shown that the lowering of serum potas-

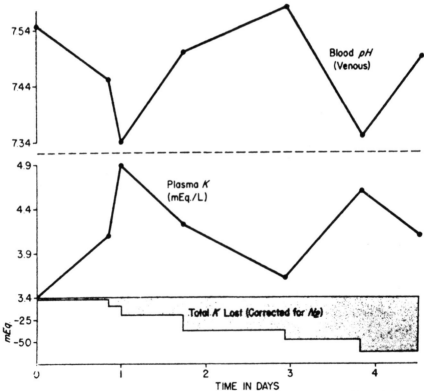

Figure 14.5. The figure shows the reciprocal relationship between pH and plasma potassium. Alkalosis is accompanied by hypokalemia. (Reproduced with permission from J. M. Burnell and B. H. Scribner.[46])

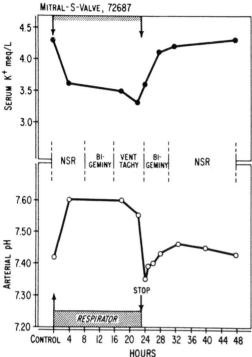

Figure 14.6. This figure shows the effect of hyperventilation with a respirator on serum potassium, arterial pH, and cardiac rhythm. When the respirator was discontinued, the serum potassium rose, arterial pH fell, and ventricular arrhythmia ceased. (Reproduced with permission from R. J. Flemma and W. G. Young, Jr.[29])

sium cannot be accounted for solely by dilution or by loss in urine or other forms of excretion. Careful studies of potassium intake and output as well as red blood cell potassium, rate of hemolysis, and serum hemoglobin have shown that much of the fall in serum potassium concentration is not accounted for by dilution or excretion. Intracellular shifts are presumably the reason for this loss of intravascular potassium. Calculations based on balance studies indicate that 25.7 ± 6.1 mg/m^2 moves into the intracellular space in the 1st hour of cardiopulmonary bypass.[30, 31] The intracellular movement is greater with serum potassium concentration more than 4.0 mg/liter, as is the excretion in the urine (Fig. 14.7). The expected intracellular shift of potassium has been studied particularly in red blood cells, skeletal muscle, and myocardium.

RED BLOOD CELLS

Chronic studies have shown that red blood cell potassium concentration reflects changes in total body potassium more readily than myocardium, liver, or skeletal muscle.[32] Clinical studies of red blood cell potassium concentration during cardiopulmonary bypass have given variable results. Kettlewells[33] found that red blood cell potassium concentration changed in the opposite direction as serum potassium. Others

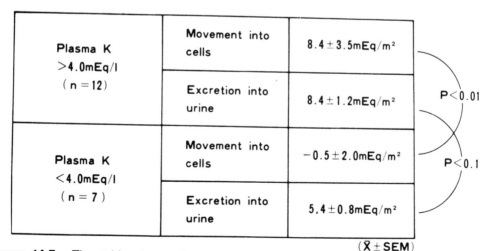

Plasma K **>4.0mEq/l** (n = 12)	Movement into cells	8.4 ± 3.5 mEq/m^2	
	Excretion into urine	8.4 ± 1.2 mEq/m^2	P<0.01
Plasma K **<4.0mEq/l** (n = 7)	Movement into cells	-0.5 ± 2.0 mEq/m^2	P<0.1
	Excretion into urine	5.4 ± 0.8 mEq/m^2	

$(\bar{X} \pm SEM)$

Figure 14.7. The table shows the calculated intracellular shift of potassium and the observed excretion in the urine during 2 hours of cardiopulmonary bypass. (Reproduced with permission from T. Abe et al.[30])

have found that red blood cell potassium remained the same or fell during cardiopulmonary bypass.[34] In Vasko's detailed study, red blood cell potassium fell with the duration of cardiopulmonary bypass. Red blood cell potassium was a poor reflection of total body potassium in these acute studies. There has been no consistent finding of an intracellular shift of potassium into the red blood cell to explain the unaccountable loss of serum potassium.

SKELETAL MUSCLE

Because skeletal muscle usually represents the largest mass of body tissue it would be a likely site for intracellular potassium to shift. Repeated observations have failed to show that skeletal muscle potassium is elevated during or after cardiopulmonary bypass.[35–38] The explanation for lowered skeletal muscle potassium include observed lowering of the extracellular potassium, increased aldosterone activity, decreased sodium pump activity, and hypotonic overhydration, including intracellular overhydration, intracellular accumulation of hydrogen ion, or change in extracellular pH.

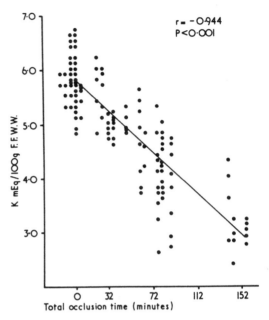

Figure 14.9. The myocardial potassium content falls progressively with increasing duration of occlusion of the coronary arteries. (Reproduced with permission from P. Taggart and J. D. H. Slater.[42])

MYOCARDIAL POTASSIUM

Myocardium has been studied as a possible site for intracellular shifting of potassium, although the mass of myocardium is not great enough to account for the unaccountable loss of serum potassium. In experimental animals and clinical studies, loss of myocardial potassium has been observed repeatedly following cardiopulmonary bypass[38–41] (Fig. 14.8). The same mechanism postulated for skeletal muscle potassium changes may apply to myocardium. Ischemic myocardium loses potassium more readily. Loss of myocardial potassium is greater with increasing periods of myocardial ischemia[41–43] (Fig. 14.9).

MECHANISMS OF INTRACELLULAR SHIFTS OF POTASSIUM

Although the site of intracellular shifting of potassium has not been determined by studies of red cells, skeletal muscle, or myo-

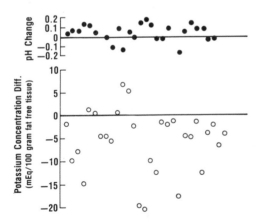

Figure 14.8. The graph shows the difference between prebypass and postbypass measurements of pH and myocardial potassium in individual patients. Myocardial potassium concentration most commonly falls. (Reproduced with permission from A. K. Mandal et al.[38])

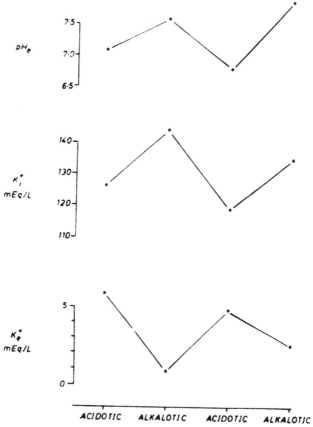

Figure 14.10. The figure shows the relationship between the acidosis and alkalosis of intracellular and extracellular potassium and extracellular pH. Intracellular potassium rises as extracellular potassium falls with alkalosis. (Reproduced with permission from M. S. Barnard et al.[27])

cardium, potent forces which have been shown to influence intracellular shifts of potassium are operating during cardiopulmonary bypass. These factors include hypothermia, alkalosis, glucose-insulin metabolism, effect of adrenergic drugs or aldosterone, Gibbs-Donnan effects, and manganese phosphate metabolism.

Hypothermia

Clinically and experimentally, serum potassium falls with a decrease in body temperature. Serum sodium may rise as serum potassium falls with hypothermia. This response to hypothermia is diminished by adrenalectomy.[44] In clinical studies, the depression of serum potassium in infants

was greater in infants cooled to 26°C than in those cooled to 32°C. This reversible change in potassium with cooling and rewarming are not well understood.

Alkalosis

Varying degrees of alkalosis are commonly observed following cardiopulmonary bypass.[45] The contributing factors include hyperventilation, use of bicarbonate, and the alkaline load of citrate in bank blood.[29] Alkalosis decreases the serum concentration of potassium in relation to intracellular stores. Alterations in pH may cause changes in serum potassium up to 3 mg/liter.[46] Amiloride, a diuretic with potassium-retaining properties, has been shown to diminish the alkalosis and hypokalemia that accompanies cardiopulmonary bypass.[47] Experimental studies show that intracellular potassium increases and extracellular potassium falls as pH rises with alkalosis[27,28] (Fig. 14.10).

Effect of Glucose and Insulin on Potassium

Serum glucose rises and serum insulin falls in response to cardiopulmonary bypass.[48] The combined effect of glucose and insulin is to cause the intracellular transport of glucose. The glycogen which is formed from intracellular glucose is deposited with an obligatory amount of potassium. Supplemental glucose and insulin increase the level of myocardial potassium during cardiopulmonary bypass.[38-40] Diabetics are particularly prone to hyperkalemia with use of cold potassium cardioplegia, presumably due to defective intracellular transport of potassium.

Endocrine Effects

The increased levels of cortisol, aldosterone, and epinephrine during cardiopulmonary bypass may have important effects on serum potassium. Cortisol and aldosterone cause increased excretion of potassium in the urine. Epinephrine affects an increased rate of potassium uptake by skeletal muscle.[49] Blocking the beta-adrenergic effects with propranolol may lead to hyperkalemia during cardiopulmonary bypass. Beta blockade with propranolol inhibits the uptake of potassium by skeletal muscle, but does not inhibit the hepatic release of potassium by beta-adrenergic stimuli.[50]

Gibbs-Donnan Effects

Experimental study in dogs showed that addition of potassium alone to the priming solutions of the pump oxygenator was insufficient to prevent hypokalemia, whereas the addition of protein as well prevented the hypokalemia.[51] This response was predicted from a mathematical model. One of the factors that determines the concentration of plasma potassium is the concentration of negatively charged protein molecules. The negatively charged protein molecules must be accompanied by positively charged charged ions, including potassium, to maintain electrical neutrality. Thus, with hemodilution the concentration of potassium falls in response to the dilutions of negatively charged proteins. The addition of albumin to the priming solution diminishes this effect.

Duration of Perfusion

The duration of cardiopulmonary bypass may have important effects on the magnitude of change of serum potassium. Short periods of cardiopulmonary bypass are associated with more severe hypokalemia than larger periods of cardiopulmonary bypass.[52] Others have noted a progressive rise in serum potassium with duration of bypass that is not related to urine volume, urine potassium concentration, pH or oxygen consumption.[53] Presumably hemolysis and possibly the cellular loss of potassium are factors that contribute to the rise in serum potassium after the initial fall with the initiation of cardiopulmonary bypass.

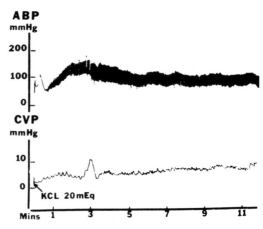

Figure 14.11. The injection of 20 mg potassium chloride is accompanied by a rise of arterial blood pressure (*ABP*) during cardiopulmonary bypass without a significant change in central venous pressure (*CVP*). (Reproduced with permission from K. A. Vasko et al.[25])

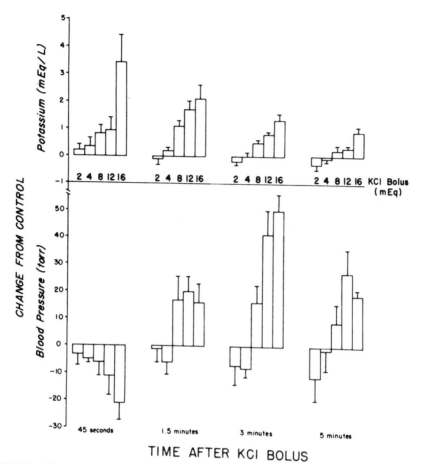

Figure 14.12. The change in serum potassium and blood pressure is shown after the injection of 2 to 16 mg KCl. Increasing doses of KCl are accompanied by increasing rise in blood pressure. (Reproduced with permission from A. J. Schwartz et al.[55])

POTASSIUM REPLACEMENT DURING CARDIOPULMONARY BYPASS

Serum potassium concentrations are routinely monitored during cardiopulmonary bypass. Protocols have been developed for potassium replacement during cardiopulmonary bypass.[6, 9, 54] Most protocols recommend a sliding scale dose of potassium based on serum potassium. The dose response of each patient is useful in determining subsequent doses. Because hyperkalemia is a dangerous event during cardiopulmonary bypass, we prefer frequent small boluses of potassium rather than continuous infusion. We determine the level of serum potassium before each bolus. Rises in systemic vascular resistance have been observed with injection of boluses of potassium[25] (Fig. 14.11). Studies of the dose response of systemic vascular resistance to boluses of potassium have shown that significant changes in systemic vascular resistance are uncommon with boluses less than 8 mEq. With boluses greater than 8 mEq, an initial fall in systemic vascular resistance followed by a rise is common[55] (Fig. 14.12). We have not observed systemic vascular effects of potassium using boluses up to 6 mEq.

References

1. Lown B, Black H, Moore FD: Digitalis, electrolytes and the surgical patient. Am J Cardiol 6:309, 1960.
2. Maginn RR, Willman VL, Cooper T, Hanlon CR: Digitalis tolerance following extracorporeal circulation. Surg Forum 12:196, 1961.
3. Ebert PA, Jude JR, Gaertner RA: Persistent hypokalemia following open-heart surgery. Circulation 31:I137, 1965.
4. Nonoyama A, Miyamoto I, Katsuda H, et al: The change in digitalis tolerance after open heart surgery. Jpn Circ J 31:1151, 1967.
5. Surawicz B: Role of electrolytes in etiology and management of cardiac arrhythmias. Prog Cardiovasc Dis 8:364, 1966.
6. Dieter RA, Neville WE, Pifarre R: Hypokalemia following hemodilution cardiopulmonary bypass. Ann Surg 171:17, 1970.
7. Selmonosky CA, Flege JB Jr: The effect of small doses of potassium on postoperative ventricular arrhythmias. J Thorac Cardiovasc Surg 53:349, 1967.
8. Walesby RK, Goode AW, Bentall HH: Nutritional status of patients undergoing valve replacement by open heart surgery. Lancet 1:76, 1978.
9. Lockey E, Longmore DB, Ross DN, Sturridge MF: Potassium and open-heart surgery. Lancet 1:671, 1966.
10. Morgan DB, Mearns AJ, Burkinshaw L: The potassium status of patients prior to open-heart surgery. J Thorac Cardiovasc Surg 76:673, 1970.
11. Cooperman LH, Strobel GE Jr, Kennell EM: Massive hyperkalemia after administration of succinylcholine. Anesthesiology 32:161, 1970.
12. Weintraub HD, Heisterkamp DV, Cooperman LH: Change in plasma potassium concentration after depolarizing blockers in anaesthetized man. Br J Anaesth 41:1048, 1969.
13. Walton JD, Farman JV: Suxamethonium, potassium and renal failure. Anaesthesia 28:626, 1973.
14. List WF: Serum potassium changes during induction of anaesthesia. Br J Anaesth 39:480, 1967.
15. Bozer AY, Ilicin G, Apikoglu A, Karamehmetoglu A, Saylam A: Serum electrolyte changes during extracorporeal circulation. Jpn Heart J 13:195, 1972.
16. Regensburger D, Paschen K, Fuchs C: Veranderungen des Electrolyt- und Säure-Basen-Haushaltes bei Operationen mit kardio-pulmonalem Bypass unter Hamodilution. Thoraxchirurgie 20:473, 1972.
17. Kirsh MM, Morales J, Kahn DR, et al: Effect of extracorporeal circulation on total body potassium. Arch Surg 101:500, 1970.
18. Marcial MB, Vedoya RC, Zerbini EJ, Verginelli G, Bittencourt D, do Amaral RG: Potassium in cardiac surgery with extracorporeal perfusion. Am J Cardiol 23:400, 1969.
19. Walker WF, Watt A: The metabolic response to cardiac surgery. Br J Surg 54:311, 1967.
20. Moffitt EA, White RD, Molnar GD, McGoon DC: Comparative effects of whole blood, hemodiluted, and clear priming solutions on myocardial and body metabolism in man. Can J Surg 14:382, 1971.
21. Johnston AE, Radde IC, Steward DJ, Taylor J: Acid-base and electrolyte changes in infants undergoing profound hypothermia for surgical correction of congenital heart defects. Can Anaesth Soc J 21:23, 1974.
22. Johnston AE, Radde IC, Nisbet HIA, Taylor J: Effects of altering calcium in haemodiluted pump primes on sodium and potassium in children undergoing open-heart operations. Can Anaesth Soc J 19:517, 1972.
23. Patrick J, Sivpragasam S: The prediction of postoperative potassium excretion after cardiopulmonary bypass. J Thorac Cardiovasc Surg 73:559, 1977.
24. Cohn LH, Angell WW, Shumway NE: Body fluid shifts after cardiopulmonary bypass. J Thorac Cardiovasc Surg 62:423, 1971.
25. Vasko KA, DeWall RA, Riley AM: Hypokalemia. Physiological abnormalities during cardiopulmonary bypass. Ann Thorac Surg 15:347, 1973.
26. Wilson GM, Dunn FG, McQueen MJ, Kerr IC, Thomson RM: Comparison of intravenous bumetanide and frusemide during open heart surgery. Postgrad Med J 51:72, 1975.
27. Barnard MS, Saunders SJ, Eales L, Barnard CN: Hypokalaemia during extracorporeal circulation. An experimental study. South Afr Med J 40:1132, 1966.
28. Barnard MS, Saunders SJ, Eales L, Barnard CN: Hypokalaemia during extracorporeal circulation. Lancet 1:240, 1966.
29. Flemma RJ, Young WG Jr: The metabolic effects of mechanical ventilation and respiratory alkalosis in postoperative patients. Surgery 56:36, 1964.
30. Abe T, Nagata Y, Yoshioka K, Iyomasa Y: Hypopotassemia following open heart surgery by cardiopulmonary bypass. J Cardiovasc Surg 18:411, 1977.
31. Abe T: Influence of cardiac surgery using cardiopulmonary bypass on metabolic regulation. Jpn Circ J 38:13, 1974.
32. DeWall RA, Roden TP, Kimura M: Red blood cell potassium as an index of total body potassium. Angiology 21:211, 1970.
33. Kettlewell M: Potassium changes after open heart surgery. Br Heart J 32:557, 1970.
34. Merin G, Viskoper JR, Borman JB, Cotev S: Red blood cell potassium and serum potassium during open-heart surgery. Isr J Med Sci 6:736, 1970.
35. Sumida S, Kamegai T: Effects of various priming solutions upon extra- and intra-cellular water and electrolytes following hemodilution technique of extracorporeal circulation. A new priming solution "LMDAS." Jpn Circ J 32:21, 1968.
36. Neville WE, Balis JU, Talso PJ, Pifarre R, Dieter R: Postbypass histochemical alterations following overinfusion of noncolloids. J Trauma 8:827, 1968.
37. Muller C, Lutz H, Schmitz W, Reiss F: Elektrolytveränderungen bei herzoperationen mit eigenblutverdünnungsperfusionen. Thoraxchirurgie 16:264, 1968.
38. Mandal AK, Callaghan JC, Dolan AM, Sterns LP: Potassium and cardiac surgery. Ann Thorac Surg 7:428, 1969.
39. Mandal AK, Callaghan JC, Sterns LP: Changes in

intracellular potassium resulting from extracorporeal circulation. Surg Forum 19:137, 1968.

40. Mandal AK, Prasad K, Dolan AM, Callaghan JC, Sterns LP: Energy dependent changes in myocardial potassium during extracorporeal circulation. Surg Forum 20:184, 1969.

41. Taggart P, Slater JDH: Significance of potassium in genesis of arrhythmias in induced cardiac ischaemia. Br Med J 4:195, 1971.

42. Taggart P, Slater JDH: The possible significance of ionic gradient changes associated with cardio-pulmonary bypass surgery. Clin Sci 38:26P, 1970.

43. Taggart P, Slater JDH: Some effects of bypass surgery on myocardial and skeletal muscle electrolytes and their clinical importance. Br Heart J 31:393, 1969.

44. Munday KA, Blane GF, Chin EF, Machell ES: Plasma electrolyte changes in hypothermia. Thorax 13:334, 1958.

45. Krohn BG, Urquhart RR, Magidson O, Tsuji HK, Redington JV, Kay JH: Metabolic alkalosis following heart surgery. J Thorac Cardiovasc Surg 56:732, 1968.

46. Burnell JM, Scribner BH: Interpretation of the serum potassium concentration in patients with acid-base imbalance. Surg Forum 7:71, 1956.

47. Hocking MA, Bain WH: Effect of amiloride on metabolic alkalosis and hypokalaemia after cardiopulmonary bypass surgery. Br Heart J 36:597, 1974.

48. Nuutinen LS, Mononen P, Kairaluoma M, Tuonenen S: Effects of open-heart surgery on carbohydrate and lipid metabolism. J Thorac Cardiovasc Surg 73:680, 1977.

49. Todd EP: Potassium kinetics during cardiopulmonary bypass. In *Pathophysiology and Techniques of Cardiopulmonary Bypass*, edited by JR Utley, Vol. 1. Baltimore, Williams & Wilkins, 1982, pp. 182–190.

50. Bethune DW, McKay R: Paradoxical changes in serum-potassium during cardiopulmonary bypass in association with non-cardioselective beta blockade. Lancet 2:380, 1978.

51. Henney RP, Riemenschneider TA, DeLand EC, Maloney JV: Prevention of hypokalemic cardiac arrhythmias associated with cardiopulmonary bypass and hemodilution. Surg Forum 21:145, 1970.

52. Yokoyama M, Fojikura I, Yokoyama K, Sakakibara S: Transient hypopotassemia and ECG changes following hemodilution perfusion. Arch Surg 104:640, 1972.

53. Lampard JR, Couves CM: Observations of serum potassium in patients undergoing cardiopulmonary bypass. Can Med Assoc J 102:61, 1970.

54. Babka R, Pifarre R: Potassium replacement during cardiopulmonary bypass. J Thorac Cardiovasc Surg 73:212, 1977.

55. Schwartz AJ, Conahan TJ III, Jobes DR, Andrews RW, MacVaugh H III, Ominsky AJ: Peripheral vascular response to potassium administration during cardiopulmonary bypass. J Thorac Cardiovasc Surg 79:237, 1980.

CHAPTER 15

EFFECTS OF CARDIOPULMONARY BYPASS ON LUNG FUNCTION

RICHARD M. PETERS, M.D.

In the early days of cardiopulmonary bypass (CPB), pulmonary complications caused a significant percentage of deaths.[1] In the past 25 years, during which time CPB has become commonplace, the incidence of pulmonary complications has fallen but still remains a problem.

The early writers described the postpump lung, a lung with interstitial edema, perivascular hemorrhages, and miliary atelectasis.[2, 3] With prolonged periods of bypass, intraalveolar hemorrhage and vascular congestion are present. Electron microscopic studies show increased numbers of polymorphonuclear cells and swelling of endothelia and the type I cells of alveolar lining, the same morphology as seen after shock or trauma.[4] With the recognition of the syndrome of acute respiratory distress (ARDS), the pump lung took its place as one form of ARDS. It is now generally agreed that ARDS is pulmonary edema due to increased capillary permeability.[5, 6] There is not agreement about the etiology of ARDS, most probably because it has many etiologies.

Chenoweth and coauthors[7] have pointed out that the consequences of release of complement-derived anaphylactotoxins C3a and C5a act as spasmogens. They stimulate the release of mast cell histamine, contract smooth muscle, and increase vascular permeability, the combination that is found in the "post pump syndrome." They used radioimmunoassays to quantitate C3a and C5a in human plasma of patients undergoing CPB. C3a was more than 15 times preoperative level, but C5a was not changed. On reperfusion of the lungs there was apparent sequestration neutrophils. The amount of sequestration was increased directly with time of aortic cross-clamping and duration of CPB. They found that nylon in the oxygenator and oxygen bubbles both produced time-dependent generation of C3a. The failure to find C5a was attributed to its binding by a single pass through the circulation. The oxygen-blood interface probably denatures protein, which activates complement. The plastics in the oxygenator are a more potent stimulus than the oxygen bubbles. If blood prime is used, the complement might be activated by foreign proteins. There is evidence that activation of immune systems results in increase in oxygen radicals such as O_3 and H_2O_2. These may be the agents that lead to alveolocapillary injury. This type of study has just recently been pursued. They give promise of new understanding of the cause of alveolocapillary damage.

LUNG FLUID EXCHANGE

Postperfusion lung dysfunction is characterized by excessive pulmonary capillary fluid filtration. The excessive filtration is due to capillary damage probably induced by complement release and/or the activation of the coagulation cascade.

Understanding the consequences of this injury must start with the basic equation that defines fluid exchange across the capillaries—the Starling equation.[8]

$$Q_f = K_f S \left[(P_c - P_t) - \sigma(\Pi_c - \Pi_t) \right]$$

This equation states that Q_f, the amount of fluid filtered across the capillary membrane in milliliters per minute, will rise with increases in:

1. K_f, the filtration coefficient or permeability of the membrane in milliliters per minute per millimeter of Hg
2. S, the surface area of the capillary bed
3. P_c, the capillary hydrostatic pressure in mm Hg
4. Π_t, the colloidal osmotic pressure of proteins in the interstitial fluid in mm Hg.

Fluid filtration will also increase with decrease in:

1. P_t, the tissue pressure in the interstitial space in mm Hg
2. σ, the reflection coefficient, a dimensionless number that defines the ability of the membrane to prevent passage of protein
3. Π_c, the colloidal osmotic pressure of plasma proteins in mm Hg.

The pulmonary edema seen after CPB is high permeability edema, the result of capillary damage. This type of injury increases the filtration of fluid. All of the changes in the four Starling pressures that increase filtration are multiplied by K_f, so any increase in K_f will amplify the increase in filtration caused by changes of these factors. The fall in σ associated with fall in K_f allows leakage of protein with fluid, so the difference between Π_c and Π_t is decreased, and serum proteins are less effective in preventing edema. Therefore, when K_f increases and σ decreases, small increases in P_c cause large increases in interstitial fluid. The goal during

and immediately after CPB is to prevent capillary injury which increases K_f. If K_f is increased, control of pulmonary capillary pressure must be optimal.

HEMODILUTION

On first appraisal the Starling equation seems to contradict a clear clinical impression that the incidence of the postpump lung syndrome decreased following the introduction of the technique of hemodilution. Despite a method which lowered colloidal osmotic pressure of serum and should increase fluid filtration, postpump pulmonary edema declined.[9, 10] A number of other studies have shown that the use of protein-free electrolyte solutions is at least as good as protein solutions in replacing blood loss or for oxygenator prime in CPB.[11, 12] Analysis of this apparent anachronism provides a good basis for introducing the complexities involved in interpreting the Starling equation.

The primary goal when hemodilution was first used was to reduce the amount of blood needed for priming pump oxygenators. The technique achieved this end, with an unanticipated dividend of reduction in the incidence of postpump ARDS and renal problems.[13, 14] In a series of patients studied, we found that hemodilution lowers the serum colloidal osmotic pressure (Π_c) from 16 to 8 mm of Hg (Fig. 15.1).[15] Byrick et al.[12] showed that even if protein was infused, serum protein concentration fell.

The Starling equation predicts that unless some compensatory change occurs, fall in Π_c will increase filtration across the pulmonary capillary. Since the incidence of postpump pulmonary edema went down, other factors in addition to Π_c must have changed. The work of Taylor et al.[16] has shown that the lung has an "edema safety factor," that is, that 7 mm change in net Starling force can occur without pulmonary edema. Studies from our laboratories have provided explanation of this safety factor with hemodilution.[17] A series of baboons underwent plasmapheresis three to four times to reduce colloid osmotic pressure from 19.6 mm of Hg to 4.7 mm of Hg while pulmonary capillary wedge pressure was maintained at

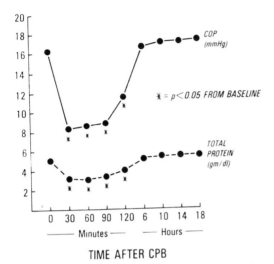

Figure 15.1. Changes in colloid osmotic pressure (COP) and plasma total protein (TP) during and after cardiopulmonary bypass. (Reproduced with permission from F. J. Menninger III et al.[15])

constant level by infusion of Ringer's lactate. None of the animals developed pulmonary edema. Since lung lymph colloidal osmotic pressure is thought to be the same as interstitial fluid colloidal osmotic pressure, the right and left lymphatic ducts were cannulated to collect pulmonary lymph and measure its colloidal pressure and volume. The apparent reasons for the lack of pulmonary edema were a seven-fold increase in lymph flow and drop in colloidal osmotic pressure of lung lymph from 16.3 to 4.7 mm of Hg (Fig. 15.2). In these experiments, the drop in II_t neutralized all but 3 mm of Hg of the 15 mm of Hg drop in II_c. The increase in lymph flow compensated for the increased fluid filtration due to 3 mm of Hg rise in net filtration force. Erdmann et al.[18] have shown that the same mechanism, dilution of lung extravascular II_t, partially compensates for rises in pulmonary capillary pressure due to left ventricular dysfunction. This study emphasizes that even in lung with intact alveolocapillary membrane, one cannot predict fluid filtration or that lung water will increase from simple measurement of the difference between serum colloidal osmotic pressure and pulmonary wedge pressure. One must include the state of the interstitium and the rate of lymph flow to predict the degree of fluid accumulation in the lungs.

Hemodilution using electrolyte solution for priming the pump oxygenator rather than priming with multiple units of blood gave a benefit that far outweighed the effects of fall in II_c. It reduced alveolocapillary damage and the resultant increase in pulmonary capillary permeability. Hemodilution also markedly reduced the complictions of intravascular coagulopathy and intravascular coagulation.[14] The reasons for these dividends are beginning to be elucidated. They are most probably multifactorial. Blaisdell[19] has presented evidence that a cause of ARDS is multiple microscopic emboli which can occur with severe trauma or multiple transfusions. Rabelo et al.[13] identified the adherence of white cells to the pulmonary capillary endothelium during CPB with subsequent endothelial and alveolar cell damage. These were not present with hemodilution.

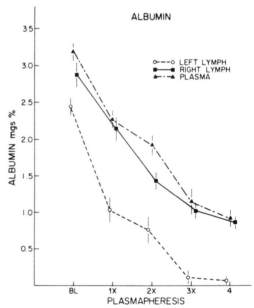

Figure 15.2. The effect of sequential plasmapheresis on albumin concentration in plasma and right and left lymph. (Reproduced with permission from C. K. Zarins et al.[17] and the American Heart Association, Inc.)

Hemodilution reduces the number of units of blood used and so the chain of events leading to alveolocapillary damage and increase in the filtration coefficient. Dilute prime does not cause pulmonary edema because the drop in the colloidal osmotic pressure of plasma proteins is compensated by drop in colloidal osmotic pressure of proteins in the interstitial fluid and rise in pulmonary lymph flow. The system can compensate for low colloidal osmotic pressure of plasma proteins if the capillary maintains its integrity.

Since ARDS is pulmonary edema due to increased capillary permeability,[5, 6] the criteria for high permeability edema are an increase in K_f and decrease in protein reflectance. In some human studies, measurement of colloidal osmotic pressure of distal bronchial aspirates has been the criterion for differentiating high permeability edema from edema due to cardiac failure.[20] If K_f is increased and σ decreased, giving protein solutions may not protect from pulmonary edema and could aggravate the problem because the protein leaks into the interstitial space and must be removed by the lymphatics before the edema can clear.

While hemodilution and control of P_c have decreased the incidence of ARDS following CPB, it has not eliminated it. As noted above, complement is activated by the nylon in the oxygenation by oxygen bubbles. When pump runs are long, over 2 hours, the incidence of postpump ARDS rises.[3] Longer pump runs cause more damage to blood elements, but they also may have other deleterious effects.

PULMONARY CAPILLARY HYDROSTATIC PRESSURE

While prevention of damage to pulmonary capillary is important, strict control of the level of pulmonary capillary hydrostatic pressure is critical to prevention of pulmonary edema.[21] During bypass, effective venting of the left ventricle is essential to prevent rises in pulmonary vascular pressures. There is significant evidence that transient acute rises in pulmonary capillary pressure can cause mechanical disruption of the endothelial cell junctures. The injury

results in increase in K_f which persists after P_c falls to normal levels. Pulmonary capillary hypertension results in immediate increase in fluid filtration and damage to the alveolocapillary membrane. This form of injury can be prevented. The use of vents is undoubtedly one of the major factors in the reduction of postpump pulmonary edema and rise in K_f.

Air emboli in the pulmonary circulation block flow to the embolized vessels and increase pressure in the open vessels. The result of this presumed benign form of air embolus can lead to damage to the unperfused areas of lung and increased filtration in the perfused areas.

Equally important in achieving control of P_c in patients undergoing CPB is the precise pre- and postoperative control of the left heart filling pressure and afterload. The common use of the Swan-Ganz catheter to monitor and control P_c while using vasodilators to alter afterload prevents previously unrecognized elevations of P_c above critical levels. If there is moderate increase in K_f, then effective control of P_c is of even greater importance.[6] The use of vasodilators with repeated measurements of cardiac output and P_c allows achievement of optimal levels of cardiac output at lowest possible P_c. In particular, it minimizes periods of low cardiac output and transient extreme elevations of P_c.

INTERACTING CAUSES OF ALVEOLAR COLLAPSE

When alveoli become filled with fluid, they cannot provide gas exchange. As a result, blood perfusing them does not exchange oxygen and carbon dioxide. An intrapulmonary shunt is present. There are two interacting causes of intrapulmonary shunting—interstitial and intraalveolar flooding and alveolar collapse.[20] Flooding results from alteration in pulmonary capillary permeability or from a change in the transcapillary permeability or from a change in the transcapillary pressures leading to increase in fluid filtration. Alveolar collapse results when lung volume falls below critical closing volume of airways and alveoli. The interaction occurs because interstitial edema and leakage of fluid into alveoli make alveoli more susceptible to collapse. The geometry of alveoli is such that their stability is greatest when they are dry. When fluid leaks into the alveolar lumen, it coats the surface and is sucked to the alveolar corners due to more negative surface pressure in these corners. When the corners are filled with fluid, the effective radius of the alveoli is smaller, and they collapse at a lower transmural pressure. As inflation decreases, transmural alveolar pressures decrease. The partially fluid-filled alveoli collapse at higher transmural pressure and so at higher lung volume than normal alveoli.

The cardiac surgical patient may have multiple causes of increase of alveolar collapse and consequent intrapulmonary shunting—increase in capillary permeability, increase in pulmonary capillary pressure due to left ventricular failure or infusion of an inappropriately large volume of fluid, decrease in oncotic pressure with hemodilution, and fall in lung volume due to decrease in lung compliance or alterations in chest wall mechanics. Each of these may contribute independently to collapse and fluid filling of alveoli, and all act synergistically when more than one cause is present.

Perfusion and Ventilation

During CPB, pulmonary blood flow is interrupted while bronchial flow is maintained. However, in experimental studies, perfusion of the lungs through the pulmonary artery is not protective but rather seems to be damaging. The nonpulsatile motion of flow, the sensitivity of the pulmonary vasculature to small changes in pressure, and greater injury from more exposure to toxic factors in the perfusing blood all may contribute to the injury induced by pulmonary artery perfusion. Lack of perfusion may result in decrease in manufacture of surfactant by type II cells. However, following CPB, a measurable change of surfactant has not been found,[22] and so this cause of ARDS in infants is unlikely to be an important cause of ARDS following CPB.

Following CPB, pulmonary vascular resistance (PVR) is often elevated. The elevated PVR may have multiple causes. Unless care is taken to prevent air from entering the pulmonary artery, air embolus can lead to transient obstruction of the pulmonary vasculature and increase in PVR. The same is true of microemboli from blood and other detritus, particularly from the blood aspirated with the suction. Microfilters decrease the amount of embolic material, but microfilters also remove platelets and increase pump pressure, which may damage blood elements. In studies of filters vs. no filters with transfusion, there is little evidence that the filter protects patients. The unanswered question about postshock and postperfusion increase in PVR is the role of the vasoactive substances, serotonin and prostaglandins.

While the use of the Swan-Ganz catheter and venting of the left ventricle by preventing rise in P_c has contribute significantly to lowering the incidence of postperfusion pulmonary edema and rises in shunt fraction, prevention of alveolar collapse must have equal attention. When lung volume falls below critical level, airways and alveoli close. The airways in different regions of the lungs do not close simultaneously. In the dependent portions of the lung, the effect of gravity compresses these areas, decreasing lung volume more than in the nondependent portions.[23] Therefore, the airways in the dependent portions will close at a higher total lung volume than will the airways in the nondependent areas. The closing volume of the lung is defined as the volume of lung at which airways in the dependent portions of the lung close. The closing volume decreases with age and smoking and is markedly reduced in emphysema. If lung volume remains below closing volume for a significant period of time, air will be absorbed from the alveoli and they will collapse. This fact has led to numerous studies of the effect of various means of ventilation during CPB.[24-26] Studies have compared static inflation, deflation, and ventilation during CPB. With all three methods, lung compliance falls, as does functional residual capacity (FRC)—the amount of air left in the lungs at the end of expiration—but there is no difference between the three forms. These various forms of inflation are carefully reviewed by Pennock et al.[27]

The conflicting results found in studies of various methods of ventilation during CPB probably are due to differences in methodology. Static inflation has been shown to be protective, as has continued ventilation, yet each has been shown to be deleterious. The differences may depend on the critical factor of whether the volume of gas in the lung was kept above the closing volume of the dependent airways and some oxygen was provided to the lung parenchyma. If lung volume falls so airways are allowed to close, it will lead to reabsorption of the air in the alveoli and their collapse. If interstitial and intraalveolar fluid are increased, when lung volume falls the alveoli are more vulnerable and will collapse faster. Since most studies of the various methods of inflating lungs during bypass do not measure the total lung volume, changes in lung volume could explain the discrepancies in the various studies (Fig. 15.3).

Despite the fact that there is no pulmonary artery perfusion during CPB, bronchial circulation continues. Bronchial circulation may not supply enough oxygen to provide for the oxygen needs of the lung parenchyma.[28] In patients with the types of cyanotic heart disease where bronchial circulation is increased, bronchial arteries may hyperperfuse the lungs. With lack of the pumping effect of periodic ventilation, lymph flow could fall and pulmonary water increase.

During CPB, the theoretically best method of ventilation would be to use air while maintaining lung volume at prebypass FRC level. If the inflation method is chosen, additional oxygen must be bled in during CPB. Those using the periodic inflation technic must carefully maintain functional residual volume constant. The mechanisms of alveolar collapse and alveolocapillary injury are further complicated by the problem of the role of oxygen toxicity in damage to alveolocapillary membrane. Increased levels of inspired oxygen above 50% can cause a picture similar to ARDS, and there is some evidence that prolonged use of increased oxygen at F_IO_2 of less than 0.5 can be toxic.[29] On the other hand, anoxia associated with lack of perfusion and/or ventilation of the lung can cause injury. If

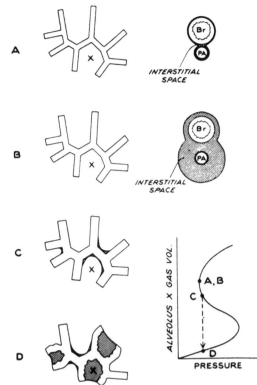

Figure 15.3. Schematic representation of fluid accumulation pattern in acute pulmonary edema. (A) Normal lung. (B) Interstitial edema in which fluid accumulated preferentially in the loose interstitial space around the conducting blood vessels and airways. (C) Early alveolar edema showing loose interstitial spaces filled and fluid overflowing into alveoli accumulating at the corners where the curvature is greatest. (D) Alveolar flooding in which individual alveoli have reached a critical configuration at which the existing inflation pressure can no longer maintain stability, and the alveolus gas volume rapidly passes to a new configuration with much reduced curvature (see *inset graph*). Final alveolus volume is much reduced. (Reproduced with permission from N. C. Staub.[20])

the cause of lung damage with release of complement is due to presence of superoxides, high oxygen concentrations will increase them.

PLEURAL CAVITIES

A simple change in operative technic, the abandonment of routine opening of the pleural cavities to afford drainage of the mediastinum, has significantly reduced pulmonary complictions.[30] Opening the pleura lowers lung volume and increases the amount of alveolar collapse. There may also be direct physical damage by handling the lung. Care to preserve the pleura intact increases lung volume during CPB and reduces the postoperative hemothorax which compresses portions of the lung. The avoidance of intrapleural chest tubes also reduces chest wall pain, a major cause of the universal postoperative decreases in all lung volumes.

POSTOPERATIVE DECREASE IN LUNG VOLUME DUE TO CHEST WALL PAIN

Most studies show that some increase in interstitial fluid in the lungs following by-

pass, which makes them stiffer, decreases their compliance. When lung compliance falls, the end-expiratory lung volume is smaller. Portions of the lung will fall below closing volume. The instability of alveoli partially filled with fluid aggravates the interacting effects of stiff lungs and low volume.

As shown in Figure 15.4, a study in our laboratories has shown a drop in lung volumes of post-CPB. Tidal volume is decreased and rate increased to maintain alveolar ventilation. The total lung volume and all of its subdivisions are reduced. Of particular significance is the fall in FRC. All of the patients in this study would have functional residual volumes below closing volume during the immediate postoperative period. The fall in end-expiratory lung volume, FRC, persists for 5 to 7 days.

At end expiration, the volume of the basilar portions of the lung in smokers and older individuals is below their critical closing volume.[31] Immobilization, particularly in the supine position, decreases end-expi-

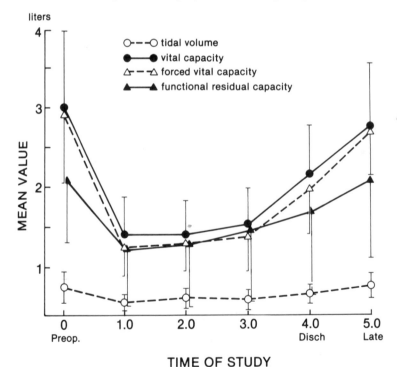

TIME OF STUDY

Figure 15.4. Postoperative changes in lung volumes in a series of patients undergoing cardiopulmonary bypass at University Hospital, San Diego. Note that lung volumes are as depressed on postoperative days 2 and 3 as on day 1.

ratory lung volume because the abdominal contents push up on rather than pull down on the diaphragm. The high diaphragm has its greatest effect on the volume of the lower lobes. CPB patients have significant incidence of lower lobe collapse. Similar changes occur with lateral thoracotomies and laparotomies. Identifying the relative contributions to postoperative pulmonary dysfunction of CPB, cardiac insufficiency, and chest wall dysfunction is next to impossible. The problem is further compounded by the frequency of preexisting degenerative lung disease in this patient population.

Shunt Fraction

Pulmonary edema leads to alveolar flooding and collapse. Since blood flow is preserved to the collapse and flooded alveoli, an intrapulmonary shunt results. Venous blood reaches the arterial circulation without any gas exchange. Delineation of the magnitude of the intrapulmonary shunt provides the most predictive measure of the degree of pulmonary dysfunction in ARDS. It defines the portion of the cardiac output going to the unventilated lung. Many clinicians use the alveolar arterial oxygen difference ($A - aO_2$) after 20 minutes of 100% oxygen breathing.[33] This test is used as an indicator of how much pulmonary blood flow is going to the collapsed and flooded alveoli. The use of $A - aO_2$ gradient can lead to serious errors. Delineation of the magnitude of the intrapulmonary shunt provides a better method. It defines the portion of the cardiac output going to the unventilated lung. Calculation of intrapulmonary shunt depends on solving a simple mixing equation. By measuring F_IO_2, arterial and venous oxygen content, shunt is calculated from the following formula:

$$Q_s/Q_t = \frac{C_cO_2 - C_aO_2}{C_cO_2 - C_vO_2}$$

where C_cO_2 is the content of oxygen that would be achieved if the patient's blood was in equilibrium with alveolar gas of the composition that would result from the measuring F_IO_2; C_aO_2 is arterial oxygen content—directly measured or calculated from PaO_2, $PaCO_2$, pH, and Hgb; and C_vO_2 is venous oxygen content—directly measured

or collected from P_vO_2, P_vCO_2, pH, and Hgb.

If either the shunt fraction increases or C_vO_2 decreases, the oxygen content and PO_2 of arterial blood will fall. The differentiation of the cause of fall in PaO_2 is critical to treatment of the post-CPB patient. Low venous oxygen content (C_vO_2), indicative of depressed cardiac output, requires treatment by adjustment of preload, afterload, and myocardial contractility; an increase in O_s/Q_t requires treatment to reexpand alveoli and decrease lung water. Since these therapies often are in conflict, precise therapy depends on precise diagnosis of the relative roles of change in Q_s/Q_t and cardiac output in depressing PaO_2.

A study of a series of ICU patients has enabled us to develop an index to predict which patients require measurement of C_vO_2 to estimate shunt fraction.[34] Using arterial blood gases and F_IO_2, the shunt is calculated assuming venous blood has an oxygen content of 4.5 volumes percent less than arterial blood. If the calculated Q_s/Q_t is greater than 0.2, mixed venous blood should be sampled to determine what portion of the decrease in PaO_2 is due to shunt and what to low C_vO_2.[34] In another study we have reviewed the shunt fractions on 50 patients undergoing CPB at University Hospital, San Diego (Table 15.1). The shunt is higher on the 2nd and 3rd postoperative days than on day 1. The interacting effects of increase in lung water, reduction of lung volumes, immobility, and failure to cough allow progressive collapse of alveoli over the first few postoperative days. These interacting effects plus probably cold injury to the phrenic nerves from cold saline in the pericardium are the cause of commonly found lower lobe atelectasis in postcoronary artery bypass patients. These patients often have added risk of increased alveolar collapse due to degenerative lung disease with increased closing volumes. Patients requiring valve replacement with elevated left heart filling presures have stiffer lungs and are more subject to increased shunt due to diffuse microatelectasis. If shunt above 0.2 is present, positive end-expiratory pressure or continuous positive pressure breathing is also indicated.

Table 15.1
Means and Standard Deviations of Shunt Fraction (Q_s/Q_t) in 50 Post-CPB Patients

	24 hour	48 hour	72 hour
All types (61)	12.93 ± 5.85	16.61 ± 7.30	16.87 ± 7.45
CABG (47)	13.40 ± 6.19	17.96 ± 7.34	17.38 ± 7.42
Valve (10)	10.90 ± 3.81	11.50 ± 5.50	16.10 ± 9.00
Valve + (4) CABG*	12.50 ± 6.45	13.50 ± 4.51	12.75 ± 5.91

* CABG, coronary artery bypass graft.

VENTILATORS

The use of ventilators to treat patients with postoperative cardiopulmonary problems first gained acceptance in post-CPB patients. In the early days, since postoperative cardiorespiratory problems were common in CPB patients, the use of ventilators to treat them led to the development of new types of respirators and wide interest in their application to treatment of all types of surgical patients. The success in assisting ventilation in CPB patients with postoperative stiff lungs or low cardiac output led to the inevitable question: would prophylactic postoperative ventilatory assistance lower the incidence of postoperative complications? Control studies have not shown any advantage in the use of prophylactic ventilation in patients without cardiorespiratory problems.[32] However, with the present popularity of narcotic anesthesia for coronary artery bypass, many patients have persistent central depression of respiration in the immediate postoperative period. These patients require ventilator support until the narcotic effect has stopped.

In the days when controlled ventilation was the method of supporting ventilation, many studies were made and criteria developed to predict the safety of removing a patient from ventilatory support. Unfortunately, the ultimate criterion was to remove the patients from support and observe them to see if they could maintain adequate alveolar ventilation. The ability to maintain adequate alveolar ventilation depended on three factors: (1) the mechanical state of the lungs—their stiffness and airway resistance; (2) the mechanical state of the chest cage—its efficiency as a chest bellows and the strength of the patient; (3) the efficiency of the lungs—the coordination of ventilation and perfusion. The postpump lung is a stiff lung with poor ventilation-perfusion coordination. It is inefficient. A debilitated patient with muscle wasting would not be able to ventilate such lungs adequately. More critical to the post-CPB patient is that a patient with low cardiac output has low respiratory muscle perfusion. They will develop respiratory failure without ventilatory support.

Weaning from Ventilator

While the patient is totally supported by a ventilator, Pa_{O_2} and Pa_{CO_2} may be normal but the patients may not be capable of supporting their own ventilatory needs. Pa_{CO_2} indicates the adequacy of alveolar ventilation[35] and Pa_{O_2} the adequacy of oxygen transfer. A post-CPB patient must be able to maintain a normal pH and Pa_{CO_2} and oxygen above 70 torr for safe, successful weaning. If Pa_{O_2} is low due to shunt, the shunt must be quantified and treated with continuous positive airway pressure (CPAP). A depressed pH without elevation of Pa_{CO_2} above 40 indicates metabolic acidosis, usually the result of low cardiac output.

Ventilator support provides assistance to the heart as well as to the lungs. By doing the work of breathing, it lowers tissue oxygen demands and thus the level of required cardiac output. Therefore, the first requirement for initiating weaning is to have a cardiac index above 2.5 liters/min. To assess the patient's strength, vital capacity, which requires patient cooperation, can be measured, but it has a wide range of values. In our laboratories, we concentrated on measures of work required to ventilate the lungs.

Unfortunately, in all such studies there was a large overlap between measured values of patients who could be weaned from the ventilator and those who could not. In a study in our laboratories[35] and one by Hilberman et al.[37] using multiple postoperative function tests, we found that the most useful criteria for predicting the success of early weaning were the preoperative pulmonary and cardiac functional status.

Despite all of these studies, for the clinician in making a decision on a patient, the ultimate test remained removal from a ventilator and subsequent measurement of Pa_{CO_2} and Pa_{O_2}. The advent of intermittent mandatory ventilation (IMV) has provided a safer solution to evaluating the need for assisted ventilation than trial without ventilation. In this mode of ventilation, the work of breathing is shared between the patient and the mechanical assist device. To test the ability of the patients to support their own ventilation, the IMV rate can be lowered and the response to the added stress evaluated. A stepwise weaning has replaced an all or nothing system.

Although studies of the efficacy of prophylactic ventilation after patients have recovered from anesthetic central depression have not shown any significant improvement and suggest that unnecessary ventilation may be harmful,[32] this does not mean that all patients can get along without ventilator support. In this regard, it is critical to understand that patients' lungs are usually better on the 1st than on the 2nd and 3rd postoperative days (Fig. 15.1).

SUMMARY

The direct pulmonary effects of CPB are hard to separate from the deficits of pulmonary function due to (1) left ventricular dysfunction requiring increased capillary hydrostatic pressure; (2) alveolar collapse resulting from lowered lung volumes caused by chest wall pain and noncompliant lungs; (3) the production of regional underventilation and edema by immobilization. CPB compromises lung function by injuring the alveolocapillary membrane, which increases filtration fraction (K_f) and decreases protein reflectance. There is no simple method to measure an increase in K_f or decrease in σ. Some investigators have measured the amount of albumin or total proteins in bronchial secretions. The protein content is elevated in patients with ARDS. These secretions must be obtained by bronchoscopy, and so the test is not a practical clinical tool. Until a clinical method of measuring K_f is available, only indirect evidence can identify whether capillary injury with rise in K_f, increased capillary hydrostatic pressure, decreased lung expansion due to chest wall dysfunction, and noncompliant lungs and immobilization are significant factors in a particular patient's post-CPB pulmonary edema. There can be no question that post-CPB pulmonary dysfunction is multifactorial. All of these factors need to be attended to protect these patients from life-theatening pulmonary complications.

The factors that are paramount in preventing post-CPB pulmonary dysfunction are:

1. Use of minimal possible number of blood transfusions. This will require reuse of cells and so some form of cell saver.
2. Keeping duration of CPB and aortic cross-clamping as short as feasible.
3. Preventing elevation of P_c by effective left heart decompression during bypass.
4. Carefully controlling filling pressure and afterload during the postoperative period.
5. Effectively controlling pain to enhance deep breathing and cough and to increase the end-expiratory lung volume.
6. Early mobilization, particularly avoiding prolonged positioning in the supine posture.
7. Avoiding excessive concentrations of oxygen by keeping Pa_{O_2} below 110 torr.
8. Teaching the patient to move in bed, take deep breaths, and cough.

References

1. Dodril FD: The effects of total body perfusion upon the lungs. In *Extracorporeal Circulation*, edited by

JG Allen. Springfield, Ill., Charles C Thomas, 1958, p. 327.

2. Asada S, Yamaguchi M: Fine structural change in the lung following cardiopulmonary bypass. Its relationship to early postoperative course. Chest 59:478, 1971.

3. Ratliff NB, Young WG Jr, Hackel DB, Mikat E, Wilson JW: Pulmonary injury secondary to extracorporeal circulation. An ultrastructural study. J Thorac Cardiovasc Surg 65:425, 1973.

4. Orell SR: Lung pathology in respiratory distress following shock in the adult. Acta Pathol Microbiol Scand [A] 79:65, 1971.

5. Brigham KL: Pulmonary edema: Cardiac and noncardiac. Am J Surg 138:361, 1979.

6. Staub NC: Pulmonary edema due to increased microvascular permeability to fluid and protein. Circ Res 43:143, 1978.

7. Chenoweth DE, Cooper SW, Hugli TE, Stewart RW, Blackstone EH, Kirklin JW: Complement activation during cardiopulmonary bypass. Evidence for generation of C3a and C5a anaphylatoxins. N Engl J Med 304:497, 1981.

8. Starling EH: On the absorption of fluids from the connective tissue spaces. J Physiol 19:312, 1896.

9. Cooley DA, Beall AC Jr, Grondin P: Open heart operations with disposable oxygenators, 5% dextrose prime, and normothermia. Surgery 52:713, 1962.

10. Neville WE, Faber LP, Peacock H: Total prime of the disc oxygenator with Ringer's and Ringer's lactate solution for cardiopulmonary bypass. Clinical and experimental observations. Dis Chest 45:320, 1964.

11. Virgilio RW, Rice CL, Smith DE, James DR, Zarins CK, Hobelmann CF, Peters RM: Crystalloid vs colloid resuscitation. Is one better? A randomized clinical study. Surgery 85:129, 1979.

12. Byrick RJ, Kay JC, Noble WH: Extravascular lung water accumulation in patients following coronary artery surgery. Can Anaesth Soc J 24:332, 1977.

13. Rabelo RC, Oleveira SH, Tanaka H, Weigl DR, Verginelli G, Zerrini EJ: The influence of the nature of the prime on post-perfusion pulmonary changes. J Thorac Cardiovasc Surg 66:782, 1973.

14. Zubiate P, Kay JH, Mendez AM, Krohn BG, Hochman R, Dunne EF: Coronary artery surgery. A new technique with use of little blood, if any. J Thorac Cardiovasc Surg 68:263, 1974.

15. Menninger FJ III, Rosenkranz ER, Utley JR, Dembitsky WP, Hargens AR, Peters RM: Interstitial hydrostatic pressures in patients undergoing CABG and valve replacement. J Thorac Cardiovasc Surg 79:181, 1980.

16. Taylor AE, Grimbert F, Rutili G, Kvietys PR, Parker JC: Pulmonary edema. Changes in Starling forces and lymph flow. In *Tissue Fluid Pressure and Composition*, edited by AR Hargens. Baltimore, Williams & Wilkins, 1981, Chap. 14.

17. Zarins CK, Rice CL, Peters RM, Virgilio RW: Lymph and pulmonary response to isobaric reduction in plasma oncotic pressure in baboons. Circ Res 43:925, 1978.

18. Erdmann AJ, Vaughan TR, Brigham KL, Woolverton WC, Staub NC: Effect of increased vascular pressure on lung fluid balance in unanesthetized sheep. Circ Res 37:271, 1975.

19. Blaisdell FW: Respiratory insufficiency syndrome: Clinical and pathological definition. J Trauma 13:195, 1973.

20. Staub NC: "State of the art" review. Pathogenesis of pulmonary edema. Am Rev Respir Dis 109:358, 1974.

21. Staub NC: Pulmonary edema: Physiological approaches to management. Chest 74:559, 1978.

22. Mandelbaum I, Giamona ST: Extracorporeal circulation, pulmonary compliance, and pulmonary surfactant. J Thorac Cardiovasc Surg 48:881, 1964.

23. West JB: Regional differences in the lung. Chest 74:426, 1978.

24. Ellis EL, Brown A, Osborn JJ, Gerbode F: Effect of altered ventilation patterns on compliance during cardiopulmonary bypass. Anesth Analg 48:947, 1969.

25. Cartwright RS, Lim TPK, Luft UC, Palich WE: Pathophysiological changes in the lung during extracorporeal circulation. Circ Res 10:131, 1962.

26. Edmunds LH Jr, Austen WG: Effects of cardiopulmonary bypass on pulmonary volume-pressure relationships and vascular resistance. J Appl Physiol 21:209, 1966.

27. Pennock JL, Pierce WS, Waldhausen JA: The management of the lungs during cardiopulmonary bypass. Surg Gynecol Obstet 145:917, 1977.

28. Barie PS, Hakim TW, Malik AB: Effect of pulmonary artery occlusion and reperfusion on extravascular fluid accumulation. J Appl Physiol Respir Environ Exercise Physiol 50:102, 1981.

29. Fisher AB: Oxygen therapy: Side effects and toxicity. Am Rev Respir Dis 122:61, 1980.

30. Sullivan SF, Patterson RW, Malm JR, Bowman FO Jr, Papper EM: Effect of heart-lung bypass on the mechanics of breathing in man. J Thorac Cardiovasc Surg 51:205, 1966.

31. Peters RM: Pulmonary physiologic studies of the perioperative period. Chest 76:576, 1979.

32. Shackford SR, Virgilio RW, Peters RM: Early extubation versus prophylactic ventilation in the high risk patient: A comparison of postoperative management in the prevention of respiratory complications. Anesth Analg 60:76, 1981.

33. Bendixen HH, Egbert LD, Hedley-Whyte J, et al: *Respiratory Care*. St. Louis, C. V. Mosby, 1965.

34. Shapiro AR, Virgilio RW, Peters RM: Interpretation of alveolar-arterial oxygen difference. Surg Gynecol Obstet 144:547, 1977.

35. Peters RM: Life saving measures in acute respiratory distress syndrome. Am J Surg 138:368, 1979.

36. Peters RM, Brimm JE, Utley JR: Predicting the need for prolonged ventilatory support in adult cardiac patients. J Thorac Cardiovasc Surg 77:175, 1979.

37. Hilberman M, Kamm B, Lamy M, Dietrich HP, Martz K, Osborn JJ: An analysis of potential physiological predictors of respiratory adequacy following cardiac surgery. J Thorac Cardiovasc Surg 71:711, 1976.

CHAPTER 16

ABDOMINAL COMPLICATIONS OF CARDIOPULMONARY BYPASS

WILLIAM B. LONG, III, M.D.

Abdominal complications of cardiopulmonary bypass are rare, occurring in less than 1% of cases. The incidence has decreased during the last decade (Table 16.1). The most common abdominal complications are gastrointestinal bleeding, acute pancreatitis, and bowel ischemia-infarction, in order of decreasing frequency. This chapter reviews the experiences of several medical centers. There appears to be a relationship between certain cardiac surgical procedures and the development of abdominal complications.

INCIDENCE OF ABDOMINAL COMPLICATIONS

In 1968 Harjola et al.[1] published a series on the subject of abdominal complications following cardiopulmonary bypass surgery. Eighteen of the 237 patients (6.6%) who underwent cardiopulmonary bypass from 1960 to 1967 by this Finnish group developed abdominal complications. Thirteen of these patients had closure of septal defects, three had aortic valve replacements, and one had saphenous vein bypass for coronary artery disease. The postoperative complications included: gastroduodenal ulceration associated with bleeding (six patients), acute gastric dilatation (four patients), prolonged ileus (three patients), cholecystitis (two patients), acute appendicitis (one pa-

tient), and acute pancreatitis (one patient). The authors did not describe any correlation between the type of operative procedure and the subsequent development of an abdominal complication.

In 1978, the Johns Hopkins group reviewed their experience with 2500 patients undergoing cardiopulmonary bypass from 1970 to 1976, and 15 patients (0.6% incidence) developed abdominal complications.[2] The authors did not break down their patient population into types of cardiac surgery performed. The abdominal complications reported were: two patients bled postoperatively from duodenal ulcers; two patients had perforated duodenal ulcers; one patient developed acute cholecystitis; two patients had infarcted bowel; one patient perforated a sigmoid diverticulum; one patient developed an acute anal fissure; and the last patient in their series received an injury to his spleen during chest tube placement. Seven of these complications (48%) occurred after aortic or mitral valve surgery.

In 1980, Wallwork and Davidson[3] of the Glasgow Infirmary, Scotland published their experience with abdominal complications following cardiopulmonary bypass. Over a 6-year period (1970 to 1975), they performed over 1000 cardiac operations requiring cardiopulmonary bypass, and had nine patients (0.85%) develop abdominal complications postoperatively. They ex-

175

Table 16.1
Abdominal Complications Following Cardiopulmonary Bypass Surgery

Surgical Center	Surgical Time Span	No. of CPB Patients	No. of Patients Developing Abdominal Complications	Incidence
Finland	1960–1967	273	18	6.6
Johns Hopkins	1970–1976	2500	15	0.6
Scotland	1970–1975	1000	9	0.9
Louisville, Ky.	1975–1980	3000	8	0.3
UCSD	1979–1981	871	8	0.9

cluded those patients who developed abdominal complications as a terminal event (*i.e.*, gastrointestinal bleeding from stress ulcer). Five of their patients developed a perforation of the intestine—four from duodenal ulcer and one from diverticula of the colon. One patient bled from a duodenal ulcer, and another had unexplained bleeding into the peritoneal cavity. Two patients developed pancreatitis.

The authors did not describe their patient population by type of surgery or the underlying disease. It is interesting to note that of the nine patients who developed postoperative abdominal complications, seven patients had mitral or aortic valve disease, and six of the patients had a preoperative history of symptoms or a history of abdominal surgery for gastrointestinal disease.

In 1980, Lucas and Max[4] at the University of Louisville reviewed 3000 patients who had undergone direct myocardial revascularization during the years 1975 to 1980. They found eight patients (0.26% incidence) who required emergency laparotomy immediately after coronary artery bypass. The authors did not describe any patients who developed abdominal complications postoperatively and who did not require or receive exploratory laparotomy. Three of their patients developed empyema of the gallbladder and underwent subsequent cholecystectomy. Two patients perforated a duodenal ulcer, and one patient perforated a sigmoid diverticulum. Two two ulcer patients had closure of the perforation, and the patient with the perforated diverticulum had a diverting colostomy and pelvic drainage. One patient underwent appendectomy for acute appendicitis, and one patient had

a laparotomy to rule out a perforated viscus, when in fact the free air noted under the diaphragm came from faulty insertion of the chest tube.

At the University of California Medical Center in San Diego, California and the VA Medical Center in La Jolla, California we received the records of 873 patients who underwent cardiopulmonary bypass surgery during the years 1979 to 1981 and found eight patients (0.9% incidence) who had developed gastrointestinal complications postoperatively.

Case 1

A 75-year-old white male with calcific aortic stenosis had an uneventful aortic valve replacement and developed nausea, vomiting, and upper abdominal pain on the 12th postoperative day. The physical examination was unremarkable. The white blood cell counts were mildly elevated. The serum amylase was normal, and an abdominal sonogram was normal. He was treated with i.v. fluids and nasogastric suction for 48 hours, and his symptoms settled. A follow-up upper gastrointestinal series was normal, and he was discharged on the 22nd postoperative day.

Case 2

A 60-year-old white male with a history of duodenal ulcer disease had a second myocardial revascularization. On the 10th postoperative day, he dehisced his sternum and bled massively from a duodenal ulcer. After stabilization, he underwent an exploratory laparotomy, truncal vagotomy, pyloroplasty, and debridement and closure of his sternal dehiscence. On the 20th postoperative day (post-CABG) he had another gastrointestinal hemorrhage and a second laparotomy with gastroenterostomy and tube duodenostomy. Thereafter, he made a slow recovery and was discharged home on the 35th postoperative day.

Case 3

A 55-year-old white male had an aortic valve replacement for aortic stenosis, and on the 7th postoperative day he developed the signs and symptoms of an acute abdomen. He had acute right lower quadrant abdominal pain, and his white blood cell count and serum amylase were elevated. He had a laparotomy which was essentially negative. He made an uneventful recovery and was discharged home 8 days later.

Case 4

A 61-year-old Hispanic male with a history of a previous aortic valve replacement for bacterial endocarditis had a second aortic valve replacement for recurrent bacterial endocarditis. Postoperatively, he had low cardiac output syndrome and developed hepatorenal failure. His abdomen became distended. He died 24 hours after surgery. Autopsy revealed intestinal infarction.

Case 5

A 29-year-old Hispanic female had an open mitral commissurotomy for mitral stenosis. She did well and was discharged on the 8th postoperative day. Two weeks later she was readmitted to the medical center for acute cholecystitis and had a cholecystectomy. She made an uneventful recovery.

Case 6

A 68-year-old white female with adult onset diabetes mellitus and coronary artery disease had an elective coronary artery bypass procedure. Six hours following surgery, she began to bleed excessively from the chest tubes and was taken back into the operating room. She was reexplored and the bleeding was controlled. She was making an uneventful recovery when, on the 6th postoperative day, she developed right up-

per quadrant pain and vomiting. An abdominal x-ray suggested a cecal volvulus and an exploratory laparotomy confirmed the diagnosis. After cecopexy, she made an uneventful recovery.

Case 7

A 4-year-old Hispanic male had a complete correction of tetralogy of Fallot. Postoperatively, he developed low cardiac output syndrome, acute renal failure, hyperkalemia, and metabolic acidosis. As a terminal event, he had a massive upper gastrointestinal bleeding and died 48 hours after surgery.

Case 8

A 73-year-old white female ruptured a dissecting ascending aortic aneurysm (Type I) and arrived at UC Medical Center *in extremis.* An aortogram revealed that the dissection had extended across the aortic valve into the right atrium. She underwent a successful aortic valve replacement and a Dacron graft replacement of her ascending aorta. Postoperatively, she continued to bleed massively from her chest tubes, and she was taken back to the operating room twice for bleeding. Her postoperative course was stormy and on the 6th postoperative day she developed right lower quadrant abdominal pain, abdominal distention, and vomiting. An abdominal x-ray showed a cecal volvulus and she underwent an exploratory laparotomy and cecal fixation. She had a prolonged recovery, but eventually was discharged.

Abdominal complications following cardiopulmonary bypass in recent years are infrequent (approximately 1% incidence), and most often are associated with aortic and/or mitral valve disease. Success with treating these abdominal complications varies with the timing of recognition and surgical intervention. In many patients, the abdominal complication is a terminal event in patients dying of pump failure.

The remainder of this chapter is concerned with an analysis and discussion of certain types of abdominal complications following cardiopulmonary bypass surgery.

GASTROINTESTINAL BLEEDING FOLLOWING CARDIOPULMONARY BYPASS

In 1968 Harjola and his colleagues[1] reported that six of their 273 patients who underwent cardiopulmonary bypass surgery developed acute gastric and/or duodenal ulcers postoperatively. Mean and Folk[5] reported that 40 of their patients developed gastrointestinal bleeding following cardiac or thoracic surgery during 1 year. Lawhorne et al.[2] reviewed 2500 patients who underwent cardiac surgery from 1970 to 1976 and found four patients who developed gastroduodenal ulceration postoperatively. Only one patient had a previous history of peptic ulcer disease. Only two patients in this group bled from their ulcers. One patient had a mitral valve replacement, and the other had a ventricular aneurysmectomy and closure of VSD. Both patients had massive hemorrhage (greater than 10 units of blood), and both were managed successfully by nonoperative measures.

Wallwork and Davidson had only one patient among 100 cardiopulmonary bypass patients develop postoperative bleeding from an acute duodenal ulcer.[3] Their patient had an emergency resection of an aneurysm of the ascending aorta, which had ruptured into the superior vena cava. The patient bled on the 14th postoperative day and subsequently underwent laparotomy, undersewing of the ulcer, vagotomy, and pyloroplasty. The patient died 3 weeks later in renal failure.

Lucas and Max[4] reported no cases of gastrointestinal bleeding requiring emergency laparotomy in the immediate postoperative period following cardiopulmonary bypass for coronary artery disease.

We reviewed our experiences with postoperative gastrointestinal hemorrhage and found only three cases in 873 patients. One patient developed gastrointestinal bleeding only as a terminal event. Another patient had a previous history of peptic ulcer disease and bled on the 10th postoperative day. The events of his hospitalization were outlined earlier in this chapter as case 2. The third patient bled following an uncomplicated aortic valve replacement.

In contrast to this infrequent experience among several medical centers, the Cleveland Clinic reported a 7-year experience (1964 to 1970) with more than 5000 cardiac surgical patients.[6] Of these, 38 patients developed acute stress ulceration of the stomach or duodenum in the early postoperative period. Not all of the 5000 patients required extracorporeal circulation, and of the 38 patients who developed acute stress ulceration postoperatively, only 22 (57.9%) had cardiopulmonary bypass. From their data, it is difficult to determine which group of surgical operations contributed the higher incidence of postoperative gastrointestinal bleeding. Nine of the 22 patients had open heart surgery for valvular heart disease; one had open heart surgery for congenital heart disease. The remaining 12 patients had myocardial revascularization while on cardiopulmonary bypass.

The authors found that 25 of the patients who had bled postoperatively had other surgical complications as an added stress to the psychological and physiological stresses of cardiac surgery. The most common complication was postoperative myocardial infarction.

Welsh et al.[7] of the Mayo Clinic reviewed their experiences with 7,333 patients who underwent open heart surgery with cardiopulmonary bypass during the period 1955 to 1969. Sixteen patients (0.22%) had significant postoperative bleeding. Only three of these patients bled prior to the cardiac surgery. Unlike the Cleveland Clinic experience, the Mayo Clinic surgeons noticed a much higher incidence of postoperative gastrointestinal bleeding in patients who underwent valve surgery than those who had undergone other types of cardiac operations.

All of the seven patients who had multiple valve operations and postoperative gastrointestinal bleeding died, as did the three patients who had had mitral valve surgery. Three of the five patients who underwent aortic valve surgery and developed postoperative gastrointestinal bleeding died.

The relationship of cardiac valvular disease and gastrointestinal bleeding is not well understood. In 1958 Heyde[8] reported his experience with 10 patients with calcific aortic stenosis and associated gastrointestinal bleeding of undetermined origin. Schwartz[9] noted a similar association. In 1961 Williams [10] analyzed 1,443 patients with gastrointestinal bleeding and found that of 95 patients with unexplained gastrointestinal bleeding, 25% of this population had an aortic valve lesion, predominantly calcific aortic stenosis. McNamara and Austen[11] reviewed their experience with 26 patients undergoing aortic valve replacement and found the same incidence of gastrointestinal bleeding (1.2%) in the group of patients with aortic regurgitation as in the group with aortic stenosis. Since Williams' report, there have been numerous reports confirming this association, but none of these reports has provided new knowledge regarding the etiology of the relationship.[7, 11, 12]

Certain clinical features separate patients who are likely to bleed following cardiopulmonary bypass from those who don't bleed.[12] First, the patient likely to bleed postoperatively has more than a 50% chance of having a previous ulcer history and a 10% chance of bleeding clinically or microscopically prior to cardiopulmonary bypass.[6, 7, 11, 12] Second, age is a factor in this surgical study, although it is not in other studies.[11] Men are more likely to develop gastrointestinal bleeding, and men have a higher incidence of valvular disease, especially calcific aortic stenosis. Statistics show that patients who bleed have longer operations and longer cardiopulmonary bypass.[6, 7, 12] They have more postoperative complications, which may cause or aggravate their tendency to bleed from the gastrointestinal tract.[7, 12]

The most common gastrointestinal lesion causing postoperative bleeding in cardiac surgical patients who have preoperative gastrointestinal bleeding is duodenal ulcer.[6, 11] For those patients who have gastrointestinal bleeding preoperatively but develop acute bleeding postoperatively, the most common finding at laparotomy is multiple gastric and duodenal ulcers, followed in frequency by hemorrhagic or erosive enteritis.[6, 7]

Anticoagulants, including aspirin, have not been proven to increase the chances for

patients to develop postoperative gastrointestinal bleeding.[7] This is true even for those patients who had known symptomatic peptic ulcer disease preoperatively. Patients requiring steroid drug therapy did not have an increased incidence of postoperative gastrointestinal bleeding.

The management of acute gastrointestinal bleeding following cardiac surgery varies among the different medical centers. The Mayo Clinic group treated 14 of 16 patients medically, and 12 patients died.[7] All of the multiple valve patients died. Only two patients were treated surgically, and one of these survived. The overall mortality for their series is 88% (13/16).

The experience at the Cleveland Clinic was considerably different.[6] The overall mortality was 23.6% Twelve postoperative cardiac patients with gastrointestinal bleeding were treated with medical measures and one died (8.2% mortalilty for medical therapy). Twenty-six of the postoperative cardiac patients with gastrointestinal bleeding were treated surgically and eight died (30.7% mortality for surgical therapy). There was no statistical difference in the success of either gastrointestinal surgery employed to stop the bleeding. Both vagotomy and pyloroplasty and gastric resection with or without vagotomy had a similar mortality in this patient population (32%).

Most of the experience with gastrointestinal bleeding following cardiopulmonary bypass surgery was gained during the period of 1965 to 1975. The use of gastrointestinal endoscopy as a means of diagnosing the source of gastrointestinal bleeding was not mentioned by any of the quoted authors.

The use of cimetidine as an agent to prevent stress ulceration has been advocated by many. None of the quoted papers employed cimetidine routinely.

In 1969 Mead and Folk[5] decreased the incidence of postoperative gastrointestinal bleeding in their cardiac and thoracic surgical patients by routinely administering an antacid down the nasogastric tube in their postoperative patients.

There are no recent reports in the literature dealing with this complication. Carrico's group[13] found that cimetidine is not

100% effective in reducing the incidence of stress ulceration in critically ill patients, and may cause harm. They found that antacid control of gastric pH was far more effective in the prevention of stress bleeding.

It is probably safe to state that patients with an ulcer diathesis who are not bleeding preoperatively and who are taking cimetidine preoperatively should continue to receive cimetidine during and following cardiac surgery. For those patients who are not symptomatic for ulcer disease and who need to undergo cardiac surgery with cardiopulmonary bypass, routine monitoring or gastric pH and titration with antacid is the best preventive therapy.

For those patients who do bleed postoperatively despite prophylactic stress ulcer therapy, intensive medical therapy should be attempted first. Those patients who continue to bleed more than 8 units of blood should have exploratory laparotomy and near total gastrectomy if multiple gastric erosions or diffuse gastritis are found.[14] For those patients who are bleeding from simple gastric or duodenal ulcer, a simple undersewing of the ulcer, vagotomy, and pyloroplasty should suffice.

ACUTE PANCREATITIS

Acute pancreatitis following cardiopulmonary bypass operations is fortunately rare but is associated with a high mortality rate. Delay in diagnosis, uncertainty of the cause, and currently poor therapy all contribute to the high morbidity and mortality. The following is a review of the literature and discussion of acute pancreatitis occurring postoperatively in patients who have undergone cardiopulmonary bypass.

Acute pancreatitis following abdominal surgery is a well-recognized, but uncommon, postoperative complication. White et al.[15] reviewed the records of 227,932 operations from 1956 to 1965 and found 70 patients developed acute pancreatitis (incidence 0.03%) during the immediate postoperative period.[15] Thirty of these patients died (42% mortality). Of the 70 patients who developed postoperative pancreatitis, 54 had abdominal surgery during which there was risk of local trauma to the pancreas, and 24 of these patients died (32% mortality). Sixteen patients had surgery during which there was no risk of local trauma to the pancreas. None of these patients had cardiothoracic surgery and/or cardiopulmonary bypass associated with postoperative pancreatitis.

Peterson et al. reviewed 22 patients treated for postoperative pancreatitis from January 1955 through June 1966 and found a 36% associated mortality.[16] Twenty percent of 22 patients had abdominal surgery and developed postoperatively acute pancreatitis for the first time. Thirty-five percent of these patients died. One patient had nonabdominal surgery—replacement of an aortic valve while on cardiopulmonary bypass, and that patient died.

Reports of postoperative pancreatitis following cardiopulmonary bypass surgery are sporadic. Harjola et al. reviewed their experience with 273 operations employing extracorporeal circulation and found only one patient with this complication—a 27-year-old female who had an aortic valve replacement.[1] She developed acute respiratory insufficiency and required ventilatory support. She developed a sigmoid volvulus on the 3rd postoperative day and acute pancreatitis on the 8th postoperative day and recovered from both complications. In 1968 Horton et al.[17] reported their experience with 168 cardiac valve replacements from 1964 to 1967 and found one patient who developed acute pancreatitis postoperatively. She had an uneventful aortic valve replacement and became hypotensive 10 days postoperatively. She developed mild abdominal distention and became anuric. Despite supportive care, she died from hemorrhagic pancreatitis on the 14th postoperative day.

In 1970 Panebianco et al.[18] reviewed their experience with 276 operations requiring extracorporeal circulation at the VA Hospital in Oteen, North Carolina between 1958 and 1969 and found eight patients who had developed pancreatitis postoperatively. In only two patients was the postoperative pancreatitis a major cause of death; the other six patients had incidental findings of pancreatitis at autopsy.

Helen Feiner[19] reviewed 182 complete autopsies performed on patients who died within 10 weeks of cardiac surgery. Twenty-nine of these autopsies revealed evidence of pancreatitis (an incidence of 16%). Thirteen patients had valvular surgery, twelve had coronary artery bypass grafting, three had aortic replacement, and one had repair of a ruptured septum and a myocardial resection. Only four patients had severe pancreatitis at autopsy, and three of the four had had valvular surgery. The other patients had mild to moderate pancreatitis as an incidental autopsy finding.

Lastly, Wallwork and Davidson[3] reviewed the records of a thousand patients who underwent cardiopulmonary bypass operations during the period of 1970 to 1975 and found only two patients who developed postoperative pancreatitis. One patient was a 65-year-old female who underwent aortic valve replacement and developed abdominal distention and hypotension immediately postoperatively. Laparotomy confirmed the clinical diagnosis of acute hemorrhagic pancreatitis, and the patient died 24 hours later. The other patient had an uneventful mitral valve replacement and was discharged 2 weeks postoperatively. She was readmitted 1 week later with abdominal distention and a high serum amylase. She received medical therapy and recovered.

Acute pancreatitis following cardiopulmonary bypass operations is relatively uncommon—1.6% approximately (Table 16.2). The association with valvular heart operations is highly significant (98%), but acute pancreatitis has been found in postoperative coronary artery bypass surgical patients, usually associated with an acute myocardial infarction.[18, 19] However, 11 of 12 of these nonvalvular patients did not have pancreatitis as a major pathological finding at autopsy.[19]

The degree of elevation of serum amylase does not always correlate with the degree of severity of acute pancreatitis. Panebianco et al.[18] measured serum amylase levels in 54 patients after cardiac surgery and cardiopulmonary bypass during the first 5 postoperative days. Eighteen patients had serum amylase levels greater than 150 Smogyi units/100 ml (Normal 80 to 160 Smogyi units/100 ml). Of the eight patients who died, only two had clinical evidence of acute pancreatitis. The other six had pancreatitis as an incidental finding at autopsy.

Hennings and Jacobson[20] studied postoperative serum and urinary amylase concentrations in the two groups of patients. One group had open heart surgery and cardiopulmonary bypass, and the other group underwent thoracotomy without extracorporeal circulation. The group who underwent cardiopulmonary bypass consisted of 12 patients, of whom eight had a valve replacement. All 12 patients had postoperative elevations of the serum amylase with an associated increase in the urinary amylase excretion and clearance rate. In four patients the serum amylase concentration rose to at least 10 times the normal level, but no patients in this group developed clinical pancreatitis. In the other group of 22 thoracic surgical patients who did not undergo extracorporeal circulation, the postoperative serum amylase concentrations did not significantly increase above

Table 16.2
Postoperative Pancreatitis in Cardiac Surgery

	Author	No. of Cases	No. with Pancreatitis*	Surgery	Outcome
1968	Harjola	273	1	AVR	L
1968	Horton	?	1	AVR	D
1968	Peterson	?	1	AVR	D
1970	Panebianco	276	8	2 MVR	D
				2 AVR,MVR	
				3 AVR	
				1 AVR with	
				graft	

*Nine of 549 is a 1.6% incidence.

the normal range, and the amylse excretion and clearance rates were less than those recorded for the cardiopulmonary bypass group. None of the patients in this group developed pancreatitis.

In a similar study, Traverso et al.[21] studied amylase-creatinine clearance ratios (ACCR) on the 1st postoperative day, and five of their six patients had normal ratios by the 2nd postoperative day. The four thoracic surgical patients did not have any postoperative elevations of the ACCR. No patient in either group developed clinical pancreatitis.

Moores et al[22] studied serum and urinary amylase concentrations in 42 patients undergoing coronary artery bypass without valvular replacement and found that no patient developed clinical evidence of pancreatitis postoperatively. Twenty-three patients had continuous perfusion with the two roller half-circle pump during coronary artery bypass and had significant elevations of serum and urinary amylase concentrations postoperatively when compared to preoperative levels. Nineteen patients had extracorporeal perfusion with a modified pulsatile heart-assist pump. Two patients had significant postoperative elevations of serum and coronary amylase concentrations, but less than those values recorded for the continuous perfusion patients. The incidence of postoperative elevations of serum and urine amylase was less for the pulsatile perfusion group (32%) than for the continuous perfusion group (70%).

The etiology of acute pancreatitis or symptomatic elevations of serum and urine amylase concentrations in patients undergoing cardiovascular surgery with extracorporeal circulation is still unclear. The most common cause of postoperative acute pancreatitis is local trauma to the organ during upper abdominal surgery. There are several studies that implicate other factors as causes of pancreatitis following cardiopulmonary bypass surgery.

Hypercalcemia associated with hyperparathyroidism has caused intravascular clotting and acute pancreatitis.[23] Johnson and Stiel[24] have reported acute pancreatitis occurring postoperatively in a patient undergoing parathyroid surgery for hyperthyroidism. Hochgelerent and David[25] described acute pancreatitis following a calcium infusion test in a patient with chronic renal disease. Other authors have noted and reported the association of hyperparathyroidism with acute pancreatitis.[26-28] Meltzer et al.[29] described a patient with hypercalcemia and multiple myeloma who developed acute pancreatitis. That patient had no previous history of pancreatic or biliary disease.

Calcium infusions are known to stimulate endocrine gland secretion but have not been associated with asymptomatic rises in serum or urinary amylase concentrations. Cardiac surgeons routinely give patients bolus doses of i.v. calcium in preparation for discontinuing extracorporeal circulation, and no one has reported any association of altered pancreatic function or acute pancreatitis with this practice. Hochgelerent and David[25] administered a calcium infusion test to evaluate parathyroid gland function in a chronic hemodialysis patient with no previous history of pancreatitis. The patient developed acute pancreatitis 4 hours following the completion of the test. The serum amylase concentration was greater than 700 units/dl, and the serum calcium level was 9.8 mg/dl. The patient responded well to medical therapy. Although there are many theories concerning the etiology of acute pancreatitis in chronic renal disease patients, the exact causes are still unknown.

Atheromatous embolization to the arteries of the pancreas may be a major cause of postoperative pancreatitis in patients having cardiac surgery. Over a 2-year period of time, Probstein et al.[30] collected 12 cases of atheromatous embolization to the pancreatic arteries from the aorta, and 10 of those patients had acute pancreatitis. In their study of organ distribution of atheromatous embolization, the pancreas ranked second only to the kidney in frequency of involvement (52%). The authors made no relationship between cardiac surgery and subsequent development of emboli.

Helen Feiner[19] studied 182 patients who died within 10 weeks after cardiac surgery and who had had complete autopsies. She found 29 patients had evidence of thromboembolism to the pancreatic arteries. Three patients had mitral valve surgery, two had aortic replacement, two had coronary artery bypass surgery, and one patient had a repair of a ruptured ventricular septum from a myocardial infarction. Only one of the nine patients had pancreatitis as a major pathological finding at autopsy.

Pfeffer et al.[13] showed experimentally that the injection of microspheres 8 to 20 μm in size into the superior pancreatic duodenal artery of mongrel dogs could produce consistently severe hemorrhagic necrotic pancreatitis within 11 hours. Larger sized microspheres produced a lesser amount of pancreatitis.

The etiology of acute postoperative pancreatitis in previously asymptomatic patients underoing cardiopulmonary bypass remains unclear. Fortunately, this clinically recognized complication is rare (<0.1% incidence in all patients undergoing cardiopulmonary bypass), but may be a major contributing factor in the deaths of those patients who died following cardiac surgery (6 to 15% incidence of pancreatitis at autopsy).[18, 19]

Extracorporeal circulation does elevate serum and urinary amylase concentrations in patients postoperatively, and the mechanism for this phenomenon is not known. Patients undergoing cardiopulmonary bypass do not seem to be at greater risk of developing postoperative pancreatitis than do other patients undergoing other types of surgery.

Transient hypercalcemia and calcium infusions have not been implicated as a cause for postoperative pancreatitis in patients who had extracorporeal circulation during cardiothoracic surgery.

Embolization of atheromatous material has been demonstrated at autopsy in patients who died following cardiac surgery.[30] There is no data incriminating any particular type of cardiovascular procedure associated with extracorporeal circulation to the subsequent development of postoperative pancreatitis secondary to atheromatous embolization. Cardiac valve surgery and congenital heart surgery are associated with a higher incidence of embolization to other organs (*e.g.*, the brain) than with other types of cardiac surgery, but these emboli are usually calcium, thrombotic emboli, or air emboli.[32, 33] Postmortem data do not exist showing thrombotic emboli or air emboli as the cause of acute postoperative pancreatitis. The origin of the atheromatous emboli as previously described may be from the aortic cross-clamp site, cannulation sites, or aortotomy.[30] More work needs to be done before these theories are proven correct or discarded.

INTESTINAL ISCHEMIA AND INFARCTION FOLLOWING CARDIOIPULMONARY BYPASS

Intestinal ischemia and infarction does occur following cardiopulmonary bypass. The incidence is very small, and only a few cases have been reported. Harjola et al.[1] had no experience with intestinal ischemia in 273 cases undergoing cardiopulmonary bypass during the later 1960s. Several years later, Johns Hopkins Hospital reported a study of 250 patients wherein two developed postoperative bowel necrosis.[2] One of these patients developed nonocclusive mesenteric vascular ischemia and ileal necrosis after an initial postoperative period with low cardiac output syndrome. The other patient had candida endocarditis, which embolized to the mesenteric vessels with resultant multiple areas of small bowel necrosis. More than 2 years later, Wallwork and Davidson[3] reported no cases of intestinal ischemia in over 1000 patients undergoing cardiopulmonary bypass operations. In 3000 patients undergoing myocardial revascularization, Lucas and Max[4] reported no instance of intestinal ischemia occurring during the postoperative period.

In a review of 873 cardiac patients undergoing cardiopulmonary bypass we found three patients who had developed intestinal ischemia postoperatively. One patient with bacterial endocarditis had low cardiac output syndrome and hepatorenal failure following an aortic valve replacement. He died 24 hours later. An autopsy revealed intestinal infarction but no mesenteric embolus. Two other patients developed cecal volvulus following cardiopulmonary bypass surgery.

Embolization to the pancreas following cardiopulmonary bypass surgery is well described by Feiner[19] and Probstein et al.[30] However, nonocclusive intestinal ischemia and infarction is more common in postoperative cardiopulmonary bypass patients.[2, 25, 36-38]

Severe cardiac failure causing nonocclusive intestinal infarction is well described by Ende. Many clinicians and investigators believe that low cardiac output causes a reflex splanchnic vasoconstriction, which in combination with the low cardiac output produces intestinal ischemia and infarction.[39-44]

Hoffman et al.[34] noted the association of massive intestinal infarction without vascular occlusion with aortic valve insufficiency. All patients were in severe heart failure at the time the intestinal infarction occurred.

It is known both clinically and experimentally that cardiopulmonary bypass produces splanchnic pooling not only in the experimental animal, but also in humans.[45] Digitalis is associated with splanchnic vasoconstriction and nonocclusive mesenteric infarction.[44]

It is, therefore, not surprising that most of the patients reported in the literature who develop intestinal infarction following cardiopulmonary bypass surgery are patients who have undergone aortic valve replacement and who have low cardiac output syndrome postoperatively. What is not clear is why there is not a higher incidence following cardiopulmonary bypass of intestinal infarction in patients who postoperatively have low cardiac output syndrome, especially those patients who require intraaortic balloon pump support and high dose adrenaline infusions to maintain blood pressure and cardiac output.

We had two cardiac surgical patients develop cecal vovulus postoperatively. The cause for this phenomenon is still speculative.

Gastrointestinal complications following cardiopulmonary bypass are rare (less than 1% approximately), and the incidence has decreased since 1965 to 1975. Postoperative gastrointestinal bleeding, pancreatitis, and intestinal ischemia-infarction are the more common complications, but cholecystitis, cecal volvulus, and appendicitis have been reported.

Most of the gastrointestinal complications seem to occur after valve surgery, rather than after myocardial revascularization. This may reflect better patient selection for myocardial revascularization than for valve surgery.

Postoperative gastrointestinal bleeding occurs most frequently in cardiac patients who were bleeding preoperatively from the gastrointestinal tract. Stress ulceration is associated with complications of cardiopulmonary bypass surgery, and its effects can be muted with modern techniques of support intensive care.

Pancreatitis following cardiopulmonary bypass surgery may well be caused by atheromatous emboli from the cross-clamped aorta and/or valve replacement. More studies are needed to confirm these associations.

Bowel ischemia and infarction are most frequently seen after cardiac valve replacement and in patients with low cardiac output. The mortality is high because of late diagnosis in patients who are already very ill.

References

1. Harjola PT, Siltanen P, Appelqvist P, Laustela E: Abdominal complication after open heart surgery. Ann Chir Gynaecol Fenn 57:272, 1968
2. Lawhorne TW, Davis JL, Smith GW: General surgical complications after cardiac surgery. Am J Surg 136:254, 1978.
3. Wallwork J, Davidson KG: The acute abdomen following cardiopulmonary bypass surgery Br J Surg 67:410, 1980.
4. Lucas A, Max MH: Emergency laparotomy immediately after coronary bypass. JAMA 244:1829, 1980.
5. Mead J, Folk F: Correspondence: Gastrointestinal bleeding after cardiac surgery. N Engl J Med 281:799, 1969.
6. Taylor PC, Loop FD, Hermann RE: Management of acute stress after cardiac surgery. Ann Surg 178:1, 1973.
7. Welsh GF, Dozois RR, Bartholomew LG, Brown AL, Danielson GK: Gastrointestinal bleeding after open heart surgery. J Thorac Cardiovasc Surg 65:738, 1973.
8. Heyde EC: Correspondence: Gastrointestinal

bleeding in aortic stenosis. N Engl J Med 259:196, 1958.

9. Schwartz BM: Correspondence: Additional note on bleeding in aortic stenosis. N Engl J Med 259:456, 1958.

10. Williams RC Jr: Aortic stenosis and unexplained gastrointestinal bleeding. Arch Intern Med 108:859, 1961.

11. McNamara JJ, Austen WG: Gastrointestinal bleeding occurring in patients with acquired valvular heart disease. Arch Surg 97:538, 1968.

12. Katz SE, Kornfeld DS, Harris PD, Yeoh CB: Acute gastrointestinal ulceration with open heart surgery and aortic valve disease. Surgery 72:438, 1972.

13. Stothert JC, Simonowitz DA, Dellinger EP, Farley M, Edwards WA, Blair AD, Cutter R, Carrico CJ: Randomized prospective evaluation of cimetidine and antacid control of gastric pH in the critically ill. Ann Surg 192:169, 1980.

14. Hubert JP, Kiernan PD, Welch JS, ReMine WH, Beahrs OH: The surgical management of bleeding stress ulcers. Ann Surg 191:672, 1980.

15. White TT, Morgan A, Hopton D: Postoperative pancreatitis—a study of seventy cases. Am J Surg 120:132, 1970.

16. Peterson LM, Collins JJ, Wilson RE: Acute pancreatitis occurring after operation. Surg Gynecol Obstet 127:23, 1968.

17. Horton EM, Murth SK, Seal RME: Hemorrhagic necrosis of small intestine and acute pancreatitis following open-heart surgery. Thorax 23:438, 1968.

18. Panebianco AC, Scott SM, Dart CH, Takaro T, Echegary HM: Acute pancreatitis following extracorporeal circulation. Ann Thorac Surg 9:562, 1970.

19. Feinder H: Pancreatitis after cardiac surgery—a morphologic study. Am J Surg 131:684, 1976.

20. Hennings B, Jacobson G: Postoperative amylase secretion. A study following thoracic surgery with and without extracorporeal circulation. Ann Clin Res 6:215, 1974.

21. Traverso LW, Ferrari BT, Buckberg GD, Tompkins RK: Elevated postoperative renal clearance of amylase without pancreatitis after cardiopulmonary bypass. Am J Surg 133:298, 1977.

22. Moores WY, Gago O, Morris JD, Peck CC: Serum and urinary amylase levels following pulsatile and continuous cardiopulmonary bypass. J Thorac Cardiovasc Surg 74:73, 1977.

23. Kelly RT, Falon WM: Hyperparathyroid crisis associated with pancreatitis. Ann Surg 168:917, 1968.

24. Johnson DC, Stiel JN: Pancreatitis following parathyroid surgery. Med J Aust 2:25, 1967.

25. Hochgelerent EL, David DS: Acute pancreatitis secondary to calcium infusion in a dialysis patient. Arch Surg 108:218, 1974.

26. Mixter CG Jr, Keynes M, Cope O: Further experience with pancreatitis as a diagnostic clue to hyperparathyroidism. N Engl J Med 266:265, 1962.

27. Warshaw AL, Heizer WD, Laster L: Pancreatic insufficiency as the presenting feature of hyperparathyroidism. Ann Intern Med 68:161, 1968.

28. Turchi JJ: Hyperparathyroidism and pancreatitis. JAMA 180:799, 1962.

29. Meltzer: Acute pancreatitis secondary to hypercalcemia in multiple myeloma. Ann Intern Med 57:1008, 1962.

30. Probstein JG, Joshi RA, Blumenthal HT: Atheromatous embolization. An etiology of acute pancreatitis. Arch Surg 75:566, 1957.

31. Pfeffer RB, Lazzarini-Robertson A Jr, Safadi D, Mixter G, Secoy CF, Hinton JW: Gradations of pancreatitis, edematous, through hemorrhagic, experimentally produced by controlled injection of microspheres into bleed vessels in dogs. Surgery 51:764, 1962.

32. Allen P: Central nervous system emboli in open heart surgery. Can J Surg 6:332, 1963.

33. Kolkka R, Hilberman M: Neurologic dysfunction following cardiac operation with low-flow, low pressure cardiopulmonary bypass. J Thorac Cardiovasc Surg 79:432, 1980.

34. Hoffman FG, Zimmerman SL, Cardwell ES: Massive intestinal infarction without vascular occlusion associated with aortic insufficiency. N Engl J Med 263:436, 1960.

35. Robertson R, Dodds WA: Mesenteric artery insufficiency complicating repair of aortic regurgitation. Can J Surg 7:269, 1964.

36. Silane MF, Symchych PS: Necrotizing enterocolitis after cardiac surgery—a local ischemic lesion? Am J Surg 133:373, 1977.

37. Hargrove WC III, Rosato EF, Hides RE, Mullen JL: Cecal necrosis after open-heart operation. Ann Thorac Surg 25:71, 1978.

38. Hill JD, Mittal AK, Kerth WJ, Gerbode F: Syndrome of acute hemorrhagic intestinal infarction and renal insufficiency following aortic valve replacement for aortic insufficiency. J Thorac Cardiovasc Surg 61:430, 1971.

39. Ende N: Infarction of the bowel in cardiac failure. N Engl J Med 258:879, 1958.

40. Ottinger LW, Austen WG: A study of 136 patients with mesenteric infarction. Surg Gynecol Obstet 124:251, 1967.

41. Berger RL, Byrne JJ: Intestinal gangrene associated with heart disease. Surg Gynecol Obstet 112:529, 1961.

42. Williams LF Jr, Anastasia LF, Hasiotis CA, Bosniak MA, Gyrne JJ: Experimental nonocclusive mesenteric ischemia. Am J Surg 115:82, 1968.

43. Britt LG, Cheek RC: Nonocclusive mesenteric vascular disease: Clinical and experimental observations. Ann Surg 169:704, 1969.

44. Boley SJ, Brandt LJ, Veith FJ: Ischemic disorders of the intestines. Curr Probl Surg 15:1–85, 1978.

45. Davidson ARG, Farthmann EH: Splanchnic probing during left heart bypass. Surg Gynecol Obstet 121:1277, 1965.

CHAPTER 17

CARDIOPULMONARY BYPASS STRATEGIES IN PATIENTS WITH SEVERE AORTIC DISEASE

WILLIAM Y. MOORES, M.D.

With the introduction of cardiopulmonary bypass, perfusion was accomplished through a peripheral artery. The femoral artery was used most often. Furthermore, it was found experimentally and clinically that venous drainage could be accomplished from a peripheral vein. Although this femoral cannulation does not provide for antigrade flow distal to the site of cannulation, its convenience led to widespread acceptance and almost universal usage until the early 1970s. Some difficulties, primarily in the form of retrograde dissections with this technique, led to the introduction and eventual widespread usage of ascending aortic cannulation. At present, aortic cannulation accomplished after a sternotomy incision is the technique most often used. Certain disease entities, especially those of the aorta, require cardiopulmonary bypass strategies that employ some type of arterial perfusion not utilizing the ascending aorta.

Central venous drainage utilizing either a single two-stage cannula or individual cannulas placed into the superior and inferior cavae is the technique of choice. Variations in this approach for venous drainage are less frequently needed. A femoral route is most commonly used for this peripheral venous drainage, although adequate drain-age can be accomplished utilizing other peripheral venous sites, such as the jugular or subclavian vein. Peripheral arterial cannulation also most commonly involves the femoral route, although other vessels, such as the iliac, subclavian, or axillary artery may be used. An understanding of the potential problems with these arterial cannulation techniques is the primary subject of this chapter.

FEMORAL ARTERY CANNULATION

Femoral artery cannulation, no longer used for the routine cardiopulmonary bypass, is used under specific conditions. A partial list would include operations on the ascending aorta, the aortic arch, repeat cardiac operations, emergency cardiopulmonary bypass prior to thoracotomy, and long-term cardiopulmonary bypass in patients with closed chest.

Unfortunately, this cannulation technique is associated with several major complications. The most catastrophic of these conditions is complete retrograde dissection, but other less life-threatening conditions, such as retrograde propagation of vascular debris and local artery obstruction, also may occur.[1-5] Femoral artery cannulae frequently

186

must be a smaller internal diameter because of small vessels than an aortic cannulae for patients of the same surface area. This may result in significantly greater blood turbulence and trauma. As with any cannulation technique, there may be local hemorrhage and hematoma at the arteriotomy site which, on occasion, may result in a pseudoaneurysm. Femoral cannulation also requires the temporary obstruction of the vessel distal to the arteriotomy site, and patients may present subsequently with signs of lower extremity ischemia.[6] A diagnostic arteriogram usually substantiates the diagnosis of a local femoral artery stenosis. The condition is most often alleviated by appropriate arterioplasty of the affected vessel. This problem usually can be avoided if the closure of the femoral arteriotomy is meticulous with avoidance of bleeding and resultant hematoma and false aneurysm formation. Even the most meticulous closure will not guarantee avoidance of this problem, as damage to the artery resulting in stenosis can occur following the insertion of a cannula which is too large, or following the occlusion of the vasa vasorum with prolonged clamping of the affected artery.[6] Patients may present subsequently with problems of distal limb ischemia. Most, if not all, of these complications can be avoided, however, if certain precautions are taken on the part of the surgeon and the clinical perfusionist.

The complication of retrograde dissection can be avoided most often by meticulous care with the insertion of the femoral cannula and by use of a cannula having the proper diameter. Even with the greatest degree of local care at the arteriotomy site, retrograde dissection can occur from a jet lesion if the cannula chosen is either too small, inserted too far into the artery, or if cardiopulmonary bypass is begun with too rapid flow. Several of these problems are illustrated in Figure 17.1. All patients must receive an adequate total body flow, but the problems of arterial damage from high velocity flow can be minimized if one avoids rapid acceleration with the institution of cardiopulmonary bypass, and if one employs femoral perfusion only in those cases

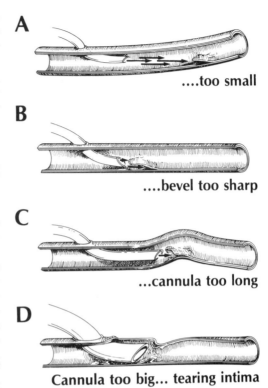

....too small

....bevel too sharp

...cannula too long

Cannula too big... tearing intima

Figure 17.1. Examples of avoidable errors in the technique of femoral artery cannulation. (*A*) Cannula is too small, giving rise to a forceful jet that can raise an intimal flap. (*B*) Cannula bevel is too sharp, causing a mechanical disruption of the intima. (*C*) Insertion of cannula with too much interarterial length, leading to damage to a tortuous iliac artery. (*D*) Cannula is too large for the femoral artery, causing a frictional disruption of the intima.

where it is possible to insert an adequate size cannula. Central nervous system complications caused by the retrograde perfusion of emboli is not unique to femoral artery cannulation, but is more frequently seen with this peripheral cannulation technique since blood is flowing in a retrograde fashion through a frequently diseased abdominal and thoracic aorta prior to reaching the cerebral circulation. The most effective safeguard against this retrograde aortic dissection is for the perfusionist and surgeon to check carefully for the presence of a pulse and adequate access to the arterial system through the cannulation port.

Coagulopathies and excessive postoperative bleeding occur with no greater frequency with femoral cannulation. The general avoidance of intracardiac suction, as well as the provision for an adequate size femoral artery cannula is important in minimizing blood trauma. Perhaps the most important factor in preventing central nerv-

ous system damage is the provision of an adequate perfusion pressure. A pressure of 60 torr is considered to be minimally acceptable, but the provision of a pressure in excess of 80 torr is probably more satisfactory and provides an additional margin of safety. This pressure should be combined with a flow of approximately 2 to 2.5 liters/m^2/min.[7] A potential disadvantage of the femoral route is that the necessity of using a smaller diameter cannula may make per-

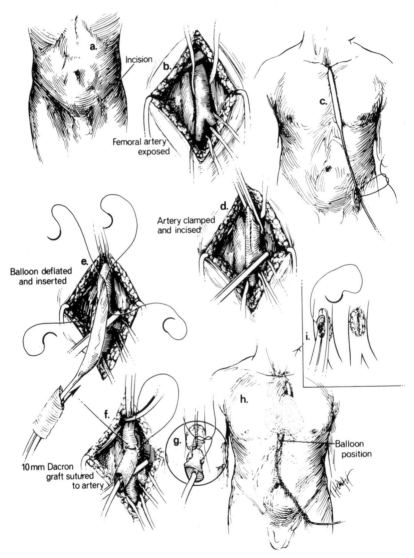

Figure 17.2. Illustration of the classic technique for the insertion of an intraaortic balloon pump. (Reproduced with permission from D. A. Cooley and J. C. Norman.[16])

fusion at these pressures and flow rates difficult to obtain.

Many cardiac surgeons will find that the most common usage of the femoral artery occurs with the provision of circulatory assistance for those patients who have compromised cardiac performance following cardiopulmonary bypass. This circulatory assistance most commonly involves the placement of an intraaortic balloon, but may employ variations in cardiopulmonary bypass. The classic technique for insertion of an intraaortic balloon pump through a graft is seen in Figure 17.2. This technique allows for the provision of distal limb flow around the catheter since no tourniquets or ligatures are placed immediately around the involved femoral artery. This technique of balloon insertion does require the performance of an end-to-side vascular anastomosis, and is most efficaciously performed in an operating room environment. The recent use of percutaneous intraaortic balloons has decreased the need for an operating room environment for balloon insertion. Furthermore, these aortic balloons are mounted on a smaller diameter catheter, which will result in better distal limb perfusion. If balloon assistance is inadequate and some type of prolonged partial cardiopulmonary bypass is to be used, then provision for distal limb flow is required; this may be accomplished either with a two-cannulae cannulation technique or with a temporary side arm graft.

Femoral artery cannulation appears to have few intrinsic advantages over the more commonly used aortic cannulation technique, but its use is required occasionally and an understanding of the problems mentioned above is imperative if the surgeon and perfusionist are to avoid these very significant problems.

AORTIC CANNULATION

Cannulation of the ascending aorta is now the most frequently used arterial perfusion technique. This technique should be used in preference to the femoral artery in those patients with severe arteriosclerosis and poor distal arteries. The use of aortic perfusion is not completely without prob-

lems, and may of the above-mentioned complications are seen occasionally. As was the case with femoral artery cannulation, many of these problems and complications occur when faulty technique is utilized. Problems analogous to those previously discussed with femoral artery cannulation include intimal damage distal to the arteriotomy site caused by a perfusion jet or a direct dissection and/or disruption of the aorta occurring at an arteriotomy site.[1] Excessive blood trauma and hematologic problems resulting in excessive postoperative bleeding can occur with both techniques if blood turbulence is not minimized. The proximity of a perfusion cannula to the cerebral perfusion has certain advantages in avoiding emboli of vascular debris; however, this technique is uniquely susceptible to the problem of carotid hyperperfusion and the direct elevation of intimal plaques in the cerebral circulation.[8] Arterial air or vascular debris from the oxygenator may also find more likely enlodgement in the cerebral circulation with aortic cannulation. Many of these perfusion problems are illustrated in Figure 17.3. The incidence of these complications can be minimized if the surgical team takes appropriate precautions. The ascending aorta is a large caliber vessel, and the surgeon should select a generous sized aortic cannula to avoid a jet lesion. Aortic disruption and/or dissection can be avoided most often by careful selection of the arteriotomy site. This same care in examining the aorta should be exercised in selecting the site for the proximal anastamoses when a saphenous vein aortocoronary artery bypass graft is being performed. The cannulation technique should provide for a completely hemostatic closure that avoids significant postoperative bleeding and the possibility of a false aneurysm. Fortunately, local arterial problems leading to dissection are rare and probably occur at a frequency of less than one in 4000 patients.[1, 8]

The special problem of carotid hyperperfusion is best avoided by taking special care to orient the cannula. This particular point is illustrated in Figures 17.3 and 17.4. The surgeon should note carefully the axis of the ascending aorta as it enters the arch and should ensure that the cannula is oriented toward the midstream of that ascending aorta rather than in a strictly vertical direction, which may, in fact, selectively perfuse the carotid artery.

As mentioned previously, it is important to avoid using a small diameter cannula. If the perfusion team has selected pulsatile flow, this problem may be aggravated further since the velocity of flow is from 5 to 10 times greater with pulsatile flow than with linear flow.

Electroencephalographic monitoring may help to determine that adequate cerebral flow is occurring. A standard encephalogram may be obtained and give useful in-

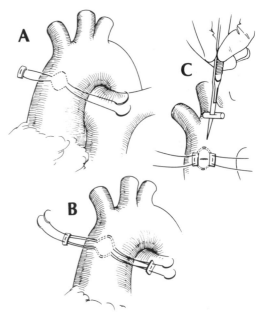

Figure 17.4. Technique of aortic cannulation using the double pledgeted suture method. (*A*) Initial pledgeted suture (note orientation perpendicular to tangent of ascending aorta). (*B*) Both pledgeted sutures in place. (*C*) Pledgeted sutures approximated with no. 11 blade being used for arteriotomy slit (note rubber catheter placed on no. 11 blade to serve as a stop).

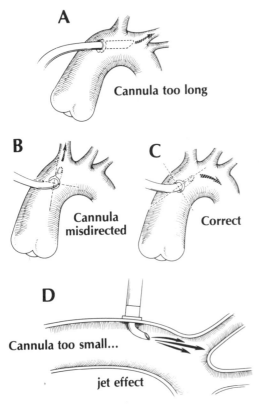

Figure 17.3. Examples of problem aortic cannulation. (*A*) Cannula is too long with extension into carotid artery and resultant hyperperfusion. (*B*) Misdirected cannula also resulting in carotid hyperperfusion. (*C*) Correct cannula oriented along the true tangent of the aorta. (*D*) Small cannula causing a jet effect with risk of raising an intimal flap.

formation regarding the adequacy of cerebral perfusion. However, we have found the use of a computerized system with a 3-dimensional graphic display to be more useful. Illustrations of this technique appear in Figure 17.5. This technique has allowed for the rapid recognition of inadequate cerebral perfusion as exemplified in these cases by cessation of pump flow with rapid and complete cessation of any electroencephalographic activities. This technique most dramatically illustrates the situation with cessation of cardiopulmonary bypass, but it is also helpful in picking up the more subtle problems of inadvertant air emboli and of plaque dislodgement.

The use of aortic cannulation is associated with problems for the cerebral circulation, but remains the preferred cannulation route. This preference is due to several obvious

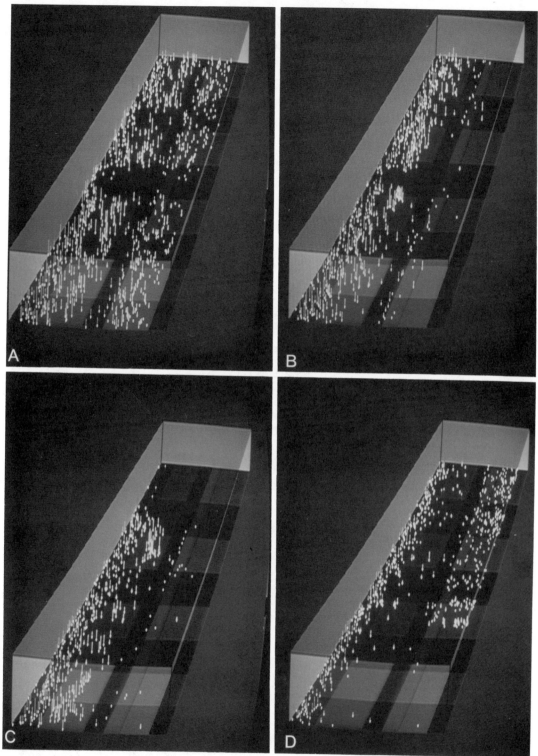

Figure 17.5. Four representative three-dimensional depictions of electroencephalograms. Frequency response is from left to right, amplitude is depicted by the height of the "trees," and time is measured from front to back (*A*) Three episodes of hypotension associated with lifting the heart. Note decreased high frequency activity in the right fields. (*B*) Sustained hypothermia at 28°C with decreased high frequency activity. "Hole" in the middle time period represents pump stoppage. (*C*) Complete cessation of activity, with discontinuation of cardiopulmonary bypass for 1 minute. (*D*) Initiation of cardiopulmonary bypass with a transient drop in blood pressure accompanied by decreased activity. (Courtesy of N. T. Smith, M.D.)

advantages. An incision in the groin area, a region generally considered unclean, is completely avoided with aortic cannulation. The flow with this cannulation is considerably more physiologic with antigrade flow and the avoidance of retrograde perfusion through a long segment of potentially diseased aorta. The problem of retrograde dissection caused by perfusion through a femoral intimal tear is completely avoided with aortic cannulation. The avoidance of peripheral cannulation also means that the risk of ischemia to the involved limb is eliminated.

COMPARATIVE COMPLICATION RATES FOR FEMORAL AND AORTIC CANNULATION

The occurrence of major and minor complications for the two cannulation techniques is summarized in Table 17.1. Examination of these data seems to support the thesis that the aortic route with a complication incidence of <0.5% is considerably safer than the femoral route with a complication incidence as high as 7%. This major difference between the two methods appears to be explainable almost entirely by

Table 17.1
Complications Associated with Femoral and Aortic Cannulation during Cardiopulmonary Bypass

| Reference | | Femoral Cannulation | | | Aortic Cannulation | | | |
	Date	No. of Cases	Complications	%	No. of Cases	Complications	%	Ref. no.
Kay et al.[9]	1966	720	0*	0	197	0	0.0	2–4
		378	28†	7.4				
Gerbode et al.[10]	1968	246	13	5.3	404	2	0.5	2–5
Roe and Kelly[11]	1969	735	9	1.2	410	0	0.0	2–6
Matar and Ross[12]	1967	160	5	3.1	198	0	0.0	2–7
McAlpine et al.[13]	1971				75	0	0.0	2–8
Flick et al.[14]	1971				1760	2	0.11	2
Salerno et al.[15]	1978	702	27	3.8	165	0	0.0	1
Daily et al.[4]	1971				1000	3	0.3	6
Taylor et al.[1]	1976				9000	3	0.03	5

* Patient's age less than 40 years
† Patient's age greater than 40 years

Table 17.2
EEG Abnormalities

| | Femoral Perfusion | | | Aortic Pressure | | |
	No. of Patients	%	Temp.	No. of Patients	%	Temp.
Normal EEG				29	34	37
	76	81	28	35	42	28
Minor EEG abnormality				6	7	37
	15	16	28	8	9	28
Major EEG abnormality				3	4	37
	3	3	28	3	4	28
Totals	94	100		84	100	

the avoidance of retrograde dissection with the aortic route. The incidence of minor bleeding problems appears to be equal using either technique, but in the case of aortic cannulation this problem probably can be avoided with the use of a purse string suture technique as illustrated in Figure 17.4.

The occurrence of encephalographic abnormalities in a population of patients perfused either through the aorta or the femoral artery is summarized in Table 17.2. This study by Flick and his associates[14] examines approximately 180 patients divided equally into two groups, one receiving aortic perfusion, the other receiving femoral artery perfusion. Although the incidence of patients having a major EEG abnormality was greater in the aortic arch perfusion group, this increase did not reach statistical significance and there appeared to be no substantive difference between the two groups in terms of maintaining a normal electroencephalogram.

CIRCUITS FOR OPERATIONS ON THE AORTA
Procedures on the Descending Aorta

The surgeon approaching dissection or disruption of the descending aorta has several options available. The arterial bed proximal to the involved segment of the aorta may provide an adequate vascular outlet so that placement of a proximal clamp will not result in an inordinately large afterload for the left ventricle. Collateral flow may also be developed adequately, and simple clamp isolation of the involved segments may allow for the conduct of resection and graft interposition. This technique is not attractive to many surgeons, and some type of shunt or partial cardiopulmonary bypass is usually utilized. In dealing with problems such as acute transection of the aorta, a heparin-bonded shunt not requiring systemic heparinization may be utilized. This shunt may incorporate the use of the apex of left ventricle to descending aorta or may use a more traditional arterial shunt with cannulation of the proximal aorta. Partial cardiopulmonary bypass using a femoral

artery to femoral vein technique is the other option. This technique utilizes cardiopulmonary bypass to provide for the circulatory needs of the lower body and requires the patient to provide the circulation and oxygenation for the upper half of the body. All of these techniques require a beating, functioning left ventricle. To avoid the incorporation of the patient's own cardiac activity into the perfusion strategy it is imperative to provide some type of partitioned bypass as illustrated in Figure 17.6 to provide for the needs of both the upper and lower circulations. Finally, a left atrial to femoral artery shunt may be utilized, which is capable of minimizing the work of the left ventricle and provides adequate oxygenation without the use of extracorporeal oxygenators.

Procedures on the Ascending Aorta

Standard cardiopulmonary bypass with an aortic cannulation site that is as distal to the aortic valve as possible may be used in many operations of the ascending aorta. If the involved artery is too extensive to allow for aortic cannulation, then some type of femoral artery perfusion will be required. These total bypass techniques offer the only appropriate perfusion strategies for dealing with this problem.

PROBLEMS OF THE AORTIC ARCH

The cardiac surgeon contemplating a procedure on the aortic arch is, perhaps, faced with one of cardiac surgery's greatest technical challenges. An examination of recent and older literature provides the reader with several possible techniques. Cardiopulmonary bypass can be avoided completely by the use of temporary bypass shunts that reroute the blood away from the aortic arch while this vessel is clamped, resected, and reconstructed. Provision for the cerebral circulation is provided through side arm grafts temporarily anastomosed to the appropriate head vessels. Cardiopulmonary bypass may be used; however, some provision for selective perfusion of the arch vessels is required. This perfusion could be provided with ap-

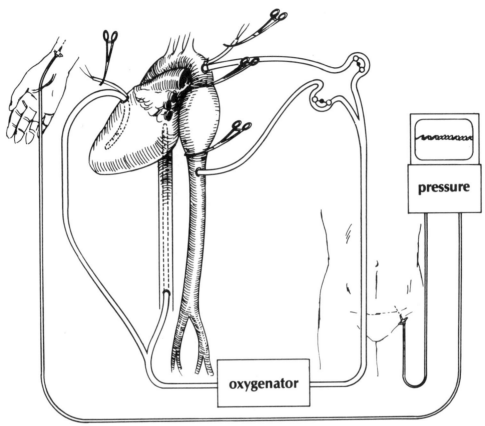

Figure 17.6. Perfusion circuit utilizing partitioned cardiopulmonary bypass with separate perfusion and pressure monitoring for the upper and lower portion of the body.

propriate side arm branches off the main arterial line, or could be provided by individual pump heads perfusing each arch vessel separately. An illustration of this technique appears in Figure 17.7. Both of these previously mentioned techniques are cumbersome and fraught with difficulty, and most surgical teams today face these problems utilizing a combination of femoral artery perfusion for support of the body and some type of hypothermic arrest to protect both the heart and cerebral circulation. Indeed, the emergence of cardioplegia and hypothermia have increased greatly the safety of dealing with these complicated problems. The myocardium can be deprived of its circulation for an extended period of time without subsequent damage. Hypothermia provides similar protection for the brain, although periods of circulatory arrest

generally should not exceed 1 hour. These two techniques have decreased the complexity of the perfusion circuits with fewer chances for poor blood flow distribution.

The selection of an appropriate perfusion circuit is crucial to the successful conduct of these operations. Of equal importance is the actual sequencing of the operative maneuvers. Patients presenting with a presumptuous diagnosis of aortic dissection or rupture must have operative strategies that will allow for the appropriate handling of the situation should exsanguinating rupture occur. This usually requires the surgeon to perform emergent bypass, frequently facilitated by actual insertion of the arterial line in a peripheral route. Aortic dissections may result in an acute life-threatening tamponade, and this problem must be anticipated with an appropriate operative approach.

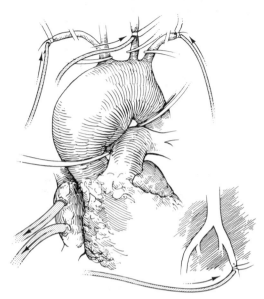

Figure 17.7. Illustration of perfusion circuit with individual perfusion of each arch artery. (Reproduced with permission from D. A. Cooley and J. C. Norman.[16])

The surgeon must take adequate care in his dissection and may want to delay or even avoid the use of anticoagulants by utilizing a shunt technique.

CONCLUSIONS

No attempt has been made in this chapter to outline the variations in operative techniques required for the successful execution of complex operations on the aorta. It is imperative, however, that the surgeon attempting to tackle these problems have an intimate knowledge of and familiarity with the various cannulation techniques so that these may be used most effectively in supporting the patient throughout his operative repair. A knowledge of the benefits of hypothermia and cardioplegia will decrease the requirements for complex, cumbersome, and complication-filled perfusion circuits, and ultimately allow a greater number of surgeons to carry out these procedures with some degree of safety and success. Unfortunately, there is no substitute for experience in dealing with these problems. Hopefully, these guidelines will prove appropri-ate in offering some assistance to all of those surgeons who must on occasion deal with these difficult situations.

References

1. Taylor PC, Groves LK, Loop FD, Effler DB: Cannulation of the ascending aorta for cardiopulmonary bypass. J Thorac Cardiovasc Surg 71(2):255–258, 1976.
2. Benedict JS, Buhl TL, Henney RP: Acute aortic dissection during cardiopulmonary bypass. Arch Surg 108:810–813, 1974.
3. Reinke T, Harris RD, Klein AJ, Daily PO: Aortoiliac dissection due to aortic cannulation. Ann Thorac Surg 18(3):295–299, 1974.
4. Daily PO, Fogarty TJ, Shumway NE: Cannulation of the ascending aorta. Ann Thorac Surg 12(1):85–88, 1971.
5. Vatayanon S, Kahn DR, Sloan H: Retrograde aortic dissection during cardiopulmonary bypass. [Report of a case with successful management.] Ann Thorac Surg 4(5):451–453, 1967.
6. Najafi H: Vascular complications of extracorporeal circulation. In *Complications of Intrathoracic Surgery*, edited by AR Cordell, RG Ellison. Boston, Little, Brown, 1979.
7. Lee WH, Brady MP: Central nervous system complications of extracorporeal circulation. In *Complications of Intrathoracic Surgery*, edited by AR Cordell, RG Ellison. Boston, Little, Brown, 1979.
8. Krous HF, Mansfield PB, Sauvage LR: Carotid artery hyperperfusion during open-heart surgery. [Report of a case]. J Thorac Cardiovasc Surg 66:118–121, 1973.
9. Kay JH, Dykstra PC, Tsuji HK: Retrograde ilioaortic dissection: A complication of common femoral artery perfusion during open-heart surgery. Am J Surg 111:464–468, 1966.
10. Gerbode F, Kerth WJ, Kovacs G, Sanchez PA, Hill JD: Cannulation of the ascending aorta for perfusion during cardiopulmonary bypass: A new technique and analysis of results. J Cardiovasc Surg 9(4):293–296, 1968.
11. Roe BB, Kelly PB: Perfusion through the ascending aorta: Experience with 410 cases. Ann Thorac Surg 7(3):238–241, 1969.
12. Matar AF, Ross DN: Traumatic arterial dissection in open-heart surgery. Thorax 22:82–87, 1967.
13. McAlpine WA, Selman MW, Kawakami T: Routine use of aortic cannulation in open-heart operations: Experience with an improved technique. Am J Surg 114:831–834, 1967.
14. Flick WF, Hallermann FJ, Feldt RH, Danielson GK: Aneurysm of aortic cannulation site. [Successful repair by means of peripheral cannulation, profound hypothermia and circulatory arrest.] J Thorac Cardiovasc Surg 61(3):419–423, 1971.
15. Salerno TA, Lince DP, White DN, Lynn RB, Charrette EJP: Arch *versus* femoral artery perfusion during cardiopulmonary bypass. J Thorac Cardiovasc Surg 76(5):681–684, 1978.
16. Cooley DA, Norman JC: *Techniques in Cardiac Surgery*. Houston, Texas Medical Press, 1975.

CHAPTER 18

POSTPERFUSION SYNDROMES, VIRAL SYNDROMES, AND BACTERIAL INFECTION AFTER CARDIOPULMONARY BYPASS

JOE R. UTLEY, M.D.

NONBACTERIAL POSTOPERATIVE SYNDROME

Within a few years after the beginning of cardiac surgical procedures employing cardiopulmonary bypass, physicians recognized that many patients developed a nonbacterial syndrome postoperatively characterized by fever with pericardial and pleural fluid. The patients with this postperfusion syndrome frequently have pericardial and pleural friction rubs, ST and T wave abnormalities on electrocardiogram, and may develop early or late pericardial tamponade. Petechei may occur with the postperfusion syndromes.[1] Between 1960 and 1965, several authors reported patients with postperfusion syndromes which included fever, splenomegaly, and atypical lymphocytes resembling infectious mononucleosis or a viral illness.[2-6] The syndrome may occur in any patient following pericardiotomy and is not necessarily associated with cardiopulmonary bypass.[7] A similar syndrome has been described after transvenous pacemaker placement.[7]

The syndrome was thought originally to be a reactivation of rheumatic fever but was soon recognized as equally common in congenital and nonrheumatic acquired heart disease. The pathogenesis of the condition in recent years has focused on the immune or viral origin of the syndrome. The syndrome does not occur in procedures not requiring pericardiotomy or myocardial manipulation, such as ductus ligation or coarctation repair. Postpericardiotomy syndrome occurs in 5 to 30% of patients undergoing intracardiac surgery. The syndrome may contribute to postoperative discomfort, delayed recovery, and prolonged hospitalization. The syndrome has been associated with development of pericardial tamponade, pericardial constriction, early occlusion of coronary saphenous vein grafts, and the development of vascular pericardial adhesions which increase the difficulty of reoperation.

These syndromes may be an activation of latent virus infection, an acquired virus infection, an autoimmune reaction, or a combination of these factors.

Viral Etiology

Kahn et al.[8] studied a group of patients who developed a postpericardiotomy syndrome and found evidence of parainfluenza virus. Evidence of virus particles in the bone marrow at the time of operation suggested that the procedure had activated the virus to produce the syndrome. The syndrome may include splenomegaly, atypical lymphocytes in the peripheral blood, and elevated heterophile agglutination titer. Some authors have considered the syndrome similar to infectious mononucleosis.[5, 9]

Immune Etiology

The development of techniques for quantitating antiheart antibodies has permitted better determination of the role of autoimmunity in the syndrome. The most thorough longitudinal study of the syndrome has been by a group of surgeons, cardiologists, and immunologists at Cornell University. They performed a prospective triple blind study in a group of over 300 patients, most of whom had procedures for congenital heart disease. They measured serum levels of heart reactive antibody preoperatively and serially postoperatively. The patients' sera were analyzed to determine the presence of antibodies to common viruses, including adenovirus, Coxsackie B virus, and cytomegalovirus. Cardiologists evaluated the patients for clinical evidence of postpericardiotomy syndrome. They found a strong correlation between the presence of antiheart antibody and postperfusion syndrome. All patients whose sera were positive for antiheart antibody had postperfusion syndrome. No patients with negative sera for antiheart antibody had the syndrome, and 5% of patients whose sera showed an intermediate level of antiheart antibody had a mild form of postperfusion syndrome. There was also a correlation with a rise in antiviral antibody titer and a rise in antiheart antibody and the occurrence of postperfusion syndrome. Patients with negative antiheart antibody titers had a 6.3% incidence of rise in antiviral titers. Seventeen percent of patients with intermediate levels of rise of antiheart antibody titers had rise in antiviral titers, and 70% of the patients with positive antiheart antibody titers had a rise in antiviral antibodies. The rise in viral antibody titers was correlated with appearance of postperfusion syndrome. The incidence of postperfusion syndrome was 70% in patients with positive titers for adenovirus, Coxsackie virus, and cytomegalovirus. The incidence of positive titers for the various viruses, including the six types of Coxsackie virus, varied during different time periods, suggesting that the virus was contemporarily acquired rather than the result of activation of a latent virus. EB virus acquired after cardiopulmonary bypass may be detected in the white cells months later. EB virus infection may be associated with postperfusion illness.[10] Myocardial trauma prior to the introduction of virus infection may increase the incidence of myocarditis.[11]

Age

There is a significant difference in the incidence of the syndrome in infants less than 1 year and children more than 2 years of age. Only 3.8% of infants less than 1 year old developed the syndrome, whereas the incidence was 35 to 38% in children more than 2 years of age and was independent of age beyond age 2 (Fig. 18.1).

Myoglobulin

Increased serum myoglobulin levels are observed in many patients after cardiac sur-

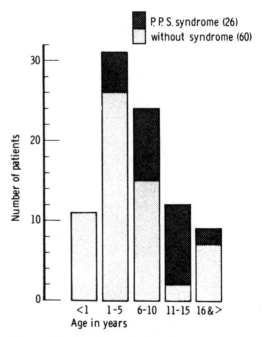

Figure 18.1. Age range of operated patients. Postperfusion syndrome is rare in infants less than 2 years of age and is most common after age 5. (Reproduced with permission from M. A. Engle et al.[61] and the American Heart Association, Inc.)

gical procedures. The appearance of cardiac antibodies are correlated with the appearance of serum myoglobulin postoperatively.[12] An experimental study in rats showed that pericardiotomy results in the early appearance of necrotic lesions beneath the epicardium. These were followed by the reappearance of myocardial antibodies. The appearance of antibodies was associated with the appearance of inflammatory lesions throughout the myocardium.[13]

Type of Operation

The incidence of the syndrome was greatest in tetralogy of Fallot and least common after repair of simple transposition by the Mustard procedure. Patients having repair of tetralogy of Fallot or ventricular septal defect closure with repair of pulmonic stenosis had 46% incidence of antiheart antibody and 33% incidence of antiviral antibody. Postperfusion syndrome is more common in patients operated upon for rheumatic heart disease.[14] Patients having the Mustard operation for simple transposition had 4% incidence of antiheart antibody and no incidence of antiviral antibody. The incidence of postpericardiotomy syndrome was 20% in all other patients. A factor in the low incidence in patients with simple transposition having the Mustard procedure is that the majority were less than 1 year of age. Patients with tetralogy of Fallot and ventricular septal defect repair had ventriculotomy and infundibular muscle resection, which may release more antigen to stimulate the antiheart antibody reaction. Their studies could demonstrate no relationship between the closure of the pericardium and the opening and drainage of the pleural spaces and the development of the postpericardiotomy syndrome. The observation that the syndrome may occur following a patient's first cardiac procedure but not following the second cardiac procedure favors an acquired virus in the pathogenesis rather than solely an immune mechanism. The working hypothesis favored by the Cornell Group is that the antibody is produced in response to myocardial injury and that more antigen sites are rendered available with more extensive injury. Increased heart-reacting antibodies and C_3 complement levels

are common after cardiac surgical procedures.[15] A recent or latent viral infection is often involved in the process, but the exact mechanism is unknown.

Mechanisms

The antiheart antibodies may affect the myocardium in a variety of ways related to production of injury and the postpericardiotomy syndrome. The antibody may be cytotoxic to myocardial cells in the presence of complement. The antibody may attach to the myocardium as a spectator without producing damage. The antibody may enhance the effect of sensitized lymphocytes in producing myocardial damage and cell death. Antibodies may attach to myocardial receptor sites and block the attachment of sensitized lymphocytes to the site[16] (Fig. 18.2). An exaggerated immune response to myocardial damage appears to be an important contributing factor in postperfusion syndrome[17] (Fig. 18.3). Decreased T cell ratios may increase the susceptibility to viral infection and postperfusion syndrome[18] (Fig. 18.4). Increased levels of IgG, IgA, and IgM have been observed in patients with postperfusion syndrome[19] (Fig. 18.5).

Other Factors

The exact consequences of complement activation, which is observed postcardiopulmonary bypass, has not been determined. Complement activation may be a contributing factor in postperfusion syndromes.[20] Other factors which have been implicated in the pathogenesis of postperfusion syndromes include reaction to blood in the pericardial space and reaction to starch powder on gloves. Postperfusion syndrome is less frequent if the pericardium is closed and drained.[21] Low serum albumin has been implicated in the pathogenesis of postperfusion syndrome. Intravenous albumin and protein alimentation has been suggested as therapy.[22] Other studies suggest that the early pleuropericardial reaction and the late acute pericarditis are not related.[23]

Treatment

Indomethacin has been shown to diminish postperfusion febrile reactions. Salicylates for milder forms of the syndrome and

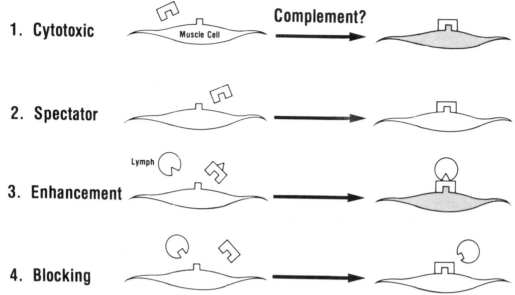

Figure 18.2. The drawing shows the various ways that antiheart antibodies may react with myocardial cells. (Reproduced with permission from M. A. Engle et al.[16])

steroids for more severe forms are the usual treatment. Coronary artery bypass occlusion has been described in association with postperfusion syndromes.[24] More aggressive treatment in patients having coronary artery bypass grafts may prevent graft occlusion due to pericardial reaction. Postoperative fever and leukocytosis has not been a reliable index of infection in cardiac surgery patients.[25,26]

CYTOMEGALOVIRUS INFECTION

Cytomegalovirus infection after cardiopulmonary bypass may induce a variety of clinical and immunological abnormalities. Patients may have fever, hepatosplenomegaly, and lymphocytosis. Hematologic and serologic abnormalities include lymphocytic leukemoid reaction, glomerulitis, anemia, erythrocyte autoantibodies, rheumatoid factor, antinuclear antibodies, cold agglutination, and cryoglobulins.[27]

The syndrome of cytomegalovirus infection after cardiac surgery may be different from that occurring in other patients perhaps related to the altered immune response after cardiopulmonary bypass.[28] Hemolytic anemia as a complication of cytomegalovirus infection has been reported following cardiopulmonary bypass.[29]

Paloheim et al.[30] found cytomegalovirus infection common after open heart procedures and uncommon after closed procedures. He postulated that the infection was due to transfusion of fresh blood.

Lang and Hanshaw[31] recovered cytomegalovirus from four patients with the postperfusion syndrome. The virus was isolated from the urine of fresh blood donors. Anti-CMV macroglobulins and complement-fixing antibody were demonstrated in all patients. The virus was associated with circulating leukocytes in all patients. He concluded that the virus was transmitted in the white cell fraction of fresh blood.

Seven of 16 heart surgery patients were studied prospectively and showed serologic evidence of CMV infection. CMV was cultured from three patients, and five of the seven were symptomatic, two were symptom-free, and only one had atypical lymphocytes. The investigators concluded CMV infection after cardiac surgery is due to fresh blood transfusion.[32]

In a later prospective study of 55 patients, 21 developed complement-fixing antibodies, seven excreted virus in the urine, four

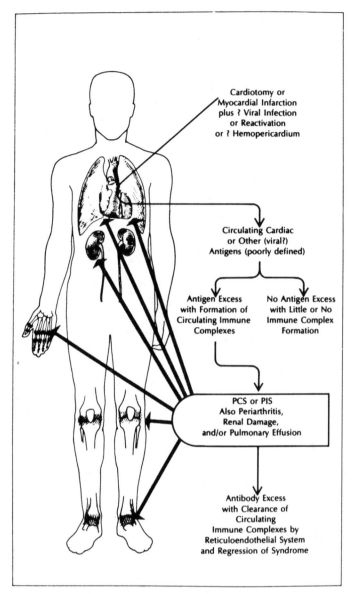

Figure 18.3. The hypothetical pathogenesis and course of PCS or PIS in relation to viral infection and the immune mechanism is shown in this drawing. (Reproduced with permission from M. H. Lessof.[17])

had atypical lymphocytes, and seven had a mild illness related to infection. There was no correlation with type of operation and CMV infection, nor was it correlated with age, sex, or season of the year. The study showed increased incidence with increasing numbers of fresh blood transfusions. Five to ten percent of blood donors are infectious with cytomegalovirus.

Prince et al.[33] found that the risk of seroconversion as evidence of cytomegalovirus infection increased with the number of

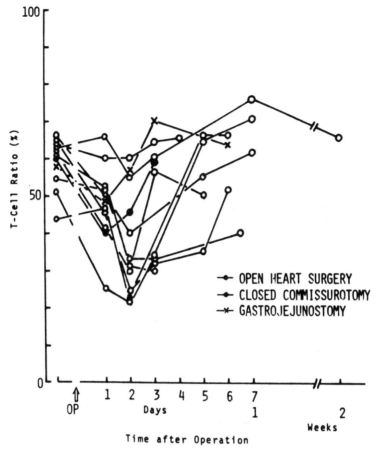

Figure 18.4. T cell ratios diminish for several days following cardiac surgical procedures. (Reproduced with permission from H. Manabe et al.[18])

transfusions used. The majority of infections are from transfusions of blood from donors who are chronic latent carriers.

BACTERIAL AND FUNGAL INFECTION

The high morbidity and mortality with bacterial infection in cardiac surgical patients make prevention rather than treatment the main concern of the cardiac surgeon.[35-38] The incidence of opportunistic bacterial and fungal infection appears to be increasing following cardiac surgery[39] (Fig. 18.6). The magnitude of the morbidity and risk of mortality when bacterial infection complicates cardiac surgical procedures is

greater than other types of procedures. The factors which increase the potential risk of infection in cardiac surgical patients include the duration of the procedure; presence of a sternal osteotomy; the use of numerous prosthetic and intravascular foreign bodies including vascular grafts, valve prostheses, pledges, and pacemakers; the postoperative immunosuppression; the aspiration of room air directly through the patient's blood stream through the cardiotomy suction and the oxygenator; the use of indwelling vascular catheters and endotracheal tubes for long periods of time; and the presence of blood, hematoma, and coagulated tissue in the area of the operation.[40] The factors which often are associated with lethal post-

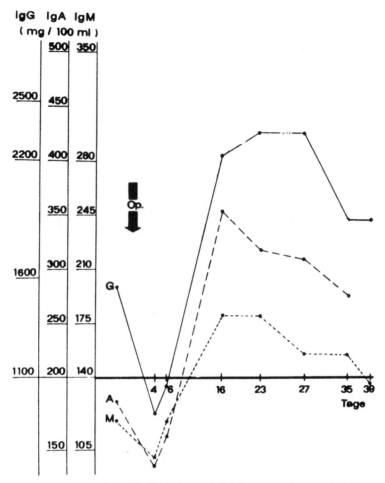

Figure 18.5. Increased levels of IgG, IgA, and IgM were observed with postperfusion syndrome. (Reproduced with permission from R. Rogos and H. Trenckmann.[19])

operative infection include preoperative bacterial endocarditis, cardiopulmonary bypass more than 3.5 hours, low cardiac output, postoperative cerebral dysfunction, and disseminated intravascular coagulation.[36]

The incidence of perioperative microbial infection has been low in most surgeons' experience in recent years. The incidence of infection was as high as 30% in earlier experience.[41] The majority of cardiac surgeons favor the use of prophylactic antibiotics to avoid the infrequent, but potentially catastrophic, infection from a virulent organism highly sensitive to antibiotics such as B hemolytic *Streptococcus*. The morbidity and risk of prophylactic antibiotic use is low.[42, 43]

Prevention

Because the cardiac surgeon is often unable to diminish the susceptibility of the wound and the patient to infection, many of his efforts are directed toward decreasing the numbers and pathogenicity of microorganisms which gain access to the patient's wounds. It is a common experience among cardiac surgeons that infections may be in groups and are not always a random event. Continuous attention to the sterility of instruments and materials, the care of the ward and the intensive care unit patients shedding bacteria, the avoiding of bacterial carrier states by the members of the operating team, and the adherence to rigid tech-

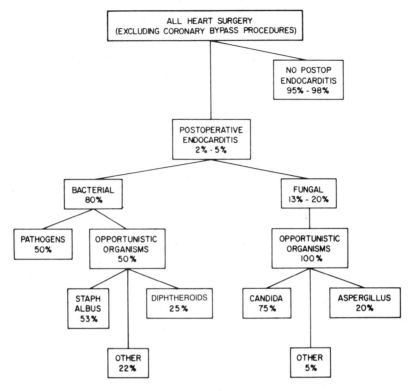

Figure 18.6. The block diagram shows the incidence of various types of infection following cardiac surgical procedures. (Reproduced with permission from R. G. Norenberg et al.[39])

nique while operating are important details. The risk of infection is proportional to the number of organisms and the virulence of organisms, as well as other local and systemic factors. Risk of infection is inversely proportional to resistance. The risk of infection following bacteremia is greatest immediately after the operation and diminishes after 6 weeks.[44]

Hughes[45] described a very extensive method for improving antisepsis with heart surgery which included prophylactic antibiotics, preoperative screening for infection, housekeeping measures, and air decontamination in the operating room. Sources of contamination may include coronary suction, heat exchanger leaks, and oxygen sources.

ORGANISMS IN CARDIAC SURGERY

Staphylococcus aureus is the most common organism causing infection following cardiac surgery. Many organisms often thought

to be nonpathogenic to man have caused infection in prosthetic heart valves. These include *Micrococcus flavus, Pseudomonas maltophilia, Oerskoviz turbata,* and *Neisseria perflara.*[46]

A wide spectrum of gram-negative organisms have been observed in postoperative infections, including *Klebsiella, Pseudomonas, Proteus, Escherichia coli, Serratia,* and *Salmonella.* Fungal organisms such as *Candida, Aspergillus,* and *Torulopsis* have also infected patients postoperatively.[46, 47] Bacteremia after cardiac surgery is due more frequently to gram-negative organisms and less frequently due to gram-positive organisms than occurred previously.[48]

Sources of Contamination

Blakemore et al.[40] cultured organisms from the pump oxygenator in 75% of his patients and found the coronary suction line to be the most common site for bacterial contamination. This observation indicates that local wound sterility and bacterial contamination of operating room air are important factors in the pathogenesis of the contamination.[46, 49] Other sources of infection include operating room personnel who are carriers of bacteria, intravenous catheters, endotracheal tubes, and pressure transducers.[50–52] Culture evidence of contamination has been observed in the intracardiac area of operation, the valve prosthesis, donor blood, excised cardiac valve, the heart-lung machine, bladder catheter, and chronic wounds in other areas of the body.[46, 53, 54] It is estimated that 1000 bacteria settle into a sternotomy wound from the air during a 2-hour operation.[46] Respirators and inhalation equipment may be a source of contamination, especially gram-negative bacteria.[50] The use of sterile disposable endotracheal tubes, suction catheters, and gloves have decreased the incidence and severity of tracheobronchial infection.[46] The incidence of bacterial contamination of glucose-containing solutions is 3 to 38%. Sixty percent of surgery gloves have unrecognized leaks[46] (Fig. 18.7).

Air is drawn through coronary suction lines at the rate of 1 to 2 cu ft/min. Ambient air in operating rooms contain 10 or more bacteria per cubic foot. Blakemore et al.[40] observed a maximum of 14 colony-forming units per cubic foot. The number of bacteria in the room air is influenced by the number of people in the room, the ventilation system, and the number of times the doors are opened.

Fifty thousand dust particles per cubic

foot were found when the operating room was not in use, and up to 824,000 dust particles per cubic foot were found during cardiac operations. He calculated that 1,200 colony-forming units would be drawn into the coronary suction lines per hour of bypass and would add one colony-forming unit per 6 ml of blood per hour.[38]

The factors which are important in preventing air contamination in cardiac surgery operating rooms include air filtration, air delivery, suction control, oxygen line control, protective clothing and masks, traffic control, aseptic control, and exclusion of a contaminated operation from the cardiac rooms.

Infection Control

When infection occurs in epidemic proportions on a cardiac surgical service, a multifaceted program must be initiated to eliminate the source of contamination. Practical considerations often preclude changing single factors sequentially. Despite the inability of such multifaceted programs to prove statistically which factors are the principal determinants of the outbreak, they have been remarkably successful in decreasing the incidence of infection. Among the factors which should be a part of a multifaceted program are operating room renovations to assure a high-flow vertical unidirectional ventilation system, improvement of barriers in gowning and draping techniques, monitoring the sterility of instruments, valves, drapes, heart-lung machine and gloves, use of local and systemic broad coverage bacteriocidal antibiotics, use of cardiac surgical operating room for only clean noncontaminated cases, admission of only clean noninfected patients to the postoperative cardiac surgery intensive care unit, and the transfer to another care unit of any patient who becomes infected. Members of the surgical team and nursing staff may be precluded from working in areas with infected and contaminated patients.[55] The training of housestaff and paramedical personnel in the importance of avoiding contamination of clothing and hands in the care of infected patients is important.[51, 56] The monitoring of techniques used for placement and care of

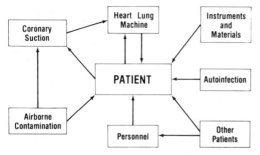

Figure 18.7. The block diagram shows the sources of infection for the cardiac surgical patient.

intravascular catheters and endotracheal tubes is important.[57] Anesthetic gas machines may be a significant source of contamination.[58] Clark et al.[57] was able to demonstrate a decrease of deep wound infection rate from 2.9 to 0.6%, and a total wound infection rate from 6.6% to 3.3%. The incidence in valve prosthesis infection fell from 5.6% to 1.4%.

The sources of contamination to the heart-lung machine include incomplete sterility of the machine itself, fluids and blood added to the machine, coronary suction, oxygenation gases, and patient and intravascular catheters. Methods to decrease bacterial contamination of the operating room were an important part of the factors which diminish infection in Carey's study.[59] Although the frequency of positive cultures from the heart-lung machine varies greatly (2 to 70%), the incidence of postoperative infection in patients with positive cultures is fortunately low and most commonly occurs when the patient has been infected preoperatively.[60]

References

1. Quintiliani R, Gifford RH: Petechiae in postcardiotomy syndromes. NY State J Med 70:2713, 1970.
2. Anderson R, Larsson O: Fever, splenomegaly, and atypical lymphocytes after open heart surgery. Lancet 2:947, 1963.
3. Wheeler ED, Turner JD, Scannell JG: Fever, splenomegaly and atypical lymphocytes. A syndrome observed after cardiac surgery utilizing a pump oxygenator. N Engl J Med 266:454, 1962.
4. Seaman AJ, Starr A: Febrile postcardiotomy lymphocytic splenomegaly: A new entity. Ann Surg 156:956, 1962.
5. Smith DR: A syndrome resembling infectious mononucleosis after open-heart surgery. Br Med J 1:945, 1964.
6. Holswade GR, Engle MA, Redo SF, Goldsmith EI, Barondess JA: Development of viral diseases and a viral disease-like syndrome after extracorporeal circulation. Circulation 27:812, 1963.
7. Kaye D, Frankl W, Arditi LI: Probable postcardiotomy syndrome following implantation of a transvenous pacemaker: Report of the first case. Am Heart J 90:627, 1975.
8. Kahn DR, Ertel PY, Murphy WH, Kirsh MM, Vathayanon S, Stern AM, Sloan H: Pathogenesis of the postcardiotomy syndrome. J Thorac Cardiovasc Surg 54:682, 1967.
9. Reyman TA: Postperfusion syndrome. Am Heart J 72:116, 1966.
10. Gerber P, Walsh JH, Rosenblum EN, Purcell RH: Association of EB-virus infection with the postperfusion syndrome. Lancet 1:593, 1969.
11. Burch GE, Colcolough HL: Postcardiotomy and postinfarction syndromes—a theory. Am Heart J 80:290, 1970.
12. Chang K, Friedman H, Goldberg H: Cardiac specific antigen and antibody in immunopathogenesis of cardiac disease. Adv Exp Med Biol 121B:335, 1979.
13. Chaturvedi UC, Mathur A, Gupta RK, Mehrotra RML: Immunopathological studies in pericardiotomised rats. J Pathol 109:345, 1973.
14. Kaplan MH, Frengley JD: Autoimmunity to the heart in cardiac disease. Current concepts of the relation of autoimmunity to rheumatic fever, postcardiotomy and postinfarction syndromes and cardiomyopathies. Am J Cardiol 24:459, 1969.
15. McCabe JC, Ebert PA, Engle MA, Zabriskie JB: Circulating heart-reactive antibodies in the postpericardiotomy syndrome. J Surg Res 14:158, 1973.
16. Engle MA, Zabriskie JB, Senterfit LB, McCabe JC, Gay WA, Read SE: Immunologic considerations in the postpericardiotomy syndrome. In *Clinical Immunology of the Heart*, edited by JB Zabriskie, Engle MA, Villareal H Jr. New York, John Wiley & Sons, 1981.
17. Lessof MH: Postcardiotomy syndrome: Pathogenesis and management. Hosp Pract 11:81, 1976.
18. Manabe H, Shirakura R, Mori T: Cardiovascular disease and immunology in cardiac surgery. Jpn Circ J 39:453, 1975.
19. Rogos R, Trenckmann H: Dysgammaglobinamie beim Postperfusionssyndrom. Allerg Immunol (Leipz) 17:38, 1971.
20. Chenoweth DE, Cooper SW, Hugli TE, Stewart RW, Blackstone EH, Kirklin JW: Complement activation during cardiopulmonary bypass. Evidence for generation of C3a and C5a anaphylatoxins. N Engl J Med 304:497, 1981.
21. Cunningham JN, Spencer FC, Zeff R, Williams CD, Cukingnan R, Mullin M: Influence of primary closure of the pericardium after open-heart surgery on the frequency of tamponade, postcardiotomy syndrome, and pulmonary complications. J Thorac Cardiovasc Surg 70:119, 1975.
22. Aronstam EM, Cox WA: A new concept of the pleuropericardial syndrome. J Thorac Cardiovasc Surg 51:341, 1966.
23. Livelli FD, Johnson RA, McEnany MT, Sherman E, Newell J, Block PC, DeSanctis RW: Unexplained in-hospital fever following cardiac surgery. Circulation 57:968, 1978.
24. Urschel HC, Razzuk MA, Gardner M: Coronary artery bypass occlusion secondary to postcardiotomy syndrome. Ann Thorac Surg 22:528, 1976.
25. Bell DM, Goldmann DA, Hopkins CC, Karchmer AW, Moellering RC: Unreliability of fever and leukocytosis in the diagnosis of infection following cardiac valve surgery. J Thorac Cardiovasc Surg 79:87, 1978.
26. DeVillota ED, Barat G, Astorqui F, Damaso D, Avello F: Pyrexia following open heart surgery. The role of bacterial infection. Anaesthesia 29:529, 1974.

27. Kantor GL, Goldberg LS, Johnson BL Jr, Derechin MM, Barnett EV: Immunologic abnormalities induced by postperfusion cytomegalovirus infection. Ann Intern Med 73:553, 1970.

28. Carlstrom G, Belfrage S, Ohlsson N-M, Swedberg J: Cytomegalovirus infection complicating open-heart surgery. Scand J Thorac Cardiovasc Surg 2:57, 1968.

29. Holt S, Kirkham N: Cytomegalovirus-induced haemolytic anaemia after cardiac surgery. Thorax 31:786, 1976.

30. Paloheimo JA, von Essen R, Klemola E, Kaariainen L, Siltanen P: Subclinical cytomegalovirus infections and cytomegalovirus mononucleosis after open heart surgery. Am J Cardiol 22:624, 1968.

31. Lang DJ, Hanshaw JB: Cytomegalovirus infection and the postperfusion syndrome. N Engl J Med 280:1145, 1969.

32. Embil JA, Haldane EV, Folkins DF, van Rooyen CE: Cytomegalovirus infection following extracorporeal circulation in children. Lancet 2:1151, 1968.

33. Prince AM, Szmuness W, Millian SJ, David DS: A serologic study of cytomegalovirus infections associated with blood transfusions. N Engl J Med 283:1125, 1971.

34. Caul EO, Mott MG, Clarke SKR, Perham TGM, Wilson RSE: Cytomegalovirus infections after open heart surgery. Lancet 1:777, 1971.

35. Engelman RM, Williams CD, Gouge TH, Chase RM Jr, Falk EA, Boyd AD, Reed GE: Mediastinitis following open-heart surgery. Arch Surg 107:772, 1973.

36. Engelman RM, Chase RM Jr, Boyd AD, Reed GE: Lethal postoperative infections following cardiac surgery: Review of four years' experience. Circulation 48(Suppl. III):31, 1973.

37. Hehrlein FW, Herrmann H, Kraus J: Complications of median sternotomy in cardiovascular surgery. J Cardiovasc Surg 13:390, 1972.

38. Ochsner JL, Mills NL, Woolverton WC: Disruption and infection of the median sternotomy incision. J Cardiovasc Surg 13:394, 1972.

39. Norenberg RG, Sethi GK, Scott SM, Takaro T: Opportunistic endocarditis following open-heart surgery. Ann Thorac Surg 19:592, 1975.

40. Blakemore WS, McGarrity GJ, Thurer RJ, Wallace HW, MacVaugh H III, Coriell LL: Infection by airborne bacteria with cardiopulmonary bypass. Surgery 70:830, 1971.

41. Goodman JS, Schaffner W, Collins HA, Battersby EJ, Koenig MG: Infection after cardiovascular surgery. N Engl J Med 278:117, 1968.

42. Antimicrobial prophylaxis: Prevention of wound infection and sepsis after surgery. Med Lett Drugs Ther 19:37, 1977.

43. Williams RW, Bradshaw MW: Prevention and treatment of infection of prosthetic valves. South Med J 69:3, 1976.

44. Carter DR, Barney JA, Lleu J, Hanna WR, Williams GR: Endocarditis after intracardiac surgery. Am J Surg 114:765, 1967.

45. Hughes RK: A method of improved antisepsis for open-heart surgery. Ann Thorac Surg 2:230, 1966.

46. Hornick RB: Source of contamination in open heart surgery. Infections of prosthetic heart valves and vascular grafts. In *Infections of Prosthetic Valves and Vascular Grafts—Prevention, Diagnosis, and Treatment*, edited by RJ Duma. Baltimore, University Park Press, 1977.

47. Jamshidi A, Pope RH, Friedman NH: Fungal endocarditis complicating cardiac surgery. Arch Intern Med 112:370, 1963.

48. Lockey E, Gonzalez-Lavin L, Ray I, Chen R: Bacteraemia after open-heart surgery. Thorax 28:183, 1973.

49. Baffes TG, Blazek WV, Fridman JL, Agustsson MH, Van Elk J: Postoperative infections in 1,136 consecutive cardiac operations. Surgery 68:791, 1970.

50. Frater RWM, Santos GH: Sources of infection in open-heart surgery. NY State J Med 74:2386, 1974.

51. Rosendorf LL, Daicoff G, Baer H: Sources of gram-negative infection after open-heart surgery. J Thorac Cardiovasc Surg 67:195, 1974.

52. Weinstein RA, Jones EL, Schwarzmann SW, Hatcher CR Jr: Sternal osteomyelitis and mediastinitis after open-heart operation: Pathogenesis and prevention. Ann Thorac Surg 21:442, 1976.

53. Kluge RM, Calia FM, McLaughlin JS, Hornick RB: Sources of contamination in open heart surgery. JAMA 230:1415, 1974.

54. Renyi-Vamos F Jr, Renyi-Vamos F Sr: Significance of asymptomatic bacteriuria in cardiac surgery. Acta Chir Acad Sci Hung 13:255, 1972.

55. Blouse LE, Lathrop GD, Kolonel LN, Brocket RM: Epidemiologic features and phage types associated with nosocomial infections caused by *Staphylococcus epidermidis*. Zentralbl Bakteriol [Orig A] 241:119, 1978.

56. Marples RR, Hone R, Notley CM, Richardson JF, Crees-Morris JA: Investigation of coagulase-negative staphylococci from infections in surgical patients. Zentralbl Bakteriol [Orig A] 241:140, 1978.

57. Clark RE, Amos WC, Higgins V, Benberg KF, Weldon CS: Surgery 79:89, 1976.

58. Craig DB: Contamination in open heart surgery. JAMA 232:19, 1975.

59. Carey JS, Hughes RK: Control of infection after thoracic and cardiovascular surgery. Ann Surg 172:916, 1970.

60. Geldof WChP, Brom AG: Infections through blood from heart-lung machine. Thorax 27:395, 1972.

61. Engle MA, McCabe JC, Ebert PA, Zabriskie J: The postpericardiotomy syndrome and antiheart antibodies. Circulation 49:401, 1974.

CHAPTER 19

THE CONDUCT OF A CLINICAL TRIAL OF AN INVESTIGATIONAL DEVICE IN 1982

RICHARD E. CLARK, M.D.

THE CRUCIAL DECADE—1950–1960

The decade of 1950 to 1960 was a period of great activity in cardiac surgery during which the animal laboratory was the keystone to a series of dramatic clinical successes. In the early part of the decade, a technique of hypothermia was developed by Bigelow and colleagues,[1] and a prosthetic heart valve for aortic insufficiency was described by Hufnagel.[2] Gibbon,[3] who had demonstrated that extracorporeal circulation was possible in 1937 using dogs, was to report the first successful clinical open heart case using total bypass.[4] Dennis et al.[5] had also developed a pump oxygenator and Clowes,[6] a left heart bypass system. Kay and Cross modified a disc oxygenator, described in 1948 by Bjork[7] and Cross et al.,[8] and DeWall et al.[9] reported success with a bubble oxygenator. Kolff et al.[10] was developing a membrane oxygenator which was given a clinical trial in 1958 by Clowes and colleagues.[11] Heat exchangers appeared,[12, 13] coronary perfusion techniques were developed, cardioplegia was used clinically,[14] and various levels of hypothermia and techniques in cooling and rewarming were reported.[15] Thus, this decade provided all of the basic types of oxygenators (screen, disc, bubble, membrane), the electric version of the roller pump of DeBakey's transfusion device,[16] heat exchangers, filters, tubing, reservoirs, cannulae, connectors, and a rapid changing array of measuring devices.

The commonalities among all the developments were the alacrity of clinical application from the time of conception and the sequence of events. The device was fabricated, tested *in vitro*, then frequently modified, retested, and used during total cardiopulmonary bypass in dogs. After three to five experiments, the same device was used in a clinical trial. During this first decade, most of the components were reusable, being made of metal. The companies that provided the hardware were few, and all major components were made on a custom basis. The hospitals performing cardiac surgery were also few in comparison to today and were limited to the university medical centers. With the growth of cardiac surgery and its constantly changing and challenging needs a new industry was created which catered to the specific needs of the cardiac surgeon and perfusionist.

The development of the private sector has been rapid and now constitutes a 300 million dollar industry. This system introduced the first practical disposable equipment, ranging initially from plastic discs to bubble oxygenator bags, to be followed by the hard shell bubble system. Metal connectors, stopcocks, filters, etc., disappeared and were replaced by similar plastic components. Today, except for the pump console and the subtending instrumentation, all components of the extracorporeal circulation are disposable.

With competition in the marketplace, the absence of standards or a regulatory body overseeing the rapidly growing industry, problems with new devices were frequent. Oxygenators failed to transfer oxygen and carbon dioxide, cleanliness of various products was a problem, filters clogged or channeled debris, integral heat exchangers lacked claimed high efficiencies in the clinical setting, and the importance of microemboli in gaseous or solid forms generated by a component or a system were not well appreciated.

Clinical trials were not carefully controlled nor conducted. The major theme was to induce well known (if possible, household) names in cardiac surgery to try a new device under the guise of "improved patient care." Several thousand patients were frequently subjected to these trials without their knowledge or consent. Too few variables were measured too infrequently to provide a sound scientific basis for judgement. One heard the coffee shop comments that "my patients do better with brand X." Rarely were concurrent control groups used to control for the rapidly changing variables in the operating room. Claims and counterclaims were hawked by the sales personnel of the perfusion industry as it entered the 1970s. Much was to change in quality control and the testing of products before clinical trials in the succeeding decade.

Various organized bodies saw the developments occurring and set forth to produce sets of voluntary standards. With respect to perfusion, the Oxygenator Standard Committee of the American Society of Artificial Internal Organs (ASAIO) was one of the first to attempt to amalgamate industry, academicians, and practitioners. Progress was slow, the debates seemingly endless, and agreements were few. Another organization, The Association for the Advancement of Medical Instrumentation (AAMI), had

been active in standards making and turned to the cardiovascular field, in part by impetus provided by The International Standards Organization. These efforts, in turn, were spurred by the grumblings of the monolithic bureaucracy of Congress which began hearing of the problems of medical devices, primarily from consumer advocate groups. After more than 2 years of hearings and floor debates over various bills and amendments, President Gerald Ford signed the Amendment to Medical Device Act of 1976 Public Law 94-295 in May of that year.

THE MEDICAL DEVICE ACT OF 1976

Classification

The Act requires that the FDA assemble "expert" panels for the purpose of classifying devices into one of three general categories. Class I devices are those that can be regulated by general controls. Class II devices are required to meet certain performance standards, and Class III devices are those that require premarket approval by the panel and the FDA before unrestricted marketing in this country. Specifically, the law notes that all life-supporting, life-sustaining, or implantable devices are to be placed in the premarket approval category. When insufficient information is available concerning the efficacy and safety of a specific device, the law requires placement in Class III.

Assignment to each category was based on an evaluation of efficacy and safety. The criteria for safety and efficacy were (1) the identification of patients for whom the device is intended; (2) the conditions of use; (3) evaluation of the benefits *vs.* the risks; and (4) the effectiveness as determined by "well controlled investigations" and "valid scientific evidence." The panels had to provide reasons for recommendation to a specific category and identify the risk and were requested to assign a priority within categories based on estimates of degree and exposure of risk.

On March 9, 1979, the FDA published the general rules applicable to the classification of all cardiovascular devices and the proposed classification list of 142 devices.

Two were recommended for general controls, with no exemptions. One hundred fourteen devices were recommended for standards, and 26 were recommended for premarket approval. The final classification differed little from that proposed.

Premarket Approval Category (Class III)

The manufacturer of a new Class III device must undertake a wide variety of *in vitro* and animal studies as initial steps. Next, based on the data obtained from such studies, the manufacturer may apply to the FDA for an investigational device exemption (IDE). An IDE is required for clinical trials for all classes of devices. The manufacturer must find investigators who are willing to undertake clinical trials of the new device, and the investigator must agree to a clinical trial protocol that must be approved by the investigator's institutional review board (IRB). Special attention must be given to the selection of the patient population, informed consent, and an assessment of the risk to benefit ratio. The FDA must respond to the IDE application within 30 days. Under the regulations, the FDA can inspect the records of the institutional review board and review the investigator's data. Additionally, punitive action can be taken against the investigator, the institution, or members of the institutional review board if the protocol is not followed or if data have been falsified.

After careful clinical trials have been conducted in several centers, an application can be made to the FDA for premarket approval. This application is read by members of the agency and presented to a specific device panel for peer review. The agency is under no legal requirement to abide by the recommendation of the expert panel. The application must embody complete reports demonstrating safety and effectiveness of performance, detail the components and principles of operations, contain a complete description of the methods, facilities, and controls used in manufacturing, demonstrate conformance to any performance standards that may exist, supply samples of the product and labeling, and provide testimony at a public hearing concerning efficacy and safety.

Performance Standards Category (Class II)

It was the intent of Congress to establish a category of regulation for devices that did not need to go through the time-consuming and highly expensive premarket approval pathway. The intent of the performance standards category was to assure the surgeon, the physician, and the public of the safety, efficacy, and reliability of a device that was not life-sustaining, life-supporting, or implanted. Class II devices would have to meet the standards 1 year after the publication of the classification and the standard. The government could adopt or adapt standards from the voluntary sector. However, the language of the Act is such that it places reliance on government agencies as the primary producers of such standards. Moreover, there is latitude in the law that will permit the FDA not only to develop performance standards but also to dictate design, compatibility of parts, testing specifications, and the variables to be measured for judgment of performance and labeling instructions concerning installation, maintenance, and operation.

General Controls Category (Class I)

General controls were devised to prevent adulteration and misbanding of devices and to prevent the manufacturing of devices prohibited by law and previously banned by the FDA. Class I devices require registration and listing with the agency and the submission of a policy concerning repair, replacement, and refund. Highly detailed records and reports concerning conformance to good manufacturing practices must be maintained.

Institutional Review Boards (IRB)

On August 8, 1978, the FDA proposed in the Federal Register a series of regulations governing institutional review boards. These proposed regulations reflected the report of the National Commission on Protection of Human Subjects which recommended a complete overhaul of the IRB system and the creation of a new Health, Education, and Welfare (HEW) office to monitor and control all IRBs through accreditation, audits, and punitive actions. The present regulations require a diversity of membership for institutional review boards, which specifically must include nonclinicians and nonscientists, *i.e.*, lawyers, clergy, consumer representatives, social scientists, and psychologists. The regulations provide for mandated inspections of the records of the IRBs to determine the appropriateness of protecting the privacy rights of the individuals at risk in a clinical trial. In addition, the audit is to review the decisions of an IRB and verify the data on which the decisions were made. It has been estimated that the cost of an institutional review board to conform to the various regulations and carry out the new responsibilities is $50,000 a year.

The Informed Consent

The informed consent is paramount in terms of federal regulation and the IRB. This document must clearly state the benefits, risks, and alternatives available to the patient. Note that the patient is entitled to a copy of the consent form. A copy of the form used for an investigational device at Washington University is included in Appendix A.

Records

Current regulations are very specific concerning record keeping. The investigational process begins with shipment of the device, usually by some registered system, and an immediate inventory of the shipment for verification of quantity, model or lot numbers, and serial numbers. Records of use must be maintained and remaining stock verified and returned after the clinical trial. Extensive special data sheets are usually supplied. If prescribed variables are not measured during clinical use, justification must be provided. If a value is incorrectly notated during a case, the principal investigator (PI) must initial the corrected value as proof that the manufacturer did not alter the data, a highly punishable offense. Copies of all records, special forms, and the informed consent must be maintained by the PI in a secure place. The PI may be called upon by an FDA inspector to open the files. Further, the manufacturer will supply a "monitor" to witness conduct of a clinical case and aid in maintaining records. The original data sheets carrying the PI's signature must be submitted to the manufacturer on a weekly to monthly basis, depending upon frequency of use.

PLAN FOR A CLINICAL TRIAL

The manufacturer usually seeks out the surgical or perfusionist group and not *vice versa*. Generally, the technical representative will make a preliminary call to ascertain interest which will then be followed by a meeting with the senior management, engineering, and sales teams. The "novel" concepts and hypothetical advantages will be pressed with little note of limitations unless these are sought by the tentative Principal Investigator (PI). A checklist is provided in Table 19.1. At this point, the PI must make a decision to explore further the prospects of a trial or not to take part and use scarce resources. Helpful in this initial decision is the Principal Investigator's insistence on use of the device in the experimental laboratory to personally determine efficacy and safety variables. Sufficient number of experiments must be performed to learn of limitations and to train personnel who might be involved in the clinical trial. If the manufacturer is unwilling to support such experiments, this author strongly suggests that negotiations should go no further. Finally, prior to preparation of an application to The Institutional Review Board, the PI should ask for a copy of the letter from the Medical Devices Branch of the Food and Drug Administration stating that an investigational device exemption (IDE) has been awarded. This will prevent the PI from wasting large quantities of time in administrative tasks should the application for the IDE be rejected by the FDA.

Planning

The first step in the plan is to obtain *all possible in vitro and in vivo data* from the manufacturer. If data are absent which the Principal Investigator considers essential, no

Table 19.1
Disclosure Subjects

Intended applications
Unsuitable applications
Specific performance limitations
   Minimum, maximum, standard deviation, mean
   Operating volume, flow rate, capacities, mass transfer, microemboli generation, protein absorption,
     coagulation studies, blood trauma
Assembly and operating instructions
Anticipated results
Prevention and counteracting problems
Materials and form of blood contacting surfaces
Warnings, dangers, contraindications
Preventive maintenance
Methods of sterilization
Recognized risks and hazards

further action should be taken until the data are provided. Much of the data may be in engineering terms which relate poorly to clinical terms. A thorough explanation must be provided by the company to the PI. Once a complete understanding has been reached of the rationale for the choice of materials, the methods used and the environmental conditions employed for fabrication, the function of the device and the possible limitations, the associated hardware necessary for operation, the investigator is prepared to develop an application to the Institutional Review Board.

It is clear that the manufacturers of new devices desire a clinical trial of their products but do not wish to support comparative trials. This distinction must be very carefully understood by the PI. The FDA requires only a carefully documented clinical experience, not scientific comparisons to existing devices to determine "worse than," "equal to," or "better than" conclusions. It is these very comparisons that are important to the clinical practitioner. If the investigator is not to become a pseudoextension of the corporate arm or a legitimized testor only, then the investigator should propose a true concurrent trial of the device in comparison to the device presently in use. Criteria of use, end points, and variables measured must be identified. Manufacturers of class III devices usually will choose three to nine primary centers, each of which is to conduct 10 or more clinical trials. If the investigator is to

be honest with his patients, the institution, and himself, he is obligated to a simultaneous "control" group. The investigator will come under considerable pressure from the manufacturer to perform consecutive cases or complete the trial in 30 days. Such rushes into adventurism are to be avoided and will provide false impressions both good and bad.

The informed consent document must be prepared carefully in accordance with the FDA and the investigator's institution. Frequently, the manufacturer will supply a sample form. Do not use this form unless it is approved by the IRB and is reprinted carrying the name of the institution, approved date of the IRB, and the name, address, and telephone number of the Chair of the IRB. After approval of the application and informed consent by the IRB, the manufacturer should submit a copy of the informed consent to the FDA for review and approval.

IRB Application

Further documentation is required for the application. Six basic issues must be addressed in the IRB application.

SUBJECTS

Identify the sources of the potential subjects, derived materials or data. Describe the characteristics of the subject population, such as their anticipated number, age, sex, ethnic background, and state of health.

Identify the criteria for inclusion or exclusion. Explain the rationale for the use of special classes of subjects, such as fetuses, pregnant women, children, institutionalized mentally disabled, prisoners, or others, especially those whose ability to give voluntary informed consent may be in question. Also, indicate if the experimental subject is to be remunerated for participation and the amount of remuneration.

RECRUITMENT AND CONSENT

Describe the recruitment and consent procedures to be followed, including the circumstances under which consent will be solicited and obtained, who will seek it, the nature of information to be provided to prospective subjects, and the methods of documenting consent.

RISKS

Describe any potential risks—physical, psychological, social, legal, or other—and assess their likelihood and seriousness. Describe alternative methods, if any, that were considered and why they will not be used.

PROTECTION

Describe the procedures for protecting against or minimizing any potential risks and include an assessment of their likely effectiveness. Include a discussion of confidentiality safeguards, where relevant, and arrangement for providing medical treatment if needed.

BENEFITS

Describe and assess the potential benefits to be gained by the subjects, as well as the benefits that may accrue to society in general as a result of the planned work.

RISK/BENEFIT

Discuss the risks in relation to the anticipated benefits to the subjects and to society.

If the application is well written, the above are carefully addressed, the proposed informed consent is complete, and the manufacturer has supplied carefully controlled *in vitro* and *in vivo* data, the application probably will be approved. The author's experience suggests that one of the strongest elements in the application that results in

approval is the requirement of personal laboratory experience within the institution prior to clinical trial.

When a Human Studies Committee (IRB) is presented with a well-conceived investigational plan involving laboratory and clinical sectors with controls in each, and the same personnel are to be used for the initial laboratory and clinical phases, the experimental plan is generally approved.

After approval of the application, the following need to be obtained by the Principal Investigator and send to the sponsor: (1) a copy of the approval letter from the IRB and (2) a copy of the current certification of licensure by the City, State, and Federal governments for the clinical chemistry, blood bank, and any other certifiable laboratories to be used in the clinical investigation.

Lastly, a final contract must be negotiated to include Principal and Co-investigators' time and effort, special requirements placed upon perfusionists and other technologists, and the time of a clinical research coordinator or secretary used for data collation and chart revision. A special fund should be established for payment of special tests required or the more frequent testing of variables than routinely required in the specific institution. Some institutions place a 20 to 50% overhead charge on any such contracts.

Conduct of the Trial of an Investigational Device for Extracorporeal Circulation

Prior to initiation of the clinical portion of the trial, a careful examination of the device should be performed in the animal laboratory. The clinical perfusionists should conduct the experiments in conjunction with all investigators. The principal objectives are three: (1) determination of the physiologic limitations and safety aspects of the device; (2) familiarity with special requirements for use; and (3) comparison to a similar device then in clinical use. A minimum of five laboratory trials should be conducted. If no long-term data are available, the investigator should consider preparing chronic animals for later complete postmortem examination. Blood coagulation effects should be examined acutely as well as the organs of each animal for evidence of hypoperfusion or regional disturbances from microemboli. The device should be torn down and critically examined with specific attention to fibrin accumulation. The same variables that are to be measured in the clinical trial should be measured in the laboratory trial, and these data should be compared to data obtained with the current device. When the Principal Investigator is satisfied that the device is at least equal to the performance of an approved device and offers no undue limitations of operation or unsafe aspects, the clinical trial may proceed.

The patients for the clinical trial must be carefully interviewed and permitted to read the complete consent form. After the patient's consent is obtained by the Principal Investigator, indications of such should be entered into both the order sheets and progress note sections of the patient's chart. These notes should contain information concerning special tests that need to be obtained preoperatively and the name and telephone number of the PI. Completed special requisition forms containing special billing codes should be left in the chart. If the Principal Investigator has met with the housestaff and nursing staff prior to the initiation of the clinical trial, the process of accurate and complete data acquisition is greatly accelerated.

The perfusionist plays a central role in the clinical trial. The perfusionist is responsible for inventory and special perfusion records and frequently must supply extensive blood gas, pH, and coagulation data. Careful notes on unusual performance characteristics of the device should be placed either on the perfusion record or maintained in a special log. These data form the basis of the perfusionist's report to the manufacturer and the FDA.

Adverse reactions must be reported within 24 hours to both the manufacturer and the IRB. These incidences most frequently involve malfunction or less than expected performance. A complete investigation of the patient and the device is required in the case of malfunction. Consultants should be used liberally to determine whether significant harm has occurred to the patient because of device malfunction and the necessary therapeutic measures required for amelioration of the untoward effects. The device should be returned the same day to the manufacturer for complete inspection.

Barring any adverse effects during the clinical trial, data sheets, each carrying the Principal Investigator's signature, should be returned promptly to the sponsor upon completion. Interim reports on adverse function, performance data, and subjective opinions and ease of operation, etc., may be required. A complete final report covering all aspects of the trial is required. A flow diagram is provided in Figure 19.1.

Benefits *vs.* Liabilities

The underlying motive of most clinical investigations is the hope that a new device may truly improve the hazards and complications of extracorporeal circulation. The elimination of these thus improves "patient care."

A combination of new knowledge, techniques, and devices has made a significant impact on the morbidity and mortality that was associated with the use of cardiopulmonary bypass. The incidences of postoperative hemorrhage, "pump lung," renal failure, and mortality have decreased remarkably in the past 10 years (Fig. 19.2). Clearly, the driving force for investigators is to continue this progress.

Other benefits accrue to the investigative team. Frequent verbal and published reports aid in the upward academic climb for the young investigator. Individual and institutional prestige and peer respect gradually accelerate the investigative efforts and bring younger minds, enthusiasm, new ideas, and increased research funds. The last is significant because private sponsored research funding must be depended upon to a far greater extent in the future than in the past because of the decay of the federal funding in the academic milieu.

The disadvantages of device testing are many. The entire process as detailed in this essay requires the repeated evaluation, presence, and direction of an experienced car-

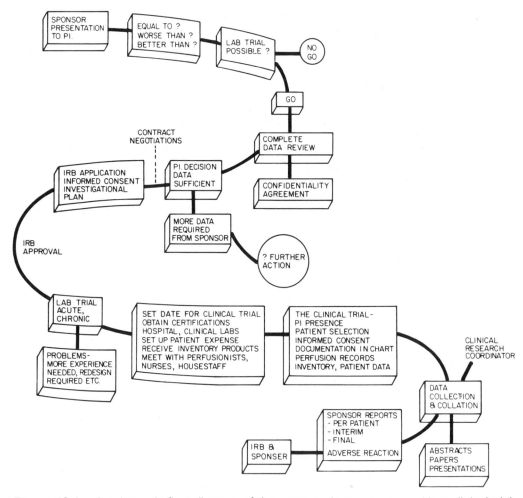

Figure 19.1. A schematic flow diagram of the steps and processes used in a clinical trial.

diothoracic surgeon for whom time is the most valuable commodity. The clinical trial of an investigational device is a highly time-consuming process, much of which is administrative in nature. This aspect, generally disliked by surgical practitioners, is the single greatest deterrent to participation.

A second strong disadvantage is the possibility that the investigator can be a testor rather than a researcher. It is all too easy to bend to the corporate desires of "try this"—instead of "study this." Manufacturers may spend years in the research and development process, fewer in "in-house" testing, and then expect a 30-day "quicky" so that they can rush the data to the FDA. Once a

device has been programmed for clinical trial, the pressure by top management and especially the marketing division to complete a clinical trial is tremendous. If the investigator is to attain stature and respect, he must investigate carefully and not unwittingly become a drone of the corporate sector.

Finally, the exacting requirements for documentation and careful records carry a potential punitive element from the FDA. Any of the data may be questioned in terms of veracity. The subsequent inquisition of patients, personnel, and the institutional review board brings grief to all involved. It is mandatory that the Principal Investigator,

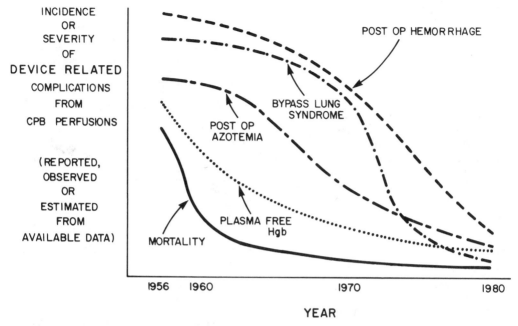

Figure 19.2. Incidence of complications of cardiopulmonary bypass perfusions over time. (Adapted from J. D. Mortensen: Final Report CPB Systems: A Study of Safety and Performance. Washington, DC, US Government Printing Office, 1981, pp. 88–89.)

who is usually a busy clinician, have a designated individual to gather, certify, and correlate the data to prevent oversight and incompleteness of documentation which produce inquiries.

SUMMARY

Historically, the trial of the new device was begun in the animal laboratory and graduated to the operating room. A review of the past problems of devices for cardiopulmonary bypass and past clinical trials suggests that a return to the methodology of the past using concurrent controls has strong merit.

The Medical Device Act of 1976 placed most new, disposable devices for cardiopulmonary bypass in Class III, which requires premarket approval. Extensive *in vitro* and animal testing must be conducted and the data approved by the FDA before a clinical trial may be initiated.

The application to the Institutional Review Board requires extensive documenta-

tion of efficacy and safety and a careful experimental protocol which contains controls. The application should carry the requirement for animal investigation before the clinical trial to familiarize the personnel and attempt to find significant limitations of the device that would preclude further investigation.

The conduct of the trial should have the Principal Investigator's personal attention, and the data from each case must be carefully reviewed and verified. The perfusionist performs a major role and is responsible for inventory, perfusion, and observational data and records. Adverse reactions must be reported within 24 hours to the Institutional Review Board and the manufacturer.

The benefits of participating in clinical investigation of new devices for cardiopulmonary bypass can be rewarding. Significant reductions in morbidity and mortality have occurred because of the persistence of surgeons and industry in seeking improvement in patient care. Carefully controlled clinical trials are difficult but demonstrate efficacy and safety and provide prestige to an investigative environment, which in turn attracts trainees and research monies, both essential to the continuation of a program of excellence.

The negative aspects are the time consumed in preparation of applications, documentation, and submission of periodic and final reports. The liabilities from untoward effects of new devices and the problems of verification are best prevented by active Principal Investigator supervision and the delegation of data collection and collation to a designated and highly trained clinical research coordinator.

References

1. Bigelow WG, Lindsay WK, Greenwood WF: Hypothermia; its possible role in cardiac surgery: An investigation of factors governing survival in dogs at low body temperatures. Ann Surg 132:849, 1950.
2. Hufnagel CA: Aortic phasic valvular prostheses. Bull Georgetown Univ Med Center 4:128, 1951.
3. Gibbon JH Jr: The maintenance of life during experimental occlusion of the pulmonary artery followed by survival. Surg Gynecol Obstet 69:602, 1939.
4. Gibbon JH Jr: Application of mechanical heart and lung apparatus to cardiac surgery. Minn Med 37:171, 1954.
5. Dennis C, Spreng DS Jr, Nelson GE, Karlson KE, Varco RL: Development of a pump oxygenator to replace the heart and lungs; an apparatus applicable to human patients: Application to 1 case. Ann Surg 134:709, 1951.
6. Clowes GHA Jr: Experimental procedure for entry into the left heart to expose the mitral valve. Ann Surg 34:957, 1951.
7. Bjork VO: An artificial heart or cardio-pulmonary machine. Lancet 2:491, 1948.
8. Cross FS, Berne RM, Herose Y, Jones RD, Kay EB: Evaluation of a rotating disc type reservoir oxygenatory. Proc Soc Exp Biol Med 93:210, 1956.
9. DeWall RA, Warden HE, Gott V, Read RG, Varco RL, Lillehei CW: Total body perfusion for open cardiotomy utilizing the bubble oxygenator; physiologic responses in man. J Thorac Surg 32:591, 1956.
10. Kolff WJ, Effler DB, Groves LK, Peereboom G, Morca PP: Disposable membrane oxygenator (heart-lung machine) and its use in experimental surgery. Cleve Clin Q 23:69, 1956.
11. Clowes GHA Jr, Neville WE, Sabga G, Shikota Y: The relationship of oxygen consumption, perfusion rate and temperature to the acidosis associated with cardiopulmonary circulatory bypass. Surgery 44:220, 1958.
12. Ross DN: Hypothermia −I, a technique of blood stream cooling. Guys Hosp Rep 103:97, 1954.
13. Brown IW Jr, Smith WW, Emmons WO: An efficient blood heat exchanger for use with extracorporeal circulation. Surgery 44:372, 1958.
14. Melrose DG, Drager B, Bental HH, Baker JBE: Elective cardiac arrest. Lancet 2:21, 1955.
15. Hufnagel CA, Conrad PW, Schanno J, Pifarre R. Profound cardiac hypothermia. Ann Surg 153:790, 1961.
16. DeBakey ME: Simple continuous-flow blood transfusion instrument. New Orleans Med Surg J 87:386, 1934.

WASHINGTON ▥ UNIVERSITY

SCHOOL OF MEDICINE

MEDICAL DEVICE

INFORMED CONSENT FOR PARTICIPATION IN RESEARCH ACTIVITIES

Participant _____ Date _____
Principal Investigator _____ Human Studies Committee
Title of Project _____ approval number _____

This form is to be typewritten, clearly defining all risks and benefits in layman's language and used only in connection with research approved by the Human Studies Committee.

1. I hereby authorize Dr. _____ and/or such assistants as may be selected by him for use now or at a later time, to perform upon me the following procedures in connection with a research project:
    (State nature of procedures, including any drugs to be administered. Identify those which are experimental.)

2. I understand the possible benefits to myself or others associated with the procedures described above. These are:
    (State the possible benefits.)

3. I understand certain hazards and discomforts might be associated with the procedures described above. These are:
    (Describe possible hazards and discomforts.)

4. I understand the following alternative procedures are available that would be advantageous to me:
    (Describe alternative procedures and advantages.)

(continued)

Appendix (Part 1)

5. I understand that the nature of the investigational device and the expected duration of its use is: *(State the nature of the device and expected duration of use.)*

6. I understand that the likely results should the procedures fail are: *(Describe results should the procedures fail.)*

7. I understand that the scope of the investigation, including the number of subjects involved, consists of: *(Describe the scope of the investigation including the number of subjects involved.)*

8. I understand that the device is being used for research purposes.

9. I understand that the investigator is willing to answer any inquiries I may have concerning the procedures herein described. All the inquiries I have at this time have been answered. I understand the confidentiality of my records will be maintained in accordance with applicable state and federal laws.

10. I understand that my participation is voluntary and that I may refuse to participate and/or withdraw my consent and discontinue participation in the project or activity at any time without penalty or loss of benefits to which I am otherwise entitled. I also understand that I may ask a question or state a concern to the University's Chairman of the Human Studies Committee, and that the investigator will, on request, tell me how to reach the Committee Chairman.

11. I understand that the University will provide immediate medical treatment in the event that a physical injury results because of my participation in this project. I also understand that no financial compensation will be paid to me by the University.

12. To the best of my knowledge I am not pregnant, and if I do become pregnant I will notify the principal investigator of my pregnancy.

13. I have received a copy of this informed consent which I have read and understand. I hereby consent to the performance of the above procedures upon me.

Parent or legal guardian's signature on particticipant's behalf if participant is less than 18 years of age or not legally competent. (Blood drawing only: Less than 17 years of age)

Participant's Signature

Auditor Witness' Signature, if witness is present

I have explained the above to the participant (or parent or guardian) on the date stated on this Informed Consent for Participation in Research Activities.

Investigator's Signature

Appendix (Part 2)

CHAPTER 20

MEDICAL/LEGAL IMPLICATIONS OF CARDIOPULMONARY BYPASS

JOSEPH M. SINDELL, L.L.B., J.D.

PROFESSIONAL NEGLIGENCE DEFINED

Malpractice has a bad connotation for the physician, and is poorly defined for the lay person. *Webster's New World Dictionary* defines malpractice as "injurious or unprofessional treatment or culpable neglect of a patient *by a physician or surgeon.*"[1] Medical professionals are not alone as subjects of malpractice claims. Attorneys have come under close scrutiny by their clients. In the past 10 years, attorneys' clients have filed thousands of claims, seeking redress for damages suffered.[2,3] Many claims have been pursued successfully to settlement against lawyers who were negligent in the manner in which they handled cases for their clients. This negligent handling includes failure to file a lawsuit or other papers within the proscribed time period; failure to prepare the case for trial; and other reasons that the courts have determined fall below the professional standards for lawyers.[4]

If physicians and lawyers seek comfort in the fact that other professionals are being held accountable for negligence, then they also should be most comfortable in knowing that judges, certified public accountants, architects, school teachers, and many other professional people are coming under review by those they serve.[5,6] However, when physicians or other medical care personnel become the subject of litigation, there is a protest heard throughout the land. This may be a cry of wolf by the insurance industry, not the medical profession. Some investigators of this phenomenon attribute this problem to the fact that the insurance industry's claimed losses are not from the payment of medical negligence claims, but from bad investments made with the premium dollars collected.[7] To its good credit, at least one medical negligence insurance carrier has reduced premiums to the policyholders, due to the reduction of claims made as a result of the institution of an effective prevention program for residents and interns.[4]

Currently, the professions of law and medicine are more understanding and considerate of each other's disciplines than in the past. Both professions are discovering that each has something to offer the other to benefit the patient and the client. The Code of Hammurabi laid down a harsh rule for the doctor committing medical negligence, "The physician who has performed a careless operation will have his hands cut off."[8,9] Maiming the doctor was not the method in ancient China where doctors were paid when their patients were kept well, not when they were sick. Believing that it was the doctor's job to prevent disease, Chinese doctors often paid the patient

219

if the patient lost his health. If a patient died, a special lantern was hung outside the doctor's house. At each death another lantern was added. Too many lanterns were certain to ensure a slow trade.[10]

Disparaging physician's abilities, physical maiming, and other antequated judicial measures have been replaced with trial by jury. In spite of the grumblings of doctors and lawyers, a body of law has emerged from professional negligence conflicts to keep the scales of justice more evenly balanced. True, the rule of law is not always black and white—it is often grey and murky. It is difficult for the law to keep abreast of new modalities in medicine that can go awry and cause damage, pain, and suffering. Should the patient who suffers the agony of a negligent act (sometimes referred to by coroners as "therapeutic misadventures") go without relief? Certainly, surgeons would prefer the present system of legal relief to the ancient Hammurabi Code.[11-13]

In this enlightened era, let us dwell upon the genesis of medical negligence claims, how to avoid becoming a defendant, and what to do when medical negligence occurs.

GENESIS OF PROFESSIONAL NEGLIGENCE CASES

Medical negligence can be understood best by examining the definition of general negligence. When the trial of a negligence case is concluded, the trial judge instructs the jury on the law to be applied to the particular case. The judge defines negligence to mean doing what a reasonable person would not do under the circumstances; or failing to do what a reasonable person would do under the circumstances. This standard definition is applied to all situations, whether the facts involve automobile collisions, defective products, poorly maintained physical premises, or hospital or medical care.[14] The jury members apply the law to the facts as they deliberate them to be and return their verdict.

Tables 20.1 and 20.2 delineate the leading causes of medical claims based on frequency and severity. This information is based upon

Table 20.1
Frequency of Medical Negligence Claims*

1. Improper diagnosis (not involving surgery)
2. Technical surgical error
3. Adverse reactions to drugs
4. Improper treatment of fractures
5. Improper anesthesiology
6. Injury to child in childbirth
7. Infection in surgical site
8. Foreign body left in patient during surgery
9. Injury from falls (during examination or while under doctor's care)
10. Employee error

* Reprinted with permission from J. W. Walker.[15]

Table 20.2
Severity of Medical Negligence Claims*

1. Injury to child in childbirth
2. Injury to mother in childbirth
3. Improper anesthesiology
4. Abandonment
5. Improper diagnosis (not involving surgery)
6. Employee error
7. Technical surgical errors
8. Adverse reactions to drugs
9. Infection in surgical site
10. Assault (generally, operating without permission)

* Reprinted with permission from J. W. Walker.[15]

a 17-year study performed in Florida from 1963 to 1980.[15]

During the 17-year period of the study, particularly within the last 2 years, the ranking of frequency and severity shifted. The study's conclusions came from a review of 10,324 closed claims upon which approximately $143 million had been paid to claimants. The study's author concluded, after ". . . review of the rank and file order of the claims, the most were preventable. In addition, there continues to be a need for obstetricians, anesthesiologists, pediatricians, and other medical specialists to document thoroughly those procedures in which they become involve."[15]

MISDIAGNOSES—A LEADING CAUSE OF LAWSUITS

A clinical study conducted by Gruver and Freis makes the need for diagnostic investigation clear. Based on 1,106 postmorten examinations of patients who had been hospitalized or treated immediately prior to death, their study sought to determine the number of cases in which the fatal disorder had been improperly diagnosed. Six percent of the cases had been clinically misdiagnosed. Sixty-four people had died of causes that were not suspected during treatment.[16] The lack of adequate medical history appeared to be the foremost reason for this appalling record. The doctors and hospital personnel had been unsuccessful in obtaining complete histories in 29 of the 64 misdiagnosed cases, and this directly resulted in misdiagnosis. A second major cause of faulty diagnosis was the tendency of some doctors to ignore certain symptoms. Gruver and Freis reported that the physician's history or progress report would clearly record an important sign or symptom, but this would be completely discarded in arriving at a diagnosis. Eighteen of the 64 patients (28%) had experienced signs or symptoms which were ignored. In carefully reviewing the charts of these 64 incorrectly diagnosed patients, it become apparent that in 10 cases (16%) there was a prejudiced viewpoint on the part of the doctor in charge. A more alert and critical approach coupled with thoroughness on the part of the responsible physician will decrease the incidence of diagnostic errors.

Misdiagnoses are natural concomitants of poor and inadequate history taking, a blasé attitude by the doctor toward the patient and his problems, and little or no communication with the patient. If communication is inadequate, it is most likely that informed consent has not been conveyed clearly, and an unhappy, uninformed patient may seek redress if there is an unsatisfactory result.

PROGRESS IN SCIENCE VERSUS DAMAGE TO PATIENTS

Negligence occurs in the everyday world, however infrequently, yet this is a difficult fact to accept. Physicians and surgeons complain that scientific progress must battle professional liability and multiple litigations. Some scientists feel that support for innovative work and experimental devices will be discouraged and progress handicapped by the worry of financial and reputational loss through litigation. Realistically, though, this has not been the case; cardiovascular procedures increase every year. The failure of a particular procedure may give rise to a new and better one. In some cases, the cutting edge to the improved approach is a medical negligence or product liability action.[17] Product liability cases have inspired manufacturers to exercise extreme caution in preparing, assembling, and marketing their products. Engineers have been prodded to consider safety in design and structure before releasing their ideas to manufacturers. They may not be motivated by fear of lawsuits, but if that fear is at least one motivating factor, the injury lawyer has performed a valuable service.

It is hoped that the combined accomplishments of law and medicine will result in a safer modern world.[14] When injury does occur, the task of determining cause and effect will be simplified as a result of greater understanding between doctor and lawyer.

MEDICAL NEGLIGENCE CRISIS— FACT OR FICTION?

A few years ago, the insurance industry succeeded in upsetting the medical profession and the public by precipitously increasing insurance premiums for professional liability coverage. There is some question as to whether there was a medical negligence crisis at all.[18] While doctors, lawyers, and others were busy complaining about the outrageous increases, the insurance lobbyists were prevailing upon legislators to pass laws eliminating jury trials; limiting the amount of recovery; reducing the time within which a medical negligence case had to be filed; creating numerous procedural steps before a complaint could be filed; setting up a list of medical and surgical procedures which eliminated the requirement that an informed consent be obtained from the patient; setting up mandatory arbitration before a claimant could file a medical negligence action in court; and other changes in the law.[19] The insurance companies wanted the best of both worlds—higher premiums and fewer claims!

Some states have declared their Medical Negligence Reform Acts to be partially or entirely unconstitutional. Denying a litigant a jury trial and limiting the amount of recovery have been declared to be in violation of the U.S. Constitution.[20] Surgical progress cannot be made by weakening or eliminating the rights of patients who resort to the courts to have their grievances adjudicated.[7] Adherence to the rule of law will protect the rights of the public and will not infringe upon or restrict the efforts of the careful, skilled cardiovascular surgeon.

GOING "BARE"—A FINANCIALLY UNHEALTHY HABIT

Suing a surgeon for professional negligence is a blow to his ego because his professional skills and reputation have been attacked. Few surgeons would operate a motor vehicle without automobile insurance, why then are some physicians practicing medicine without professional liability coverage? The high cost of insurance premiums is usually the cause. I contend that this excuse is irrelevant. The physician is playing Russian roulette with his financial security. It is too late to buy protection after the hammer strikes the bullet. The cost of defense and the payment of a verdict makes it too financially unhealthy to go "bare."

In most jurisdictions, the law prohibits informing the jury about the amount or lack of insurance coverage. It is a well-established principle that jurors consider the defendant who is a professional capable of paying the plaintiff or carrying insurance sufficient to pay the successful plaintiff. The conditions of an insurance policy with a deductible feature delineate that the insurance carrier agrees to defend and pay any verdict up to the policy limits, less the deductible. The premiums on these tailored policies are reduced in proportion to the exposure to negligence suits. Carelessness has nothing to do with intelligence, skill, or experience. *Negligence occurs in spite of these fine qualities, and must be insured against.*

SEEDS OF MEDICAL NEGLIGENCE CLAIMS

The seeds of many medical negligence cases are planted at the time of the first patient/surgeon meeting. The patient is nervous and apprehensive. The surgeon may be insensitive to the patient's personal concern about his chances of life or death. The patient sees the surgeon as his savior or his executioner, with no gradations of character in-between; the surgeon is the last stop, the final hope. In most cases, the patient has been examined by an internist and a cardiologist and undergone many tests before being seen by a cardiovascular surgeon. Pronouncements about open heart bypass surgery are sufficient to strike fear into the heart of the already stressed patient.

INFORMED CONSENT—INFORMED CHOICES

Effective communication is the key to informed choice and informed consent.[11] It is not enough that the surgeon knows the condition and methodology he plans to use in an effort to relieve the patient's symptoms. He must communicate his recommendations to the patient so the patient knows the facts and is sufficiently informed to make a knowledgable choice. I strongly recommend that the surgeon take the time to explain the benefits, risks, and the percentage of possibility of their occurrence to each patient diagnosed as needing the surgical procedure. The conversation should be in the presence of the patient, spouse, and members of the patient's family. It will take additional time to explain these issues, but it will benefit the surgeon later, when asked upon the witness stand, "Doctor, how much time did you spend with the patient and his wife when you first saw them? Did you explain the known risks and hazards of the surgical procedure to them? Did you give the patient an opportunity to ask questions? Did you explain alternative remedies that might be explored to relieve the patient's symptoms?"

The fact that the surgeon cannot predict given results in a particular surgical procedure is understandable. But failure to inform the patient of the unpredictable nature of the surgery is unforgivable and wrong—the patient has been deprived of his freedom of choice for or against the operation. The surgeon must avoid making promises of perfect results in an effort to encourage the patient to undergo the procedure.[7, 22-24] It is a terrible temptation for the surgeon to tell of operative successes and omit the failures. This is smug subjectivity; creativity is stifled and progress delayed if this practice becomes dominant in a profession. Without candid scrutiny, experience deteriorates into an exercise of repetitive errors. Neither the patient nor the physician benefits.[25, 26]

Time after time, lawyers listen to a litany of complaints from an unhappy patient who has become a raging client. Each complaint alone may have little legal efficacy, but compile the complaints, secure expert testimony that an informed consent fell below the standard of care, and you might have the genesis of a medical negligence case. Most patients would never seek legal advice if they had been properly and fully informed. The patient who is fully informed is able to make an intelligent choice. The surgeon can give the medical data, present the choices, put in his recommendations, and step out of the picture.[7] If the surgeon takes the time to do so, he will reduce the risk of medical negligence charges.

THE CAPTAIN OF THE SHIP DOCTRINE

The surgeon is the captain of the ship. Since the captain gives the orders, then the sailors or members of the team who execute those orders are an extension of the captain. The captain/surgeon remains responsible for the negligent acts of his sailors/team members—*so long as the surgeon maintains control over the activities of the team member*, thus maintaining a master-servant relationship.

In each case of employee negligence that results in a suit against a surgeon as the responsible party, the most important issue is whether or not the surgeon had *sufficient*

control over the employee to hold the surgeon responsible. Specifically, the courts will hold an operating surgeon liable for the acts of hospital employees assisting in the operation where he has assumed control of the operating room.[27] Alternately, when the doctor orders care and treatment for the patient, but has no control over which particular hospital employee carries out his order, there is no basis for finding a master-servant relationship through which the doctor could be held vicariously liable for acts of those not directly under his supervision.[28] Therefore, it is the agency theory which delineates the supervisor's responsibility for the negligent acts of subordinate personnel, when their actions are under the supervisor's control.

AVOIDING PROFESSIONAL NEGLIGENCE SUITS

Medical negligence actions can be reduced by following a few simple rules:
1. *Establish Good Physician-Patient Rapport.* Patients often complain about the lack of personal attention by the physician. It is not necessary to fawn over the patient, but compassion and understanding should be evidenced by the doctor and the staff.
2. *Diagnostic Tests.* Set aside the fear of being charged with practicing defensive medicine. Perform or order whatever tests you deem necessary and appropriate in arriving at a diagnosis.
3. *Other Consultations.* Encourage the doubting and worried patient to obtain second or third opinions. If the consulting opinion confirms the diagnosis, the original diagnosis is strengthened, and the patient feels more secure in following your advice. If the consultation is not in accord with your diagnosis, a reevaluation may be in order.
4. *Continuing Medical Education.* Medical techniques undergo rapid changes. To be current in your specialty, attend local, state, and national meetings. Attend peer review conferences. Teaching is always a great learning experi-

Table 20.3
Money Expended at Various Stages of Litigation

Number of Cases	Posture of Case	Dollars
4500	Settled without a lawsuit	$20,000,000
4050	Settled after suit filed	60,000,000
200	Jury verdicts	20,000,000
1250	Dropped or dismissed	
Total: 10,000	Total dollars paid on 10,000 claims	$100,000,000

ence. Standards of care are no longer limited to the standards in the community where the surgeon practices. The courts have adopted the national standards formulated by the specialty boards and are permitting cross-country testimony on a standard of care regardless of the locale of the suit.

5. *Medical Records.* Comprehensive, accurate, and objective medical records should be maintained, both in the office and at the hospital. A common fault is that of signing dictated medical records without reading them. Any errors should be corrected before or at

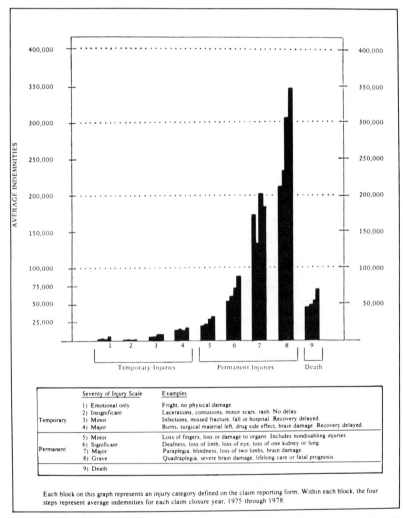

	Severity of Injury Scale	Examples
Temporary	1) Emotional only	Fright, no physical damage.
	2) Insignificant	Lacerations, contusions, minor scars, rash. No delay.
	3) Minor	Infections, missed fracture, fall in hospital. Recovery delayed.
	4) Major	Burns, surgical material left, drug side effect, brain damage. Recovery delayed.
Permanent	5) Minor	Loss of fingers, loss or damage to organs. Includes nondisabling injuries.
	6) Significant	Deafness, loss of limb, loss of eye, loss of one kidney or lung.
	7) Major	Paraplegia, blindness, loss of two limbs, brain damage.
	8) Grave	Quadraplegia, severe brain damage, lifelong care or fatal prognosis.
	9) Death	

Each block on this graph represents an injury category defined on the claim reporting form. Within each block, the four steps represent average indemnities for each claim closure year, 1975 through 1978.

Figure 20.1. Annual average indemnity by severity of injury. (Reproduced with permission from M. Sowka.[32] Copyright 1982, Connecticut Medicine.)

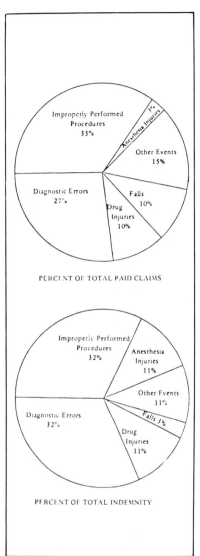

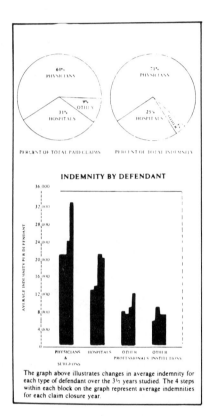

Figure 20.2. (*Left*) Distribution of claims by defendant for all years. (*Right*) Distribution of claims for all years by allegation. (Reproduced with permission from M. Sowka.[32] Copyright 1982, Connecticut Medicine.)

the time of signing. Any effort to change the medical record after a malpractice suit has been instituted is tempting, but unethical and usually disastrous.[30]

6. *Informed Consent.* The patient's right to know is a paramount consideration in avoiding professional negligence. The courts hold that the jury must determine if a surgeon obtained informed consent from the patient.[30]

THE LAWSUIT, THE VERDICT, AND THE INSURANCE COMPANIES

Coronary artery surgery was endorsed by the National Institutes of Health in December, 1980. The annual rate of coronary artery surgical procedures has risen from 50,000 in 1975 to 110,000 in 1980. Some authorities believe that the number of procedures could grow to 200,000 per year.[30] Hypothetically, let us assume that 5% of the

	Most Frequently Reported Procedures	Incidents Total	Paid	Average Indemnity	Average Severity of Injury
1	Treatment with Drugs	5687	2786	36,827	5.0
2	Physical Examination	3386	1397	43,616	5.7
3.	Emergency Room Examinations	2394	1002	32,333	5.5
4.	Other X-Ray Procedures	2062	971	19,703	4.2
5	Incision, Excision and Suture of Skin, Including Skin Grafts	2040	964	13,127	3.7
6	Hysterectomy, Abdominal (Total and Subtotal) and Vaginal	2055	960	36,036	4.7
7	Closed and Open Reductions of Fractures and Dislocations With or Without Fixation Device, Excluding Facial Fractures	2166	828	37,773	4.5
8	Operations on Teeth and Supporting Structures	1480	794	7,555	3.3
9	Inhalation and Intravenous Anesthesia Procedures	1281	716	100,573	5.7
10	Sterilizations—Male and Female	1381	647	14,954	3.1
11	Dilation and Currettage and Aspiration Currettage of Uterus	1168	564	26,870	4.0
12	All Types of Monitoring	1030	478	101,347	6.9
13	Excision of Intervertebral Disc	929	400	72,921	5.4
14	Obstetrical Procedures Excluding Caesarean Sections	866	380	69,755	4.9
15	Physical Therapy and Rehabilitation	717	358	11,940	3.7
16	Operations on the Biliary Tract Including Exploratory Laparotomy	690	347	61,716	5.0
17	Incision, Excision of Abdominal Wall and Peritoneum Including Exploratory Laparotomy	708	300	38,889	5.2
18	All types of Herniorrhaphy	671	257	33,003	4.8
19	Appendectomy	605	244	54,379	5.4
20	All types of Caesarean Sections	525	236	76,343	5.8
21	Operations on Tonsils and Adenoids	338	190	35,102	5.1
22	Insertion of Intra-uterine Device	444	177	21,191	3.6

Figure 20.3. Most frequently reported procedures. (Reproduced with permission from M. Sowka.[32] Copyright 1982, Connecticut Medicine.)

200,000 patients will seek legal assistance, claiming their procedure was negligently performed, causing injury and damage or death. At least 10% of the 10,000 will be advised that they do not have a substantial case for one or more of the following reasons: (1) the surgeon did not fall below the accepted standard of care in the performance of the surgical procedure; (2) the surgeon is not an insurer, guaranteeing a 100% recovery from all symptoms; (3) the surgeon may have been negligent, but there was no damage sustained as the direct and proximate result of the surgery; (4) the surgeon made a mistake of judgment, but was not negligent; (5) the surgeon may have been negligent, but the damages are too minimal to justify the cost of litigation; (6) there is a valid case, but the attorney is unable to obtain expert testimony that the surgeon was negligent. For these reasons, 9,000 cases remain.

Of the 9,000, 50% will probably be settled without the necessity of bringing a lawsuit. The balance of 4,500 cases will be filed in court; approximately 90% of all lawsuits are settled or dismissed prior to reaching trial. Of the approximately 450 cases that will be tried to jury verdict, at least 50% or more will result in a verdict for the physician. The plaintiff's verdicts in each of the remaining 225 cases will range from $1,000 to $4,000,000. The insurance carrier will probably appeal 50 to 75 cases, and the appellate courts may reverse 20 to 30 cases.

The tally for approximately 200 cases could total nearly $20 million. Table 20.3 describes the money expended at the various steps of litigation.

The total dollars paid on 10,000 claims represents 3% of the projected cost of the 200,000 per year coronary artery surgical procedures predicted in 1980.[31] Three percent of this $3 billion cardiovascular surgical bill is not a figure which should cause the professional negligence insurance underwriters to become overly concerned, nor is it likely that they will increase premiums out of proportion to the risks involved. The percentage of cases won by physicians has increased from 80% in 1975 to 90% in 1978.[31]

Figure 20.1 illustrates the annual average indemnity paid by severity of injury. Figure 20.2 shows the percentage of claims paid on behalf of the medical provider. Figure 20.3 shows the distribution of most frequently reported procedures.[32]

CONCLUSION

The rule of law is the most effective method for resolving medical negligence claims. The public is demanding and receiving damages for the negligent acts of physicians. Legislative efforts to change the rules of law for the benefit of one class of people (physicians) to the harm of another class (patients) have been rejected by reviewing courts as being in violation of the constitutional right to a trial by jury, the equal protection clause, and the due process of law provisions. The most common causes of negligence cases are lack of informed consent and the negligent acts of an employee/team member acting under the control of a surgeon.

Product liability and medical negligence claims have not impaired the advancement of cardiovascular surgical techniques. In some instances, the lawsuit has emphasized the faulty product or technique, opening the door to improvement and correction of the product or procedure. Statistics indicate that cardiovascular surgical procedures will cost the public $3 billion soon. It is projected that professional liability claims (for cardiovascular procedures only) will be approximately 3% of this bill. Claims can be reduced in number if surgeons keep abreast of the changes in medical and surgical techniques, fully inform their patients, keep accurate records, encourage consultations, and obtain all necessary diagnostic tests. Laws should not be passed to restrict the right to bring a medical negligence suit, rather they should be aimed at the improvement of surgical technique and the delivery of excellent medical care.

References

1. *Webster's New World Dictionary*, Second College Edition. New York, William Collins Publishers Inc., 1980.
2. Fleischman AC: Legal malpractice forum, inadequate disclosures to client: Malpractice pitfall. Colorado Lawyer Rev 9:2378, 1980.
3. Mauther W: Malpractice comes to divorce court. J Fam Law 19:263–294, 1981.
4. White E: Epidemic of suits hits lawyers. Mich Med 5:246–247, 1981.
5. His honor buys a little protection. In Los Angeles Times, pp. 1–2, 7, Jan. 25, 1982.
6. Scott P: An overview of accountants' liability. Forum 15:579–194, 1980.
7. Spence J, Roth J: Closing the courthouse door: Florida's spurious claims statute. Stetson Law Rev 10:397–426, 1981.
8. Seagle W: *Men of Law.* New York, MacMillan, 1947.
9. Wecht C: Informed consent. Forensic Sci 12, 1978.
10. Louis D: *Fascinating Facts.* New York, Ridge Press/Crown, 1977.
11. Larrabee E: *The Benevolent and Necessary Institution.* New York, Doubleday, 1977.
12. Wallechinsky D: America's first riot—the doctor's mob of 1788. In *The People's Almanac*, 1975.
13. Hostage standoff ends; police kill distraught man. In Los Angeles Times, Part I, p. 14, Feb. 6, 1982.

14. Masington R: Legal aspects of dermapathology. Am J Dermatol 2:37–38, 1980.

15. Walker JW: Medical malpractice claims, causes and prevention. J Fla Med Assoc 69:167, 1982.

16. Curran W: *Law and Medicine*, 1980.

17. Cooley D: Perspectives in cardiac surgery with personal reflections. Surg Clin North Am 58:895, 1978.

18. Sepler: Professional malpractice litigation crisis: Danger or distortion? Forum 15:493, 1980.

19. Rachlin: The effect of the Texas Medical Liability and Insurance Improvement Act on the Texas standard for medical disclosure. Houston Law Rev 17:615–641, 1980.

20. Aldano *v*. Holub, Southern Reporter, Second Series 381:231–1980.

21. Halberstam M: *A Coronary Event*. Philadelphia, J.B. Lippincott, 1976.

22. Van Geertrayden H: Ann Surg 574–609, 1956.

23. Salgo *v*. Leland Stanford Board of Trustees, Pacific Reporter, Second Series 317, 1957.

24. Beebe H: *Complications in Vascular Surgery*. Philadelphia, J.B. Lippincott, 1973.

25. Letter to the editor: Retaliatory actions in malpractice. N Engl J Med 30:1307–1308, 1981.

26. Stoffer A: Iatrogenic is not a dirty word. Chest 58, 1970.

27. Kitto *v*. Gilbert, Pacific Reporter, Second Series 570:544, 1977.

28. Adams *v*. Leidbolt, Pacific Reporter, Second Series 579:618, 1978.

30. Davidson A, Coleman A: Helpful hints to lessen risk of a malpractice suit. J Natl Med Assoc 73:218–282, 1981.

31. Cohn V: Coronary artery surgery endorsed by NIH panel. Washington Post, Dec. 6, 1980.

32. Sowka M: The medical malpractice closed claims study. Conn Med 45:91–97, 1981.

CHAPTER 21

ULTRAFILTRATION FOR CONCENTRATION AND SALVAGE OF PUMP BLOOD

ROY L. NELSON, M.D.
YEHUDA TAMARI, M.S.
ANTHONY J. TORTOLANI, M.D.
MICHAEL H. HALL, M.D.
CARMINE G. MOCCIO, M.D.

Concentration of the dilute blood in the cardiopulmonary bypass circuit by plasma water removal is a new application of ultrafiltration. We will present a brief history of ultrafiltration, its principles of operation and its advantages. In addition, we will review the clinical data gathered at North Shore University Hospital on ultrafiltration in conjunction with cardiopulmonary bypass (CPB).

DEVELOPMENT AND EARLY USES OF ULTRAFILTRATION

Ultrafiltration dates back to 1929 when Brull[1] constructed the first ultrafilter from filter paper and collodian and connected it in-line to the internal carotid artery of a dog. In 1952, Lunderquist et al.[2] reported on the use of ultrafiltration in the treatment of edema. More extensive clinical use was described by Kobayashi and colleagues[3] in 1972. Since then ultrafiltration has been widely used for the removal of excess of plasma water, in conjunction with renal dialysis, or as an alternative to it.[4-6] The first reported use of ultrafiltration to concentrate the blood remaining in the heart-lung machine was by Romagnoli and associates[7] in 1976. In that study, 700 cc of blood with a mean hematocrit of 21% was ultrafiltered for 11 minutes, producing a final hematocrit of 31%. In 1979, a group headed by Darup[8] included an ultrafiltration device in the CPB circuit in 10 patients with reduced renal function. Ultrafiltration removed 3.4 liters of plasma water during 4 hours of CPB, maintaining the plasma proteins at 5.4 gm%. In 1981, Hopeck and colleagues[9] used ultrafiltration during CPB on 35 patients. They were able to reduce the fall in hematocrit as well as decrease positive fluid balance associated with CPB when compared to patients who did not undergo ultrafiltration.

INDICATIONS FOR THE USE OF ULTRAFILTRATION

Concentration of blood components during cardiopulmonary bypass requires balancing diuresis against fluid administration. Insufficient natural diuresis can be augmented by diuretics. However, forced diuresis still may be insufficient, especially when crystalloid cardioplegia is employed or in the presence of renal insufficiency. When plasma water is extracted by the kidneys, its rate of removal is not easily controlled, and the obligatory potassium loss may potentiate or exacerbate cardiac rhythm disturbances. The rate of water removal is readily controlled when the extraction is done by ultrafiltration.

Transfusion of dilute residual pump blood may cause circulatory overload in patients with normovolemic anemia. For these patients, the pump blood should be concentrated prior to transfusion. Presently, the most popular method to concentrate blood during open heart surgery is centrifugation.[10] The method yields concentrated washed red blood cells. It has the following drawbacks:

1. Discards noncellular blood components
2. Removes platelets
3. Is cumbersome and bulky
4. Requires a large pump prime volume for use during CPB

In contrast, a small, disposable ultrafilter may be used on or off bypass. It controls the rate and quantity of plasma water removed. The device increases the concentration of red blood cells as well as those elements discarded in the centrifugation process.

PRINCIPLES AND CONCEPTS OF ULTRAFILTRATION

In ultrafiltration, as blood flows along a porous membrane, plasma water, electrolytes, and small molecules driven by a hydrostatic pressure difference, are separated from blood by passage through the membrane. The difference is achieved by positive pressure on the blood side and/or negative pressure on the nonblood (dialysate or ultrafiltrate compartment) side of the membrane. The sum of the two pressures is the transmembrane pressure (TMP). The formula for transmembrane pressure is as follows:

$$TMP = \frac{Pi + Po}{2} + Pu$$

Pi is the inlet pressure; Po is the outlet pressure, and Pu is the negative pressure in the ultrafiltrate compartment.[11] This is obtained by applying a partial vacuum and is the primary force for ultrafiltration. The negative pressure is between -200 and -700 torr. The inlet and outlet pressures tend to be low, less than 100 torr, and are due to resistances across the ultrafilter. To increase the positive pressure in the blood compartment (Po) a screw clamp can be used on the outlet tubing.

Ultrafiltration devices can be characterized by their ultrafiltration coefficient (K_{uf}), which is the ultrafiltration rate divided by the TMP.

$$K_{uf} = \frac{\text{ultrafiltration rate}}{\text{TMP}} \quad (\text{ml/hr/mm Hg})$$

The ultrafiltration rate (Qv) is related to the ultrafiltration coefficient of the device (K_{uf}), the protein oncotic pressure of the blood ($\prod p$) and TMP so that

$$Qv = K_{uf} (TMP - \prod p).$$

The factors that determine the ultrafiltration rate are as follows:

1. Transmembrane pressure
2. Blood flow rate
3. Depth of pores (membrane thickness)
4. Number of pores (membrane surface area)
5. Diameter of pores (membrane composition)

The ultrafiltration rate increases linearly at low transmembrane pressures, becomes curvilinear as pressure increases, and finally plateaus. Further increases in TMP do not produce any increase in the ultrafiltration rate (Fig. 21.1). For different ultrafiltration membranes and materials, the values on the ordinate and on the abscissa will be different, although the shapes of the curves are similar. The plateau is due to an accumulation of proteins adjacent to the membrane surface.[12] Higher flow rates increase the shear rate which moves the protein away from the membrane surface towards the center of blood flow.[13, 14] Consequently, increase in blood flow rate raises the ultrafiltration rate by decreasing protein accumu-

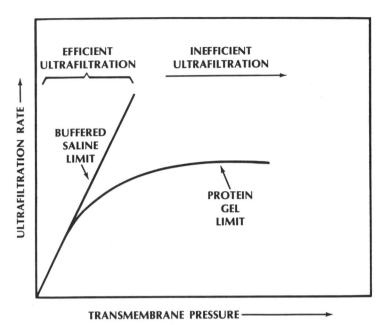

Figure 21.1. Relationship between ultrafiltration and transmembrane pressure. At low transmembrane pressure the relationship between ultrafiltration rate and transmembrane pressure is linear for both blood and crystalloid solutions. However, for blood, with increasing transmembrane pressure, the relationship becomes curvalinear and then reaches a plateau. The plateau is due to the formation of a protein-gel layer at the membrane interface that impedes ultrafiltration. Efficient ultrafiltration takes place on the linear aspect of the curve. Note that when the ultrafiltration rate is determined using a nonprotein-containing solution, the relationship between ultrafiltration and transmembrane pressure remains linear. The *in vitro* determinations of ultrafiltration rate using crystalloid solutions do not reflect clinical performance but may be used to compare devices.

lation at the membrane surface. The ultrafiltration rate of nonprotein solution is linear at all TMP and, therefore, does not reflect blood ultrafiltration. However, it is useful for approximate comparisons between membranes or devices. Proteins inhibit ultrafiltration by: (1) increasing the distance between the blood and the membrane (protein boundary layer); (2) reducing the TMP (see formula).

In the process of ultrafiltration, all molecules smaller than the smallest pores in the membrane are present in equal concentrations on both sides of the membrane. Molecules larger than the largest pores cannot cross the membrane at all, and their concentration on the blood side increases in proportion to the water removed[15] (Fig. 21.2). The removal of molecules larger than the

smallest pores and smaller than the largest pores depends upon the sieving coefficient of the membrane for that molecule. This coefficient is the ratio of the concentration of the substance in the ultrafiltrate to that of the blood. It is a measure of membrane porosity. A molecule with a coefficient of 1 is found in equal concentrations on both sides of the membrane, while a molecule with a coefficient of 0 cannot cross the membrane at all and is found only on the blood side. For removal of plasma water from the cardiopulmonary bypass circuit during and after operation, a membrane that has a low sieving coefficient for small molecules will maintain increasing concentrations of both small and large molecules on the blood side of the membrane.[16] For example, if the membrane has a sieving

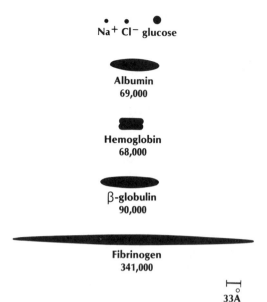

Figure 21.2. Plasma component size. Ultrafiltration membranes generally have a pore size of 25 to 35 Å. Electrolytes such as sodium and chloride and small molecules such as glucose can pass freely while larger molecules, as illustrated by albumin, hemoglobin, and fibrinogen will be trapped on the blood side of the ultrafiltration membrane. Their concentration will increase in direct proportion to the water removed.

coefficient near 0 for albumin, then albumin and all molecules larger than albumin will be conserved, and ultrafiltration will increase their concentration.

Finally, ultrafiltration depends on the membrane characteristics: thickness, number, and diameter of the pores (Fig. 21.3).

CHOICE OF ULTRAFILTERS

For ultrafiltration, porous membranes can be formed into sheets used to construct parallel plate types of ultrafilters or into hollow fibers for capillary type ultrafilters (Fig. 21.4). The sheets are deformable and need a support structure for rigidity. Consequently, the parallel plate devices tend to be slightly larger than the hollow fiber devices. The latter need no external support.[17] A comparison of all the hollow fiber dialyzers currently marketed, including ultrafiltration rates, has been placed in table form

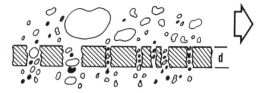

EXTRACTION RATE = • Number and Size of Pores
• Depth of Pores
• Transmembrane Pressures
• Shear Rate

Figure 21.3. Illustrated is a cross-section of a semipermeable ultrafiltration membrane. The ultrafiltration rate is related to the number, diameter, and the depth of the pores as well as the transmembrane pressure. In addition, the blood flow rate determines the shear rate. Increasing the shear rate augments ultrafiltration.

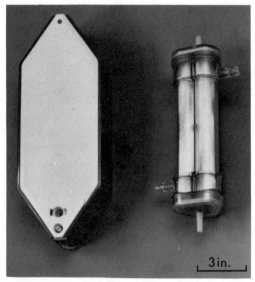

Figure 21.4. Types of ultrafiltration devices. On the *left* is an example of a parallel plate and on the *right* a hollow fiber ultrafiltration device. The former are, in general, somewhat larger and have a slightly higher priming volume. The hollow fiber devices are smaller and have a lower priming volume (see Appendices A and B).

by Sigdell[18, 19] (Appendix A). Henderson et al.[20] believes that the hollow fiber design may prove to have a more stable blood flow path, and this will maintain higher shear rates to maximize ultrafiltration. However, it would appear that for ultrafiltration, both parallel plate and hollow fiber devices can serve equally well.

For ultrafiltration in conjunction with cardiopulmonary bypass, Harvey markets a hollow fiber device manufactured by Cordis Dow made of regenerated cellulose and marketed under the name of Hemoconcentrator. Bentley is investigating a Gambro parallel plate device called the Continuous Blood Processor (CBP). Data on the use of these devices in conjunction with cardiopulmonary bypass is limited.

ULTRAFILTRATION AND CARDIOPULMONARY BYPASS

Ultrafiltration depends on blood flow and transmembrane pressure, both of which may be precisely controlled. However, there is a maximum transmembrane pressure that should not be exceeded. Using the Tri Ex-3 artificial kidney or the Hemoconcentrator the maximum transmembrane pressure is 750 torr and for the Continuous Blood Processor, it is 500 torr. The recommended blood flow rates are between 200 and 300 cc/min.

Blood for the ultrafiltration device can be taken either from the venous or arterial sources within the cardiopulmonary bypass circuit (Fig. 21.5). A venous source is not recommended for the following reasons: (1) There may be air bubbles in venous blood which can plug some of the fibers of the hollow fiber devices. (2) Off bypass, in the absence of venous return, withdrawal would be difficult.

Arterial blood from the coronary perfusion port or the arterial tubing (between the oxygenator and the pump head) provides bubble-free blood on or off bypass but does require an additional pump head. Blood

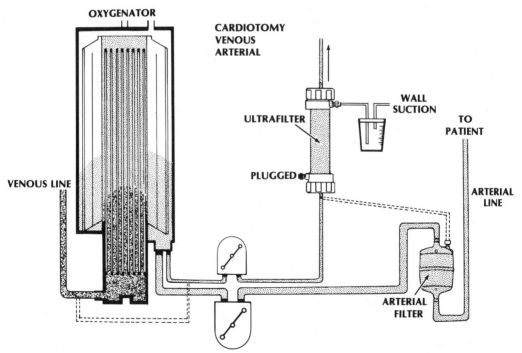

Figure 21.5. Cardiopulmonary bypass circuits including ultrafilters. Illustrated are the possible sources of blood for the ultrafilter. Blood can be taken from the coronary perfusion port and passed through the ultrafilter. Alternative sources of blood include, on the *left*, the venous line, and on the *right*, the arterial filter. Potential return sites include the cardiotomy reservoir, venous line, and arterial line. When a membrane oxygenator is used blood should be taken from the venous reservoir.

taken from the arterial line between the pump head and the arterial filter or from the arterial filter itself requires arterial blood flow and is only applicable on bypass. In addition, when the arterial filter is used as a source, the blood flow rate through the device is variable. A low blood flow rate combined with a high negative pressure could clot the ultrafilter. Also, when blood is pumped through the ultrafilter using the arterial pump head, there will be large variations in pressure and blood flow and consequently in the ultrafiltration rate.

Return of blood to the arterial side of the circuit carries the risk of air emboli, while return to the priming port of the oxygenator may create bubbles or foam. In addition, blood returned to this port may channel and not mix. This can cause recirculation and result in increased hemolysis. Although concentrated blood can be returned to the venous line, the readily available connectors in the cardiotomy reservoir make this the logical blood return site. When the reservoir is positioned above the ultrafiltration device, the outflow resistance increases. This, in turn, increases transmembrane pressure, and therefore, ultrafiltration rate.

We recommend that blood be taken from the coronary perfusion port and returned to the cardiotomy reservoir (Fig. 21.6), with a clamp between the pump and the device to avoid backflow when the pump is off.[21]

CLINICAL EXPERIENCE WITH ULTRAFILTRATION PROCEDURE

In the first 150 cases, we monitored both inlet and outlet pressures, as well as the negative pressure applied to the ultrafiltrate compartment. With the Tri Ex-3 and wall suction, we had a negative pressure in the ultrafiltrate compartment of −400 torr. The inlet pressure was 40 torr; the outlet pressure was 20 torr; and the transmembrane pressure 430 torr. We employed an arterial blood line manufactured for dialysis which contained drip chambers and pressure monitoring lines to measure the inlet and outlet pressures. The anaeroid manometers employed were protected by small in-line filters. When indicated, ultrafiltration was employed during bypass. After the operation,

the dilute blood was circulated in a closed loop mode and measurements performed before and after plasma water removal. The blood was maintained heparinized; samples of arterial blood were taken and flow established through the ultrafilter. The crystalloid priming solution was discarded, and the blood outlet was connected to the oxygenator. Finally, the vacuum source was connected to the ultrafiltrate outlet port. Flow rate through the device was 250 to 300 cc/min, and the ultrafiltration rate was 33 cc/min. When the oxygenator content was reduced 50%, the vacuum was discontinued and then the blood flow was stopped. The blood outlet from the ultrafilter was connected to a transfusion bag. Blood was pumped into the bag with the device inverted and the blood outlet facing down to completely empty the ultrafilter. The transfusion bag was weighed, thoroughly mixed, and another set of samples obtained.

A pretransfusion blood sample was obtained 30 minutes after the patients arrived in the Surgical Intensive Care Unit. Transfusion was completed within 60 minutes; 30 minutes later additional samples were obtained. Protamine was given to neutralize the heparin. Creatinine clearance (12 hour) was determined preoperatively and again on the 1st postoperative day. Sixty matched control patients were employed for evaluation of blood utilization.

Data was analyzed by Student's paired t-test using the Statistical Package for the Social Sciences (SPSS, Ed. 2, New York, McGraw Hill) and a Burroughs 6800 Computer.

One hundred patients were studied after bypass to define the effects of ultrafiltration on the blood without including the patient as a variable. Results are summarized in Table 21.1. Ultrafiltration concentrated the red blood cells, plasma proteins, and platelets. This was reflected in the 85% increase in hemoglobin, 91% increase in albumin, and 102% increase in fibrinogen (a measure of clotting factor concentration). The platelet count rose 57%, while function, measured by aggregation, was unchanged with ADP (2 μm). It decreased with Ristocetin and collagen and increased with epinephrine. Consequently, the concentration of

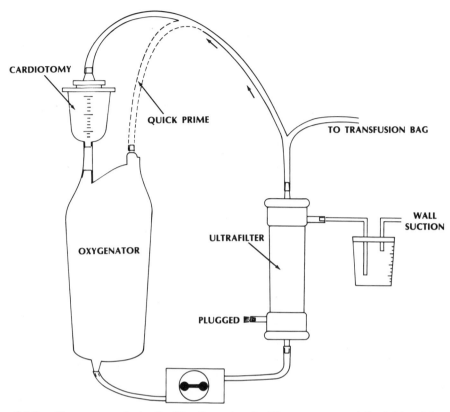

Figure 21.6. Recommended ultrafiltration circuit. We recommend that blood be taken from the oxygenator coronary perfusion port. A separate roller pump pushes the blood through the ultrafilter. The blood return site is the cardiotomy reservoir. The circuit can be used both on and off bypass. In addition, it enables the operator to exercise precise control over the rate of blood flow and ultrafiltration.

functional platelets increased. The mean corpuscular hemoglobin and the mean corpuscular volume underwent statistically significant changes, but these were clinically insignificant. When compared with the albumin concentration, there was a loss of 6% in red blood cells and 18% in platelets. We must conclude that red blood cell loss was due to hemolysis, since plasma hemoglobin rose 254% and LDH increased 122%.

Although there were statistically significant changes in potassium, CO_2, chloride, and glucose following ultrafiltration, these changes were clinically insignificant. The sodium and blood, urea, nitrogen (BUN) were unchanged and the osmolality decreased from 274 to 272 mOsmoles. There were no complications following transfu-

sion, and postoperative creatinine clearance was not significantly altered (95.3 ± 10.1 preop *vs.* 84.8 ± 4.9 ml/min postop). Transfusion of concentrated pump blood increased the patient's red blood cell, hemoglobin, and hematocrit levels, as well as the white blood cell count. Serum albumin rose 18% following transfusion. In addition, there were increases in plasma hemoglobin, lactate dehydrogenase (LDH), and fibrinogen. Blood utilization decreased from 4.8 ± 0.3 to 2.8 ± 0.2 units/case, a difference of 2.0 ± 0.2 units/case.

RECOMMENDED PROCEDURES

1. All ultrafiltration devices require flushing with a minimum of 500 cc of saline

Table 21.1
Effects of Ultrafiltration on the Blood*,†

		Pump		Patient	
		Pre	Post	Pre	Post
RBC	$(\times 10^6)$	2.13 ± .04	3.94 ± .10*	3.14 ± .06	3.60 ± .08*
Hb	(gm%)	6.8 ± 0.1	12.3 ± 0.3*	9.7 ± 0.2	11.0 ± 0.1*
Hct	(%)	19.0 ± 0.3	35.1 ± 0.8*	28.1 ± 0.4	31.4 ± 0.4*
MCV	(m^3)	89.4 ± 0.4	89.1 ± 0.4*	89.6 ± 0.4	89.7 ± 0.4
MCH	(gm)	32.0 ± 0.2	31.4 ± 0.2*	31.3 ± 0.3	31.4 ± 0.2
WBC	$(\times 10^3)$	8.8 ± 0.4	14.9 ± 0.7*	12.0 ± 0.7	13.6 ± 0.7*
Platelets	$(\times 10^3)$	125.6 ± 4.5	197.3 ± 10.1*	149.7 ± 6.2	147.7 ± 5.9
Glucose	(mg%)	198 ± 9	161 ± 8*	189 ± 6	201 ± 6*
Chloride	(mEq/liter)	104.8 ± 0.4	96.5 ± 0.7*	105.7 ± 0.4	105.3 ± 0.3
CO_2	(mEq/liter)	22.4 ± 0.3	17.8 ± 0.3*	23.1 ± 0.2	23.3 ± 0.2
Potassium	(mEq/liter)	5.0 ± 0.1	5.4 ± 0.1*	4.1 ± 0.1	4.3 ± 0.1
Sodium	(mEq/liter)	140.4 ± 0.3	140.5 ± 0.3	140.5 ± 0.5	140.9 ± 0.2
BUN	(mg%)	15.1 ± 1.1	13.4 ± 0.5	14.6 ± 0.5	14.7 ± 0.5
Osmolality	(mOsmoles)	274.0 ± 3.3	272.0 ± 3.3*	275.7 ± 2.5	279.5 ± 1.3
Albumin	(gm%)	3.0 ± .01	5.7 ± 0.2*	3.4 ± 0.1	4.0 ± 0.1*
LDH	(units/liter)	294 ± 14	682 ± 33*	300 ± 11	406 ± 16*
Pl Hb	(mg%)	52.1 ± 3.7	183.9 ± 11.8*	29.3 ± 2.4	48.8 ± 5.9*
Fibrinogen	(mg%)	137.0 ± 6.5	277.3 ± 13.6*	192.6 ± 7.1	220.7 ± 6.9*

* All values are mean ± standard error of the mean. *, $p \leq 0.01$, by paired Student's test.
† Abbreviations used are: Pump Pre, pump blood before concentration; Pump Post, pump blood after concentration; Patient Pre, patient before transfusion; Patient Post, patient after transfusion; WBC, white blood cells; RBC, red blood cells; Hb, hemoglobin; Hct, hematocrit; Pl Hb, plasma hemoglobin; MCV, mean corpuscular volume; MCH, mean corpuscular hemoglobin.

prior to use. The initial saline wash is later discarded. We prefer flushing the ultrafilter, then maintaining it filled with crystalloid.

2. The device should be mounted on a holder which is attached to a pole on the pump console.

3. After flushing, the blood inlet port is connected to the coronary perfusion port via a roller pump. If a membrane oxygenator is used, the blood inlet line can be connected to the venous reservoir. The blood outlet line is connected to the inlet port on the cardiotomy reservoir or the quick prime port on the oxygenator.

4. The ultrafiltrate inlet port of the device is occluded; the outlet port is connected to a vacuum source via a drainage bottle that measures the ultrafiltrate. The device can be primed and debubbled at the same time as the extracorporeal circuit.

5. During the use of the device, the appearance of any blood in the ultrafiltrate is evidence that membrane integrity is lost. Ultrafiltration should cease, and the device should be discarded.

6. During use, blood flow should not exceed 300 cc/min.

7. Vacuum should only be applied when there is blood flowing through the device so that there is a gradual buildup of vacuum in the system. The process is reversed to discontinue ultrafiltration: First, the vacuum is removed, and then the blood flow is discontinued. The maximum transmembrane pressure of the device should not be exceeded. The lot number of the device should be recorded.

An ultrafilter in the bypass circuit effectively and inexpensively removes excess water while conserving and concentrating blood components and red blood cells. The device maintains a stable degree of hemodilution in the presence of infusions of diluting fluid. At the end of cardiopulmonary bypass, hemodilution can be reversed. The ability to return concentrated platelets and plasma proteins to the patient provides long-term benefits in terms of hemodynamic stability, since the oncotic pressure is maintained. In addition, the concentrated levels of platelets, proteins, and fibrinogen could prove beneficial in reducing postoperative bleeding.[22,23] Ultrafiltration is not associated with any clinically significant changes in the electrolyte composition.

Our experience has led us to the conclusion that the technique is facile, safe, and effective. We believe that the device should be employed routinely whenever cardiopulmonary bypass is used.

References

1. Brull L: Realization de l'ultrafiltration *in vivo.* C R Soc Biol (Paris) 99:1605, 1928.
2. Lunderquist A, Alwall N, Tornberg A: On the artificial kidney: XXI. The efficacy of the dialyzer-ultrafilter intended for human use. Including a preliminary report on treatment of oedemic patients by means of ultrafiltration. Acta Med Scand 143:307, 1952.
3. Kobayashi K, Shibata M, Kato K: Studies on the development of a new method of controlling the amount and contents of body fluids (extracorporeal ultrafiltration method: ECUM) and the application of this method for patients receiving long-term hemodialysis. Jpn J Nephrol 14:1, 1972.
4. Lynggard F, Nielsen B: Rapid fluid extraction with the Gambro ultradiffuser. Artif Organs 2:134, 1978.
5. Henderson LW: Pre vs. past dilution hemofiltration. Clin Nephrol 11:120, 1979.
6. Ing T, Chen WT, Daugirdas JT: Isolated ultrafiltration and new techniques of ultrafiltration. Kidney Int 18:877, 1980.
7. Romagnoli A, Hacker J, Keats AS: External hemoconcentration after deliberate hemodilution. Annual Meeting of the American Society of Anesthesiologists, extracts of scientific papers, 1976.
8. Darup J, Bleese N, Kalmar P: Hemofiltration during extracorporeal circulation. Thorac Cardiovasc Surg 27:227, 1979.
9. Hopeck JM, Lane RS, Schroeder JW: Oxygenator volume control by parallel ultrafiltration to remove plasma water. J AMSECT 13:267, 1981.
10. Hauer JM, Thurer RL, Dawson RB: *Autotransfusion.* New York, Elsevier North Holland, 1981.
11. Spreiter SC, Levy LA, Wong ES: In vitro evaluation and clinical application of membrane dialyzers as pure ultrafilters. Trans Am Soc Artif Intern Org 24:448, 1978.
12. Darson WJ Jr, Pizzicone VB, Ferdman MH: Quantitation of membrane—protein-solute interactions during ultrafiltration. Trans Am Soc Artif Intern Org 24:155, 1978.
13. Solomon BA, Gastino F, LySaght MJ: Continuous flow membrane filtration of plasma from whole blood. Trans Am Soc Artif Intern Org 24:21, 1978.
14. Forstrom RJ, Bartlet K, Blackshear PL Jr: Formed element deposition onto filtering walls. Trans Am Soc Artif Intern Org 21:602, 1975.
15. Jaffrin MY, Butruille Y, Granger A: Factors governing hemofiltration (HF) in a parallel plate exchanger with highly permeable membrane. Trans Am Soc Artif Intern Org 24:448, 1978.
16. Mylius UV, Streicher E, Schneider HW: Capillary membrane for hemofiltration. J Dial 1:715, 1977.
17. Hone PW, Ward RA, Mahony JF: Hemodialyzer performance: An assessment of currently available units. J Dial 1:3, 1977.
18. Sigdell JE: Comparison of hollow fiber dialyzers. Artif Organs 5:401, 1981.
19. Sigdell JE: Addendum. Artif Organs 6:77, 1982.
20. Henderson LW, Callon CR, Ford CA: Kinetics of hemodiafiltration. II. Clinical characterization of a new blood cleansing modality. J Lab Clin Med 85:372, 1975.
21. Tamari Y, Nelson RL, Tortolani AJ: Comparison of circuits incorporating ultrafiltration devices into cardiopulmonary bypass circuits. Submitted for publication to JECT, 1982.
22. Nelson RL, Tamari Y, Tortolani AJ: Hemoconcentration by ultrafiltration following cardiopulmonary bypass. Surg Forum 33:253, 1982.
23. Nelson RL, Tamari Y, Tortolani AJ: A new method for concentration and salvage of pump blood. Presented to the Symposium "Pathophysiology and Techniques of Cardiopulmonary Bypass" sponsored by the Cardiothoracic Research and Education Foundation, San Diego, 1982.

Appendix A
Hollow Fiber Dialyzers*

Manufacturer	Model	Surface Area (m²)	Fiber Material	UFR (ml/hr/torr)	TMP (torr)	Length (mm)	DIA (mm)
Asahi	AM-10	1.1		3.5	500	215	60
	AM-10L	1.1		2.7		215	60
	AM-10H	1.1		4.3		215	60
	AM-20	1.6		4.7	500	243	65
	AM-20L	1.6		3.0		243	65
	AM-30	2.1		6.8		243	75
	AM-30L	2.1		4.0		243	75
	AM-03	0.3		0.5		178	36
	AM-05	0.5		1.0		215	60

Appendix A
Hollow Fiber Dialyzers*

Manufacturer	Model	Surface Area (m²)	Fiber Material	UFR (ml/hr/torr)	TMP (torr)	Length (mm)	DIA (mm)
	AM-06	0.6		1.5		215	60
Braun	Diacap	1.4	Cuprophan	3.1	500	285	64
Cobe	HF 130	1.2	Cuprophan	2.7	600	270	60 × 60
	HF 150	1.5	Cuprophan	3.6	600	270	60 × 60
Cordis Dow	0.6D	0.6	Regenerated cellulose	1.1	750	215	77
	1.3D	1.3	Regenerated cellulose	1.9	500	215	77
	1.8D	1.8	Regenerated cellulose	2.4	500	267	77
	2.5D	2.5	Regenerated cellulose	3.6	500	267	89
	3500	0.9	Cellulose acetate	3.2	750	215	77
	4000	1.4	Cellulose acetate	4.2	750	255	77
	Duo-Flux	1.8	Cellulose acetate	20	750	267	77
Cordis Dow "C-Dak"	1.3	1.3	Regenerated cellulose	2.4			
	1.8	1.8	Regenerated cellulose	3.6			
	135	1.35	Saponified cellulose ester	2.1			
Dasco	Multi-cap	1.1	Cuprophan	2.5	600	250	65
Extracorporeal	TriExL	0.9	Cuprophan	2.7	750	193	70
	TriEx1	1.0	Cuprophan	3.3	750	193	70
	TriEx2	1.3	Cuprophan	4.3	750	240	75
	TriEx3	1.6	Cuprophan	5.3	750	240	75
Fresenius (MTS) "Hemoflow"	C 0.8	0.8	Cuprophan	2.9	500	250	69
	C 1.0	1.0	Cuprophan	3.6	500	250	69
	C 1.3	1.3	Cuprophan	4.7	500	250	69
Fresenius "Hemoflow"	D1	0.6	Cuprophan	3.8			
	D2	1.1	Cuprophan	6.3			
	D3	1.6	Cuprophan	7.0			
	D6	2.0	High-flux Cuprophan	14.6			
Gambro "GF"	120-L	1.1	Cuprophan	2.4	500	220	57
	120-M	1.2	Cuprophan	3.5	500	220	57
	120-H	1.2	Cuprophan	4.5	500	220	57
	180-M	1.8	Cuprophan	5.7	500	255	67
	180-H	1.8	Cuprophan	7.5	500	255	67
Hospal (Disscap)	Disscap	1.1	Cuprophan	3.0	500	230	56
	080	0.6	Cuprophan	2.7		200	
	110	1.1	Cuprophan	3.7		200	
	140	1.4	Cuprophan	4.8		200	
Inphardial (Fidial)	1	0.9	Cuprophan	3.7	600	234	68
	2	1.2	Cuprophan	4.5	600	234	68
	3	1.2	Cuprophan	3.2	600	234	68
	4	1.6	Cuprophan	6.0	600	304	68
	HF	1.0	Cuprophan	11.0	600	234	68
Kawasumi	KF 1	0.8	Cuprophan	3.0	500	275	
	KF 1	1.0	Cuprophan	3.6	500	275	103 × 50
	KF 1	1.2	Cuprophan	4.3	500	275	

Appendix A
Hollow Fiber Dialyzers*

Manufacturer	Model	Surface Area (m²)	Fiber Material	UFR (ml/hr/torr)	TMP (torr)	Length (mm)	DIA (mm)
Kuraray	KF 1	1.5	Cuprophan	5.3	500	275	117 × 56
	KF 1	0.7	Cuprophan	3.0	500	275	103 × 50
	KF 11	1.2	Ethylene vinyl alcohol copolymer	3.5	500	325	67
	KF 101	0.7	Ethylene vinyl alcohol copolymer	2.4	500	255	67
	KF 101	1.0	Ethylene vinyl alcohol copolymer	3.7	500	325	67
	KF 101	1.3	Ethylene vinyl alcohol copolymer	4.3	500	380	67
Kawasumi/ Kuraray	KF-1N	0.6	Cuprophan				
	KF-1N	0.8	Cuprophan				
	KF-1N	1.0	Cuprophan				
	KF-1N	1.2	Cuprophan				
Kuraray	KF-11	0.8	Cuprophan	2.8			
	KF-11	1.0	Cuprophan	3.5			
	KF-11	1.5	Cuprophan	5.0			
	KF-11N	0.8	Cuprophan				
	KF-11N	1.0	Cuprophan				
	KF-11N	1.2	Cuprophan				
Nikkiso	Alpha 11	1.1	Cuprophan	3.0	500	250	100 × 63
Nipro (NF)	NF-C 11	1.1	Cuprophan	4.2	500		
	NF-C 13	1.3	Cuprophan	5.0	500		
	NF-C 16	1.6	Cuprophan	5.7	500		
	NF-C 16	1.6	Cuprophan	5.7	500		
	NF-C 21	2.1	Cuprophan	8.0	500		
	NF-D 11	1.1	Cuprophan	3.2	500		
	NF-D 13	1.3	Cuprophan	3.7	500		
	NF-D 16	1.6	Cuprophan	4.6	500		
	NF-D 19	1.9	Cuprophan	5.4	500		
	H 9	0.9	High-flux Cuprophan	13.0	500		
	H 11	1.1	High-flux Cuprophan	15.9	500		
	H 13	1.3	High-flux Cuprophan	18.8	500		
	H 16	1.6	High-flux Cuprophan	23.1	500		
Nipro (NF)	E 11	1.1	Eccentric type Cuprophan	3.9	500		
	E 13	1.3	Eccentric type Cuprophan	4.6	500		
Nipro (Niprizer)	C 110	1.1	Cuprophan	4.2	500	218	65
	C 180	1.8	Cuprophan	6.9	500	275	73
	D 150	1.5	Cuprophan	4.3	500	275	73
	H 90	0.9	High-flux Cuprophan	13.0	500	218	65
	H 150	1.5	High-flux Cuprophan	21.7	500	275	73
	C 130	1.3	Cuprophan				
	D 90	0.9	Cuprophan				
	D 110	1.1	Cuprophan				
	NAC-07	0.7	Cellulose acetate				
	NAC-09	0.9	Cellulose acetate				
	NAC-11	1.1	Cellulose acetate				
	NAC-13	1.3	Cellulose acetate				
	NAC-15	1.5	Cellulose acetate				

Appendix A
Hollow Fiber Dialyzers*

Manufacturer	Model	Surface Area (m²)	Fiber Material	UFR (ml/hr/torr)	TMP (torr)	Length (mm)	DIA (mm)
	NAC-17	1.7	Cellulose acetate				
Organon	11F100	1.0	Cuprophan	3.0		310	75
(Nephross)	16F160	1.6	Cuprophan	2.8	500	310	75
	Lento	0.7	Cuprophan				
	Andante	1.0	Cuprophan				
	Allegro	1.4	Cuprophan				
SMAD	100.2	1.0	Cuprophan	2.9			
(MP)	125.2	1.25	Cuprophan	3.6			
	100.1	1.0	Cuprophan	4.0			
	140.1	1.35	Cuprophan	4.9			
SORIN	SD-1	1.3	Cuprophan	4.8	500	235	65
(Spiraflo)	SD-2	1.0	Cuprophan	3.3	500	235	65
	SF-08	0.8	Cuprophan	2.7	500	235	65
	SF-06	0.6	Cuprophan	2.0	500	235	65
Tecnodial	50 C	1.0	Cuprophan	4.3		255	72
(Tecno)	50 C	1.5	Cuprophan	5.5		255	72
Teijin	TF-15	1.6	Regenerated cellulose	3.3	500		
Terumo	TH-10	1.0	Cuprophan	2.9	500		
(Clirans)	TH-13	1.3	Cuprophan	3.2	500		
	TH-15	1.5	Cuprophan	4.2	500		
	TE-07	0.7	Cuprophan	2.8	500		
	TE-10	1.0	Cuprophan	3.7	500		
	TE-15	1.5	Cuprophan	5.2	500		
	TH-16S	1.6	Cuprophan		500		
Toray	B1	1.15	Polymethyl methacrylate	10	500	240	73
(Filtryzer)	B1-M	1.36	Polymethyl methacrylate	15	500	247	85
	B1-L	2.10	Polymethyl methacrylate	45	500	247	85
	B2	1.15	Polymethyl methacrylate	3.9	500	240	73
	B2-M	1.36	Polymethyl methacrylate	4.7	500	247	85
Travenol	CF1200	1.3	Cuprophan	2.5		255	76
	CF1500	1.5	Cuprophan	4.0		255	76
	CF2300	2.3	Cuprophan	4.1		350	76
	CF12.11	0.8	Cuprophan	3.1		250	58
	CF15.11	1.1	Cuprophan	4.2		250	58

* Abbreviations used are: UFR, ultrafiltration rate; TMP, recommended transmembrane pressure.

Appendix B
Parallel Plate Dialyzers

Manufacturer	Model	Surface Area (m²)	Membrane Material	UFR (ml/hr/torr)	TMP (torr)	Priming Vol.
Rhone-Poul-enc	RP6		Polyacrylonitrate			
	H12-10		Polyacrylonitrate	20	250	
Gambro Lun-dia	Minor 13.5	0.51	Cuprophan	1.75	500	68
	Plate 11.5	1.25	Cuprophan	5.7	500	129
	Plate 17	1.25	Cuprophan	2.5	500	115
	Major 11.5	1.70	Cuprophan	8.0	500	169
	Major 17.0	1.70	Cuprophan	3.5	500	138
	Ultradiffuser	1.86	Cuprophan		500	270
	Plate High Flux	1.2	Cuprophan-HDF	10.5	400	205
	Major High Flux	1.7	Cuprophan-HDF	15.0	400	205

INDEX